UNMET NEED IN

PSYCHIATRY

Problems, resources, responses

This innovative book considers ways to resolve the imbalance between the demand and supply of mental health services. Treatment services in most countries reach only a minority of people identified as suffering from a mental disorder. Few countries can provide adequate health services for all the mentally ill, yet none has developed a rational system to decide who should be treated.

The questions are clear. Could we develop a staged treatment process to reach all in need? If not, how do we decide who to treat? What should the criteria be for deployment of scarce treatment resources? How do we determine such criteria? What are the ethical implications of applying such criteria?

In this pioneering work, an international team of eminent psychiatrists, epidemiologists, health administrators, economists, and health planners examines these questions. The result will inform and encourage all concerned with the equitable provision of mental health care.

Professor Gavin Andrews is Professor of Psychiatry, Director of the Clinical Research Unit for Anxiety Disorders, and Director of the World Health Organization Collaborating Centre for Mental Health and Substance Abuse at St Vincent's Hospital, the University of New South Wales, Sydney, Australia.

Professor Scott Henderson is Director of the National Health and Medical Research Council's Psychiatric Epidemiology Research Centre at The Australian National University in Canberra, Australia.

T0312089

UNMET NEED IN
PSYCHIATRY

Problems, resources, responses

Edited by

Gavin Andrews

and

Scott Henderson

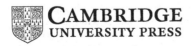
CAMBRIDGE
UNIVERSITY PRESS

CAMBRIDGE UNIVERSITY PRESS
Cambridge, New York, Melbourne, Madrid, Cape Town, Singapore, São Paulo

Cambridge University Press
The Edinburgh Building, Cambridge CB2 2RU, UK

Published in the United States of America by Cambridge University Press, New York

www.cambridge.org
Information on this title: www.cambridge.org/9780521662291

First published 2000
This digitally printed first paperback version 2006

A catalogue record for this publication is available from the British Library

Library of Congress Cataloguing in Publication data
Unmet need in psychiatry : problems, resources, responses / [edited by] Gavin Andrews and
Scott Henderson.
    p. cm.
  Includes index.
  ISBN 0 521 66229 X hardback
  1. Mental Health Services – Utilization Congresses.   2. Medical care – Needs Assessment
Congresses.   3. Mental Illness – Epidemiology Congresses.   I. Andrews, Gavin.   II.
Henderson, Scott, 1935–   .
  [DNLM: 1. Community Mental Health Services Congresses.   2. Health Services Needs and
Demand Congresses.   3. Mental Disorders – Therapy Congresses.   WM 30 U603 2000]
RA790.5.U565   2000
362.2–dc21
DNLM/DLC
for Library of Congress   99–25835 CIP

ISBN-13 978-0-521-66229-1 hardback
ISBN-10 0-521-66229-X hardback

ISBN-13 978-0-521-02723-6 paperback
ISBN-10 0-521-02723-3 paperback

Contents

Contributors

Editors

Gavin Andrews
Professor of Psychiatry, School of
Psychiatry, University of New South
Wales at St. Vincent's Hospital, 299
Forbes Street, Darlinghurst, NSW,
2010, Australia.

Scott Henderson
Director, National Health and Medical
Research Council, Psychiatric
Epidemiology Research Centre, The
Australian National University,
Canberra, ACT, 0200, Australia.

Technical Editor

Malinda Jarry
World Health Organization
Collaborating Centre for Mental Health
and Substance Abuse, 229 Forbes
Street, Darlinghurst, NSW, 2010,
Australia.

Authors

Margarita Alegría
Professor and Director of the Center
for Sociomedical Research and
Evaluation, Graduate School of Public
Health, Medical Sciences Campus,
University of Puerto Rico, PO Box
365067, San Juan, Puerto Rico,
00936-5067.

Gavin Andrews
Professor of Psychiatry, School of
Psychiatry, University of New South
Wales at St. Vincent's Hospital, 299
Forbes Street, Darlinghurst, NSW,
2010, Australia.

Mattias Angermeyer
Professor, Department of Psychiatry,
University of Leipzig, Johannisallee 20,
D-04317, Leipzig, Germany.

James C. Anthony
Professor, Johns Hopkins University,
624 North Broadway, 8th Floor,
Baltimore, Maryland, MD-21205, USA.

Annette Beautrais
Principal Investigator, Canterbury
Suicide Project, Christchurch School of
Medicine, PO Box 4345, Christchurch,
New Zealand.

Paul Bebbington
Professor of Social and Community
Psychiatry, Department of Psychiatry
and Behavioural Sciences, University
College London Medical School,
Archway Campus, Whittington
Hospital, Highgate Hill, London, N19
5NF, United Kingdom.

Rob Bijl
Trimbos-instituut, Netherlands
Institute of Mental Health and
Addiction, PO Box 725, 3500 AS
Utrecht, The Netherlands.

Philip Burgess
Associate Professor, Mental Health
Research Unit, Private Bag 11,
Parkville, VIC, 3052, Australia.

Jean Marc Cloos
Centre Hospitalier de Luxembourg, 4,
rue Barblé, 1210 Luxembourg.

Wilson M. Compton
Assistant Professor of Psychiatry,
Washington University School of
Medicine, 40 North Kingshighway,
Suite 4, St Louis, Missouri, MO-63108,
USA.

John E. Cooper
Emeritus Professor of Psychiatry,
University of Nottingham, 25 Ireton
Grove, Attenborough, Nottingham,
NG9 6BJ, United Kingdom.

John R. M. Copeland
Professor and Head, Department of
Psychiatry, Royal Liverpool University
Hospital, Liverpool, L69 3GA, United
Kingdom.

Linda Cottler
Professor of Epidemiology,
Department of Psychiatry, Washington
University School of Medicine, 40
North Kingshighway, Suite 4, St. Louis,
Missouri, MO-63108, USA

Renee M. Cunningham-Williams
Research Assistant Professor of Social
Work in Psychiatry, Department of
Psychiatry, Washington University
School of Medicine, 40 North
Kingshighway, Suite 4, St. Louis,
Missouri, MO-63108, USA.

Tracey Davenport
Research Assistant, Academic
Department of Psychiatry, St. George
Hospital and Community Health
Services, 7 Chapel Street, Kogarah,
NSW, 2217, Australia.

Ellie Fossey
Lecturer, School of Occupational
Therapy, La Trobe University, Health
Sciences 3, Bundoora, VIC, 3038,
Australia.

Heinz Häfner
Director, Schizophrenia Research Unit,
Central Institute of Mental Health, J5,
D-68159 Mannheim, Germany.

Wayne Hall
Professor of Drug and Alcohol Studies,
Executive Director, National Drug and
Alcohol Research Centre, University of
New South Wales, Sydney, NSW, 2052,
Australia.

Carol Harvey
Senior Lecturer, Department of
Psychiatry, The University of
Melbourne, Royal Park Hospital,
Private Bag 3, Parkville, VIC, 3052,
Australia.

Steven G. Heeringa
Director, Survey Design and Analysis,
Institute for Social Research, University
of Michigan, Room 1006, 426
Thompson Street, Ann Arbor,
Michigan, MI-48106-1248, USA.

Scott Henderson
Director, National Health and Medical
Research Council, Psychiatric
Epidemiology Research Centre, The
Australian National University,
Canberra, ACT, 0200, Australia.

Ian Hickie
Professor of Community Psychiatry,
School of Psychiatry, University of New
South Wales, Director, Academic
Department of Psychiatry, St. george
Hospital and Community Health
Services, 7 Chapel Street, Mogarah,
NSW, 2217, Australia.

Caroline Hunt
Lecturer, School of Psychiatry,
University of New South Wales at
St. Vincent's Hospital, 299 Forbes
Street, Darlinghurst, NSW, 2010,
Australia.

Ernest Hunter
Professor of Public Health (Mental Health), Department of Social and Preventative Medicine, North Queensland Clinical School, University of Queensland, PO Box 1033, Cairns, QLD, 4870, Australia.

Sonia Johnson
Senior Lecturer in Social and Community Psychiatry, Department of Psychiatry and Behavioural Sciences, University College London Medical School, 48, Riding House Street, London, W1N 8AA, United Kingdom.

Anthony F. Jorm
Professor and Deputy Director, National Health and Medical Research Council, Psychiatric Epidemiology Research Centre, The Australian National University, Canberra, ACT, 0200, Australia.

Peter Joyce
Head of Department, Department of Psychological Medicine, Christchurch School of Medicine, P.O. Box 4345, Christchurch, New Zealand.

Charles T. Kaelber
Chief, Diagnosis and Disability Assessment Program, Services Research and Clinical Epidemiology Branch, Division of Services & Intervention Research, National Institute of Mental Health (NIMH), Parklawn Building, Room 10C-16, 5600 Fishers Lane, Rockville, MD-20857, USA.

Heinz Katschnig
Professor, Department of Psychiatry, University of Vienna, Wahringer Gurtel 18-20, A-1090, Vienna, Austria.

Ronald C. Kessler
Professor, Department of Health Care Policy, Harvard Medical School, 180 Longwood Avenue, Boston, MA-02115-5899, USA.

Bohdan Kolody
Professor of Sociology, San Diego State University, San Diego, CA-92182, USA.

Annette Koschera
Research Assistant, University of New South Wales at St. George Hospital, 7 Chapel Street, Kogarah, NSW, 2217, Australia.

Helen Lapsley
Economist, School of Health Services Management, University of New South Wales, Sydney, NSW, 2052, Australia.

Morven Leese
Statistician, Section of Community Psychiatry (PRiSM), Special Hospitals Case Register Research Unit, Institute of Psychiatry, De Crespigny Park, London SE5 8AF, United Kingdom.

Elizabeth Lin
Assistant Professor, Department of Psychiatry, University of Toronto; Research Scientist, Health Systems Research Unit, Clark Institute of Psychiatry, 250 College Street, Toronto, Ontario, M5T 1R8, Canada.

Kurt Maurer
Senior Scientist, Schizophrenia Research Unit, Central Institute of Mental Health, J5, D-68159 Mannheim, Germany.

Graham Meadows
Senior Lecturer, Department of Psychiatry, University of Melbourne, Royal Park Hospital, Private Bag 3, Parkville, VIC, 3052, Australia.

Roger Mulder
Senior Lecturer, Department of Psychological Medicine, Christchurch School of Medicine, PO Box 4345, Christchurch, New Zealand.

Steve Muller
Centre Hospitalier de Luxembourg, 4, rue Barblé, 1210 Luxembourg.

William E. Narrow
Senior Advisor for Epidemiology, National Institute of Mental Health (NIMH), 31 Center Drive, Suite 4A52 (MSC 2475), Bethesda, MD-20892-2475, USA.

Vikram Patel
Senior Lecturer, Institute of Psychiatry (King's College), University of London, and MacArthur Fellow, Sangath Society, Goa, India.
Sangath Centre, 48 Defence Colony, Porvorim, Goa 403521, India.

George Patton
Professor of Adolescent Health, Department of Paediatrics, University of Melbourne, Centre for Adolescent Health, 2 Gatehouse Street, Parkville, Victoria, 3052, Australia.

Harold Alan Pincus
Deputy Medical Director; Director, Office of Research, American Psychiatric Association, 1400 K Street NW, Washington, DC, 20005, USA.

Rene G. Pols
Senior Consultant Psychiatrist, Flinders Medical Centre: Senior Lecturer in Psychiatry, Flinders University of South Australia, GPO Box 2100, Adelaide, SA, 5001, Australia.

Charles B. Pull
Professor of Psychiatry, Centre Hospitalier de Luxembourg, 4, rue Barblé, 1210 Luxembourg.

Donald S. Rae
Statistician, Biostatistics & Data Management Unit, Division of Intervention & Services Research, National Institute of Mental Health (NIMH), Parklawn Building, Room 10-102, 5600 Fishers Lane, Rockville, MD-20857, USA.

Beverley Raphael
Director, Centre for Mental Health, New South Wales Health Department, Locked Bag 961, North Sydney, NSW, 2059, Australia.

Jean Reggers
Centre Hospitalier Universitaire de Liège, Belgium.

Darrel A. Regier
Associate Director for Epidemiology and Health Policy Research, National Institute of Mental Health (NIMH), 31 Center Drive, Suite 4A52 (MSC 2475), Bethesda, MD-20892-2475, USA.

Wendy Reich
Research Associate Professor, Division of Child Psychiatry, Washington University School of Medicine, 40 North Kingshighway, Suite 4, St. Louis, MO-63108, USA.

Kathy Rourke
Patient Research Coordinator, Washington University School of Medicine, 40 North Kingshighway, Suite 4, St. Louis, MO-63108, USA.

Agnes Rupp
Chief, Financing and Managed Care Research Program, Division of Intervention and Services Research, National Institute of Mental Health (NIMH), Parklawn Building, Room 10C-06, 5600 Fishers Lane, Rockville, MD-20857, USA.

Norman Sartorius
Professor of Psychiatry, Hopitaux Universitaires de Genève, H.U.G., Département de psychiatrie, 16-18 Bd de St Georges, CH-1205 Genève, Switzerland.

Michael Sawyer
Associate Professor, Department of
Psychiatry, University of Adelaide;
Director, Research and Evaluation
Unit, Division of Mental Health,
Women's and Children's Hospital, 72
King William Road, North Adelaide,
SA, 5006, Australia.

Mike Slade
Lecturer in Clinical Psychology with
the Department of Psychology and the
Section of Community Psychiatry
(PRiSM), Institute of Psychiatry, De
Crespigny Park, London SE5 8AF,
United Kingdom.

Arnaud Sztantics
Centre Hospitalier de Luxembourg, 4,
rue Barblé, 1210 Luxembourg.

David T. Takeuchi
Professor, Dept of Sociology, Indiana
University, 744 Ballantine Hall,
Bloomington, IN-47405-6628, USA.

Maree Teesson
Lecturer in Drug and Alcohol Studies,
National Drug and Alcohol Research
Centre, University of New South
Wales, Sydney, NSW, 2052, Australia.

Graham Thornicroft
Professor of Community Psychiatry,
Section of Community Psychiatry
(PRiSM), Institute of Psychiatry, De

Crespigny Park, London SE5 8AF,
United Kingdom.

T. Bedirhan Üstün
Chief, Epidemiology, Classification and
Assessment Unit, Division of Mental
Health and Prevention of Substance
Abuse, World Health Organization,
Room L3.19, CH-1211 Geneva 27,
Switzerland.

Harvey Whiteford
Director of Mental Health,
Commonwealth Department of Health
and Family Services, Canberra, ACT,
2601, Australia.

Kay Wilhelm
Associate Professor of Psychiatry,
School of Psychiatry, University of New
South Wales; Head, Consultation
Liaison Psychiatry Unit, St. Vincent's
Hospital, Victoria Street, Darlinghurst,
NSW, 2010, Australia.

Hans-Ulrich Wittchen
Head, Clinical Psychology and
Epidemiology, Max Planck Institute of
Psychiatry, Kraepelinstrasse 10,
D-80804 Munich, Germany.

Deborah A. Zarin
Deputy Medical Director; Associate
Director, Office of Research, American
Psychiatric Association, 1400 K Street
NW, Washington, DC, 20005, USA.

Preface

The 25 years from 1955 was the period when psychiatry came of age. Effective medications for the common mental disorders, such as schizophrenia and the affective and anxiety disorders, became generally available for the first time. Community attitudes towards the mentally ill, and the confidence of patients being treated with the new drugs, enabled people in many countries who would otherwise be nursed in hospital to live in the community and receive their treatment there. The focus of psychiatry moved to the general hospital and to ambulatory care, exactly as in the rest of medicine. Primary care physicians were increasingly expected to recognize and manage people with mental disorders, exactly as they did for people with physical disorders. Psychiatry and the mental health services felt excited and were exciting.

A series of epidemiological studies published in the 1960s showed that the number of people in the community who met criteria for a mental disorder far exceeded the number who were receiving attention from the specialist mental health services, from primary care physicians, or from any other segment of the health service. It was not that the majority of those untreated were afflicted only by mild or transient disorders, for in some studies significant numbers of people with serious and disabling mental disorders went untreated. The introduction of the psychotropic drugs and the move to community care had been politically easy – both steps saved money for either the state or the private insurer. Attempts to widen the reach of mental health services were not easy for, it was claimed, it would not be cost-effective to invest more health dollars in mental health unless it were to pay for cost-effective treatments. The World Bank and World Health Organization project on the Burden of Disease suggested that as no country could afford to provide services for all citizens who required them, services should be rationed according to the burden of a disease and the cost-effectiveness of treatment for it, a strategy that quite overlooked the rights of citizens to shelter, primary care and emergency care when ill. Either way, there was little discussion in either the clinical or health economics literature of how one might manage scarcity and triage services in some equitable way.

The World Psychiatric Association's Section of Epidemiology and Public Health has held a scientific symposium almost every two years since the first in Aberdeen, Scotland, in 1969. Some years the symposia are general, and at other times are focused on a problem of particular importance. In 1995, the Section Committee, meeting in New York, asked us to convene a meeting in Sydney, Australia, in late 1997, the meeting to be focused on 'The Unmet Need for Treatment'. With this topic in mind, and with the intention of preparing a book on the topic, we deliberately invited members of the Section and other key scientists to consider preparing papers to address the problem and to come to the Sydney meeting to present them. This book is the result of asking this group of invited scientists to address the following topic: treatment services in most countries reach only a minority of the people who epidemiologists identify as having a mental disorder. Few countries could afford to provide health services to all citizens who meet criteria for a mental disorder, yet no country has developed a rational system to decide who should be treated. The questions are clear: if everyone with a diagnosis needs treatment, could we develop a staged treatment process so that the available skills in the community and in the health services can be organized to reach all in need? If not everyone with a diagnosis needs treatment, how do you decide who does? Should we use diagnosis, disablement, or likelihood of treatment success to deploy scarce health services? Do we have sufficiently reliable estimates of the prevalence, comorbidity, disablement, treatment effectiveness, and of the direct and indirect costs of illness to do this? If we had such data, would it be ethical to triage people in this way?

Now read on . . .

Part I

Unmet need: defining the problem

Assessing needs for psychiatric services

Norman Sartorius

Life is becoming more complicated by the day. In times past, when asked how much should be invested in providing services for a particular mental or physical illness, we could provide an estimate of the number of people who had such an illness. Then we could state how many personnel, drugs and beds are necessary for appropriate care and how they should be used. It is still possible to do this today but, in many settings, it will no longer be correct.

There are several reasons for this. First, the needs of the patients, the needs of the community and the needs of the government only partially overlap. For example, governments are particularly interested in avoiding high costs for disease control, while the community places a high premium on diminishing or preventing disturbance to the normal ways of societal functioning. Patients and their families are more insistent that quality of life, before and during treatment, is an important criterion of treatment acceptability. Consultation between these three groups, therefore, emerges as a necessary part of the estimation of needs.

Second, it has gradually become accepted that the notion of calculating needs, outcomes or costs by using averages is misleading. Average (demographic) citizens, average reactions to treatment, and average outcomes are often not applicable in individual cases.

People are different whether well or ill. They belong to different cultures, have different personalities, physical constitutions and personal histories, all of which makes them perceive their diseases in a specific manner. They cope with the consequences of diseases in individual ways, and thus require different types of help. Some of them do not want anyone to help them; others want more help than could sensibly be expected given the impairment or suffering that their disease produces. Some of them do not want help from a health service; if convinced that their disease is a consequence of someone's magical influence they may prefer to seek the help of traditional healers, exorcists or others that deal with black magic.

Third, the needs of the health professions play a particularly important, yet neglected, role in planning health services and assessing and providing care for a sick population. Health workers, for example, will not take jobs in places where their children might not get acceptable schooling. In some countries, this keeps the density of health care agents in rural areas low and, in turn, affects the expression of demands for, and availability of, care in a rural population.

Fourth, it has become clear that plans made to cover long periods must be vague, addressing only overall objectives and goals. The notion that a five-year plan should be precise and include operational details, as was promoted in countries of Eastern Europe, lost much of its attraction when it became clear that services in those countries did not develop in accordance with the plans, and that the making and announcing of those plans had served mainly political purposes. These reasons and others – unforeseen political changes, methodological problems in the planning and evaluation process, incompetence of planners because of insufficient training – have led to an increasing recognition that the previous standardized ways of planning are not very useful. In many countries during the late 1970s and early 1980s this type of planning has resulted in the gradual disappearance of planning institutes, planning departments in the ministries of health, and planning courses in public health training programs.

More recently, planning and evaluation services have regained strength under the pressure of economic factors (expressed mainly as the wish of governments to reduce the costs of care) and the population's insistence that they receive more care of better quality.

This new wave of planning is, however, different from previous versions in that it has begun to define the three key elements of planning in a new way:

1. Investment is measured in terms of *total expenditure* – not only the money spent to build services or pay health personnel, but also implicit expenses such as the time that relatives spend looking after sick members of their family.
2. The main indicator of health care productivity is now assessment of *outcome* in terms of improved health, whereas it used to be assessment of improvement in the *process of providing health care*.
3. The definition of needs for health services are changing. Previously the best indicator was thought to be the total number of people in the population with the disease in question. There are now four parts to defining the needs for health care services: (1) the need for health care should consider the expressed demands of the community; (2) the needs of the health professionals' quality of life should be assessed and addressed; (3) the need for health care must consider the availability of effective and ethically acceptable solutions; and (4) the health sector's involvement must depend on how much the solution lies within the health sector's competence and responsibility.

The consideration of these four elements raises several unresolved issues:

1. *Whose need is the most relevant?* The demands expressed by people

affected by a disease are not necessarily the same as those of their families. As previously mentioned, planning for health services has become less popular because of disparities between the expressed needs of those who are sick, their families, and the community. It is imperative to consult all those concerned when needs are defined. In theory, this sounds reasonable; the difficulty lies in applying the process, which requires all concerned to learn new ways of behaving.

2. *Are demands linked to disease, illness or sickness?* The English language has the luxury of having three terms that can be used for the three aspects of a morbid condition: *disease* corresponds to a specific pathological substrate and a specific course and outcome of the condition; *illness* corresponds to the subjective experience of the morbid condition; and *sickness* corresponds to the societal recognition that the disease prevents an individual from contributing to society. Psychiatrists – and other health workers – have to deal with *diseases* and *illnesses* in their clinical practice and with *sicknesses* when they are acting as agents of society. Illnesses, diseases, and sicknesses are not exactly the same. People sometimes feel more ill than their disease warrants in terms of average values; sometimes people have diseases that do not make them feel ill; and sometimes the term sickness is used to describe individuals who do not feel ill and have no demonstrable pathological substrate for their condition. What then is a 'true' intervention? – the one that responds to a disease? or to an illness? or to a sickness? or to all three?

3. *What is an effective intervention?* A problem becomes a need when there is an effective and ethically acceptable intervention that can be performed by the health services. It is therefore necessary to define an effective intervention. There is a growing consensus that the value of interventions should be assessed on the basis of the results of scientific investigations. This does not resolve everything. Sometimes, interventions deal with the disease or its consequences in totality; sometimes, they can only deal with part of the problem caused by a disease. Different interventions may be effective for different parts of the disease problem. The question that arises is whether the gains of using the different interventions (each dealing with a different part of the disease problem) are equivalent – but equivalent from whose point of view? The population? The population in general, or the population affected by the disease? Alternatively should experts, for example experts on the social impact of disease, be invited to advise? For a long time, psychiatrists have valued interventions by how well they relieve symptoms. Their patients might have preferred a treatment with fewer side-effects, even if that meant a less complete relief of symptoms. The population might have been particularly keen to see the application of treatments or other interventions that reduce disability, diminish dependence on others, or eliminate public disturbance. The three groups have different agendas.

There is also confusion about who is responsible for the implementation of some interventions. When the intervention requires knowledge and skills unique to health service staff, the issue is easy to resolve; unfortunately, for many diseases the situation is not that clear-cut. For example, as science has not yet provided an answer to dementia, should health staff decline to be involved with the problems faced by people with this disorder? Yet families need help in dealing with, say, the symptom of fecal incontinence, which is a consequence of the dementia. Should health care staff become involved in the provision of incontinence pads and the education of carers as to how to persuade the demented person to wear them? At one level this can be seen as preventing decubitus ulcers, a proper concern of medicine, but at another level the supply of incontinence pads and education about their use could well be the responsibility of aged care services generally. Similarly, if a person with a chronic psychosis fails to take medication because they cannot live in settled accommodation, is it the responsibility of the health service to provide and pay for suitable accommodation? The boundaries between health and education, health and child-care services, between health and housing or health and the criminal justice services are often unclear in an individual case, and much negotiation is required to ensure that each service can apply the majority of their budget to their main task. In the case of medicine this is the intervention against disease, but a broad view is likely to prove more beneficial than a narrow one.

The second issue concerning the assignment of responsibility is of a more profound nature. It concerns the justification for any medical intervention intended to help people who have a disease. Recently this issue has become confused. It has been said that disease must be treated because it will save society money. By spending several thousand dollars to cure a disease, the argument goes, the individual, freed from disease, will be able to contribute financially to society for many years, which will amply repay the investments made. Of course, the argument is flawed: it is not certain that the person who had the disease will find or maintain a job and contribute to society. There is no guarantee that the same individual will stay free of disease and that the State will not have to spend more money on his/her health. It is not certain how long a person who has been cured of a disease will live and receive retirement benefits; and so forth.

However, even if the economic argument were not flawed, it should never become the main reason for providing health care. Care for the sick members of a society is an ethical imperative, even if significant amounts of money are spent and not recouped. This consideration is important because it moves the burden of deciding whether a particular person merits care from the health system to the political arena. The task of the health care specialist is to provide the best possible treatment or support for those members of society who are not well: the political structure of the country has to decide on the total amount of money that will be spent on health.

With these considerations in mind it is possible to propose that needs for health care be defined as, '*the agglomerate of those demands of people having a health problem, their families and their communities to which the health care system can respond by an effective intervention. In this context, effective interventions are those that have a predictable and significant positive effect on the problem and are acceptable to the individuals who have the problem and to those who care for them.*' This definition would allow a pragmatic assessment of needs for care and is cast in the spirit of seeking an alliance between patients, their families, their communities and the health care system. Its acceptance would avoid the pitfall of deciding that illness without an organic substrate is not a legitimate reason for seeking and obtaining help. Similarly, it would avoid equating epidemiological estimates of the prevalence of mental disorders with needs, regardless of the capacity of the health sector to respond to it. It underlines the need to assess interventions scientifically and ensures that only those interventions that are effective are used. It also implies that it is the health sector's responsibility to decide which of the interventions should be applied on ethical and scientific grounds, while the decision not to provide the best treatment remains in the political domain.

2

Unmet need: a challenge for governments

Harvey Whiteford

Governments around the world are struggling to find ways to improve the health status of their populations. Priorities change within and between countries; however, modern public health programs and clinical medicine now offer more than can be bought by historically set health budgets. When this is combined with the considerable unmet need for health services, including mental health and substance-abuse services, the politicians and the government departments responsible for health have an unenviable challenge.

The general population, health professionals and consumer groups all routinely demand new or better health services. In my experience, politicians generally try to do what they believe the electorate wants and respond to these demands. At the same time, they are wary of the disproportionate influence of vested interests, but do acknowledge that these groups are often well organized and skillfully use the media to apply pressure to governments. So usually there are demands for more money, and for a greater slice of the available public or private payers' budget for health care. There has been little public debate on how much a country should spend on health versus, for example, education, law and order or defence. How do we know if the Organization for Economic Co-operation and Development (OECD) average of around eight percent of gross domestic product (GDP) is right? The most successful national example of expanding health expenditure is the USA. This experience clearly shows that doubling the proportion of the GDP a country spends on health services does not, by itself, fix that many problems. It shifts the cut-off point where funding is stopped, but does not change the fundamental problem of how governments allocate scarce resources and respond to unmet need.

Most western countries can point to their form of national health insurance as a safety net. Many of these are reasonably accessible to people with mental illness; even those that are not are slowly moving in that direction. For example, amendments to the US Public Health Service Act and the 1996 Mental Health Parity Act, passed at a time when the USA is trying to rein in its health expenditure, are steps toward requiring parity in insurance coverage for mental illness in that country.

However, once the ability to purchase basic health services is removed as a barrier, funders such as governments and health insurance companies become more involved in deciding which services are to be paid for. Using price signals such as consumer copayments can limit demand, but the supply and consumption of health services notoriously fail to meet the criteria required for market forces to act as effective controls. People with chronic illness are especially vulnerable. Some countries such as Australia have effectively used supply-side controls, including limiting the number of medical practitioners, to contain costs.

To reduce the pressure for increased funding, governments and other third-party payers try to squeeze more out of the existing funding by increasing the efficiency and effectiveness of services. This is not simply a matter of containing health care costs. It involves changing funding incentives and difficult structural reform of the service delivery system. It involves stopping or reducing inefficient or ineffective services, many cherished by vested interests, and introducing new ways of financing and providing services. The unfortunate lack of routinely collected outcome data has seriously compromised this reform. As a result, cost reduction, as opposed to quality and health gain, has driven the microeconomic reforms. Services can be denied because of their cost, regardless of their effectiveness.

Unfortunately, the heat generated in the health reform debate between consumers, professionals, governments, and funders has shed little light on the matter. The Oregon experience (Haas & Hall, 1992) and debates within the UK National Health Service (Calman, 1994) are notable exceptions. One of the problems has been the different perspectives and languages used by clinicians, funders, and consumers. Health professionals have been trained to deal with individuals who present for treatment. Their aim is to provide the best care for those patients who manage to see them, and they base their professional standing on achieving and maintaining high-level clinical skills. This is, of course, appropriate and the tradition is centuries old. Clinicians tend not to think about those patients who cannot see them or do not present.

A clinician's decision to undertake one particular type or occasion of service is also a decision not to undertake another. The cost of giving up this next best alternative, the opportunity cost, does concern governments and third-party payers. Rational decision-making about which services should be provided is needed, especially in regard to people whose need will be unmet (McGuire, Henderson & Mooney, 1988). To make these decisions, governments, professionals, health service managers and society as a whole need to be better informed about who is and who is not receiving services. The US Epidemiologic Catchment Area and National Comorbidity Surveys, and epidemiological surveys in the UK, Canada, Australia and other countries are providing crucial data on these matters.

While all countries ration public goods and services, it is politically unpalatable that large numbers of people with serious health problems are not receiving care. As well as needing to respond to this unmet need for humane reasons, government economists know that one of the determinants of the economic health of a country is the health status of its population. The rising burden of neuropsychiatric disease is now well documented (Murray & Lopez, 1996). The debate is not purely academic.

So the challenge for governments is to influence the allocation of scarce resources on a rational basis to optimize the health status of the population for both humane and economic reasons. It has been suggested, I believe with merit, that the burden of illness on the individual and society (measured for example by quality- or disability-adjusted life years) combined with treatment efficacy could be used to inform these decisions (Andrews, 1997). This would mean that disorders with high prevalence, mortality or disability that respond to effective treatments would receive funding, with those interventions demonstrating the greatest health gain for the lowest cost being highly prized.

Who receives care in the health system of the future will continue to depend on the way the system is organized and financed, as well as on the specific training of the clinicians in the system. Inevitably pressure groups promoting areas of special interest and media 'shroud waving' will distort resource allocation. Nevertheless, the debate must be conducted openly and publicly. Epidemiological data on both met and unmet need is crucial to the debate so that we can scrutinize the true opportunity costs of what we are currently providing in health care.

References

Andrews, G. (1997). Managing scarcity: a worked example using burden and efficacy. *Australasian Psychiatry*, **5**, 225–7.

Calman, K.C. (1994). The ethics of allocation of scarce resources: a view from the centre. *Journal of Medical Ethics*, **20**, 71–4.

Haas, M. & Hall, J. (1992). The rationing of health care: should Oregon be transported to Australia. *Australian Journal of Public Health*, **16**, 435–40.

McGuire, A., Henderson, J. & Mooney, G. (1988). *The Economics of Health Care*, pp. 102–15. New York: Routledge and Kegan Paul.

Murray, C.J.L. & Lopez, A.D. (eds.) (1996). *The Global Burden of Disease: A Comprehensive Assessment of Mortality and Disability From Diseases, Injuries and Risk Factors in 1990 and Projected to 2000*. Cambridge, MA: Harvard University Press.

3

Meeting the unmet need with disease management

Gavin Andrews

Half to three-quarters of the people identified in epidemiological surveys as meeting criteria for a mental disorder do not report receiving treatment. All mental health professionals are busy and there is usually no prospect of an increase in the available labor force. So what should be done? One view is that scarce health resources should be offered to those who are sickest. The techniques for ranking diseases by the burden of mortality and morbidity they generate are well advanced. However, if we focus on the sickest, we risk running out of resources before we maximize any health gains. Wouldn't it be better to identify the diagnosis/treatment pairings that offer the greatest prospect of reducing mortality and morbidity, that is, the greatest health gain, and deploy our resources accordingly? This would certainly impact on health, but what if maximizing health gains means that some severely ill people must go untreated? We must develop a mechanism to prioritize the delivery of health care to maximize the attainable health gains, while still attending to the chronically sick. Yet it is this balance between care and cure, between equity and efficiency, that is so difficult to achieve. Thankfully, there is a further alternative to this scenario of chronic shortage. We could supplement the expensive medical model with a public health disease management approach to emphasize primary prevention, community education, and patient self-help by using books and the newer interactive technologies via the automated telephone and Internet. Sadly for doctors, but fortunately for sufferers, the doctor–patient relationship is not essential if one has effective and proven treatments. And psychiatry has many effective treatments that could be delivered without the need for a physician to be involved. We do need to use all possible resources.

The problem

Met need is defined as the proportion of people with a disorder who see a health professional. It will be a considerable overestimate, for many seeing a health professional will not be correctly diagnosed, or get appropriate treatment, and will not have their need for a reduction in the burden of their disease met. *Unmet need* is the proportion of people who meet criteria for a disorder and do not see a clinician. Again it is an overestimate, for some who meet criteria will not be sufficiently distressed or disabled to seek or want treatment and some, who are disabled, will choose not to get treatment. The decision to seek treatment is a complex matter driven by ease of access, by the severity and chronicity, and the disability produced by the disorder, and by the perception that treatment will be effective. *Met un-need* refers to people who have no current mental disorder and yet are consulting clinicians for mental problems. Again it is an overestimate, for some may not currently meet criteria simply because of the good treatment they are now receiving.

At present mental health services everywhere are overwhelmed by the demand for treatment. The unmet need appears considerable and the discontent among consumers and carers is palpable. If all clinicians diagnosed accurately and only practised evidence-based medicine, if patient attendance was only determined by severity and treatability and no services went to well people with minor concerns, could all needs be met and would the level of unmet need become zero? Probably yes, at least in an established market economy with well developed mental health services, and with some use of nonmedical systems of delivery – at least that is the thesis of this chapter.

A word of warning. Unmet need and met un-need are evocative terms that suggest that need is a finite phenomenon. Unfortunately human needs are infinite, and the needs of our patients for cure, relief and comfort, and of their therapists to provide these services, are no exception to this rule. The human capital approach to estimating the burden of disease is more conservative, preferring to focus on the reduction of mortality and the lessening of disability as needs which can and should be met by an efficient health service. The problem is that the number of procedures that health services can deliver is legion, ranging from prevention, through cure and relief, to comfort and support for those with intractable disorders. At one level the problem has always appeared to be the management of scarce resources, but at another level the problem in established market economies is one of plenty, of choosing which of the many alternatives to fund. Therefore, we will propose criteria, on the basis of burden of disease and gains from treatment, for choosing which services to provide, and will discuss care for those who are ill, but for whom few gains can be expected.

An efficient health service should focus on health gains by maximizing the met need and minimizing met un-need and, if there is still a shortfall of services, prioritize services to maximize the health gains – a 'greatest good to the greatest number' type of argument. It seems obvious to say that:

1. An efficient health service should favor treatments that generate health gains over treatments that do not, even if clinicians want to conduct such treatments. Evidence-based medicine is endorsed by most health services.

Everyone forgets that once you have persuaded clinicians to practise in new and effective ways you also have to dissuade them from practising in old and ineffective ways. In Australia, health services still pay for staff to learn drama therapy, simply because stopping such procedures will be an unwelcome decision, whereas encouraging evidence-based medicine faces little entrenched opposition. There are insufficient funds to have both effective and noneffective therapies being offered in parallel. Being a good manager means making hard decisions but, even so, we always underestimate the tribal and reactionary nature of medicine. A telling example is the orthopedic surgeons' victory over the US Agency for Health Care Policy and Research in respect to spinal-fusion surgery, a procedure that the Agency had said was not of proven benefit (Deyo, Psaty, Simon, Wagner & Omenn, 1997).

2. An efficient health service would prefer simple treatments over complex procedures of comparable effectiveness. Yet we often move funds from proven community procedures to complex hospital procedures, or deploy resources to unusual or difficult cases, forgetting that by so doing we deprive many more people, who might have been simply and cheaply treated in the community, from access to any treatment at all. Clinicians like the challenge of the very difficult case and ignore the costs of their preoccupation with highly technical medicine. For example, a pediatric hospital in Brazil (World Bank, 1993) eventually closed the intensive care unit and redirected the funds to community health posts. The intensive care unit had saved babies, but the community strategy of using the same money to identify high-risk children and treat them earlier resulted in a one-third reduction in infant mortality rates in the neighborhoods where the health posts had been established.

3. An efficient health service should prefer prevention and education-for-self-care over direct patient care. For example, there are good data about the value of identifying highly anxious children and using educational programs to teach parents and children how to cope with anxiety, so that the lifetime risk of disabling anxiety and depressive disorders is lessened (Roth & Dadds, 1999). Unfortunately every patient wants personal treatment and every clinician wants to treat patients, even though indirect measures may be more effective. The United States Public Health Service (1995) estimated that only one-sixth of the improvement in life expectancy over the past 50 years was due to clinical medicine and that much of the remainder was due to public-health-type changes. Yet the expenditure is biased in exactly the opposite way.

Mental health services spend considerable sums on clinician-favored treatments, on costly hospitalization, and spend virtually nothing on prevention or health education (Andrews, 1992). A good mental health system should do better than this, it should educate the community to prevent the disorders that are preventable, and treat and cure the people who are most disabled by their illness, focusing resources on the most treatable, and do so with community-based clinicians who practise evidence-based medicine. Would that be enough to meet the unmet need? Let us look at the data.

The US, Canadian, and UK epidemiological surveys

The number of people who meet criteria for a mental disorder and the associated health service utilization rates have been determined in a number of large population studies. The 1981–85 Epidemiologic Catchment Area (ECA) studies (Regier et al., 1993) used the Diagnostic Interview Schedule for DSM-III among people aged 18 and over and reported that 20% had met criteria for a mental disorder in the past 12 months, although following a restricted second wave this was revised to 28%. The disorders enumerated were cognitive impairment, affective disorders, anxiety disorders, substance-use disorders, schizophrenia, and antisocial personality disorder. For met need, the percentage of people with a diagnosis who were seen by the health services was 29% and the proportion varied according to severity of disorder. For unmet need, the percentage not seen was therefore 71%. For met un-need, the percentage of people consulting a mental health provider who did not meet criteria for a mental disorder was 45%, a figure that surprised many.

The 1990 National Comorbidity Survey (NCS, Kessler et al., 1994) used a changed Composite International Diagnostic Interview (CIDI) for DSM-III-R, modified with initial probes and commitment procedures, to identify a similar range of disorders (except for the omission of obsessive compulsive disorder (OCD) and cognitive impairment) in people aged 15–54. Twenty-nine percent of this population were reported to meet criteria for one or more disorders in that year. Met need was a low 21%, and unmet need a high 79%. Nearly half the services were delivered to people without diagnoses: 45% went to met un-need, and the probability of this inappropriate consulting was significantly correlated with high income (Kessler et al., 1997) – perhaps a manifestation of the ability to rent-a-friend. The 1990 Canadian survey (Lin, Goering, Offord, Campbell & Boyle, 1996) used the same methodology as the NCS study. The 12 months prevalence of any disorder was significantly lower (18%) and the service utilization figures different. Met need prevalence was 35% and was associated with being on public assistance, an indirect indicator of disablement. Unmet need prevalence was 65%. Met un-need prevalence was a low 28%, and one-third of these apparently well consultees had a lifetime history of mental disorder. The low met un-need rate was attributed to a match, among Canadians, between morbidity and the perception of need for care.

The UK Household survey (Jenkins et al., 1997) used a checklist to identify a similar range of disorders to the ECA studies among people aged 16–65.

The ICD-10 classification was used, and bipolar disorder, personality disorder, and cognitive impairment were not ascertained. No figure for the number meeting criteria for any mental disorder in the previous 12 months is available, but we estimate that the one year prevalence would have been about 24%. Service utilization data for met and unmet need are not yet available and data for met un-need were not collected. The World Health Organization and Harvard University have established an International Consortium of Psychiatric Epidemiology which, by pooling the data from a large number of international surveys, is able to explore inter-country similarities and differences in prevalence rates and health delivery systems (see Chapter 7). It is regrettable that the UK survey did not use the CIDI, which is now the standard world instrument, to enable the UK results to be compared with the results from other countries. All of us are poorer for their decision.

The Australian National Survey of Mental Health and Well-Being

The Australian Survey of Mental Health and Well-Being was a household survey of 10,600 adults aged 18 to 90 that attained an 80% response rate (Australian Bureau of Statistics, 1998). These data do allow consideration of many of the issues raised by the contributors about meeting need in terms of case identification, chronicity, disability, and service utilization. An early paper in medical care (Hulka, Kupper & Cassel, 1972) explored the reasons why people seek medical help. The majority of the variance in that study was explained by the seriousness and chronicity of the symptom complex, by the resulting disability, and by the perception that the doctor could help. However, medical knowledge and treatment are not organized in terms of symptoms, but in terms of diagnosis of the underlying construct or disorder that is probably responsible for the symptoms and likely to indicate the effective treatment. This book is organized around disorders. Patients suffer symptoms and while they certainly want relief from those symptoms, mostly they want diagnosis and treatment for the underlying disorder so that the symptoms will not return. Diagnosis is therefore the appropriate focus.

Case identification

The Australian Survey used the computerized 12 months Composite International Diagnostic Interview (CIDI 2.1) to identify the 16 common ICD and DSM affective, anxiety, and substance-use disorders in an average of 20 minutes interview time. Screening interviews for cognitive impairment (Mini-Mental State Examination or MMSE) and for ICD-10 personality disorder, neurasthenia and psychosis, and for disability and health service utilization took an additional 20 minutes of interview time. The interview

Table 3.1. Twelve month prevalence of ICD-10 disorders

Disorder	Prevalence (%)
Any anxiety disorder	10.9
Any affective disorder	7.2
Any substance-use disorder	7.7
Any personality disorder	6.1
Any neurasthenia disorder	1.5
Any cognitive impairment	1.3
Any psychosis	0.5
ANY DISORDER	23.3

Note: Prevalences (percent of adults in Australia) from CIDI data rescored and weighted by the inverse probability of being interviewed, exclusion criteria not applied.

proved acceptable, and only rarely were data missed or the interview terminated prematurely. The main concern in surveys is the accuracy of the diagnostic interviews, but there is also a real problem with the correspondence between the ICD and DSM classifications. This could bias the results of research, and materially influence estimates of unmet need, depending on which classification is used to identify cases (Andrews, Slade & Peters, 1999). We also have severe reservations about the ability of people to recall the details of illnesses that occurred many years ago (Andrews, Anstey, Brodaty, Issakidis & Luscombe, in press). Therefore, unlike previous surveys using the CIDI, we chose to only ask about symptoms to identify diagnoses in the past 12 months, and then to ask when the disorders first began and were last present. The latter question allows determination of one month prevalences and provides some estimate of chronicity during the previous 12-month period, an informative step, as Regier et al. (Chapter 4) point out. The prevalences of meeting criteria for an ICD-10 disorder in the previous 12 months are displayed in Table 3.1. They appear lower than the ECA and NCS estimates but the detail remains to be examined. Exclusion criteria were not applied, so the prevalences of some individual disorders will reduce when they are applied, although the total will not change.

The strongest finding in the survey was the drop in prevalence of mental disorders with age, down from 31% in the 18- to 24-year-old age group to 6.5% in the 75-plus age group, with the substance-use and personality disorders virtually disappearing, and cognitive impairment appearing. It is nice to know that as you get older you get saner, even if less cognitively intact. It is concerning that the group with the highest morbidity are the young, who are least likely to seek help.

One month prevalence

Much of the discussion about who should be treated has presumed that the one in four or five adults who meet criteria for a mental disorder in the previous 12 months are candidates for current treatment. This may be an error. While some mental disorders are chronic others are transient, and the extent of this remission is usually underestimated. Regier et al. (Chapter 4) noted that only 56% of people who met criteria for a disorder during a particular year were symptomatic at the end of that year. The present survey asked about symptoms in the previous year, and when those symptoms met criteria for a mental disorder the respondent was asked, 'When was the last time you had symptoms like . . . '. Thus we can use these data to calculate the proportion of people who met criteria for each mental disorder who report symptoms of that disorder this month. Sixty percent did so, a figure virtually identical to the ECA estimates. Thus, while the 23.3% of the adult population met criteria for an ICD-10 mental disorder sometime that year, only 14.1% reported the relevant symptoms that month. We did not ask about duration for schizophrenia or cognitive impairment but scored them as conditions that would continue throughout the year. The chronicity of the other disorders varied by diagnosis. We found that 82% of people with personality disorder or neurasthenia who had met criteria during the year were currently affected. This figure was 60% for people with an anxiety disorder, 54% for those with an affective disorder, and 34% for those with a substance-use disorder. Thus, we have data on chronicity that reflect what most of us believe about the disorders – personality and somatoform disorders are chronic, depression and substance use are more episodic, and anxiety disorders occupy some middle ground.

Disability

In the Hulka et al. (1972) study, disability followed seriousness and chronicity of symptoms as reasons why people would seek help. Throughout this book some authors have stressed the importance of directing services to those that are most disabled, as though reducing the unmet need is a matter of rationing care and directing it to those most in need. The National Survey established the frequency of mental and physical disorders in the Australian adult population, and the extent of the disability and service use generally, and then disability and service use associated with each disorder. The SF12 disability scale (Ware, Kosinski & Keller, 1996) and two questions on disability adapted from the NCS (Kessler & Frank, 1997) were asked of everyone before any disorders were identified. The two questions were, 'Beginning yesterday and going back four weeks, how many days out of the past four weeks were you totally unable to work or carry out your normal activities

Table 3.2. Average, total and proportion of disability days by current prevalence for each diagnostic group

	1-month prevalence %	Disability days (mean)	Disability days (total) ('000,000)	Proportion of total %
Anxiety disorders	6.5	9.0	7.8	31
Affective disorders	3.9	11.6	6.0	24
Personality disorders	5.0	8.0	5.3	21
Neurasthenia	1.2	14.7	2.4	10
Substance-use disorder	2.5	6.4	2.2	9
Cognitive impairment	1.3	6.1	1.1	4
Schizophrenia	0.4	7.3	0.4	2
Any mental disorder	14.1	7.6	14.4	100

Note: The effect of cormorbidity with other mental and physical disorders was not controlled.
1-month prevalence: % of adult population.

because of your health?' *and* 'Apart from those days, how many days in the past four weeks did you have to cut down on what you did, or did not get as much done as usual because of your health?' The sum of these is called disability days. When the presence of a disorder seemed likely, respondents were asked the disability days question with respect to the group of symptoms just elicited. Later in the interview, when all disorders had been identified, respondents completed the Brief Disability Questionnaire (Von Korff, Üstün & Ormel, 1996) and, if they had met criteria for two or more disorders, they were asked to complete the relevant questions again with respect to their main complaint.

Half of the population was well, and did not meet criteria for any mental or physical disorder in the past 12 months. Comorbidity between physical and mental disorders and within mental disorder groups was common. Twenty-eight percent met criteria for a physical disorder but not for a mental disorder, 13% met criteria for a mental disorder but not for a physical disorder, and 10% met criteria for both. These were one year prevalence data, but even in the one month prevalence data it was also common to meet criteria for more than one mental disorder. As is evident from Table 3.2, many of those who met criteria for a mental disorder met criteria for additional disorders from other groups. We did not control for comorbidity in the disability measures in Table 3.2. We have previously used data from a large pilot survey to model the effect of this comorbidity (Andrews, Sanderson & Beard, 1998). In that study a picture consistent with the data in Table 3.2 emerged whatever disability measure one used (disability days, SF12 disability scale or Brief Disability Questionnaire scores). Neither was the picture influenced by whether one considered people with one disorder only, people identified by their nominated main complaint, or the importance of classes of disorder, as determined by regression analysis in which the effect of mental and physical comorbidity was controlled.

Diagnosis does not always disable. Only one-third of people with a mental disorder reported any disability days in the previous 28 days. The average number of disability days reported varied by diagnosis, with neurasthenia and affective disorders the most disabling, and cognitive impairment and substance-use disorders the least. Disability days is a transparent measure, good for illustrating discussions, but it lacks good psychometric characteristics. However, the mental health factor scores of the SF12 disability scale, which do have acceptable psychometrics, showed an almost perfect group rank order correlation with the data presented on disability days ($r = 0.97$). The total number of disability days reported by people with mental disorders was considerable: 14.4 million days per month for a population of 13.4 million adults. People interested in the human capital approach to costing disease should take note.

In these data, the anxiety and affective disorders, which are closely related disorders (Andrews, 1996), account for 55% of the disability attributed to mental disorders. On the other hand, the seemingly more severe disorders, such as cognitive impairment and schizophrenia, account for less than 10% of the disability. Surely the psychoses are more disabling than is suggested by the disability days data? Schizophrenia and cognitive impairment are relatively rare disorders and even if they produced complete disablement, the total disability days attributed to them would be half that generated by the more common anxiety and affective disorders. The best estimate, from the companion Australian survey of low-prevalence disorders, is that schizophrenia accounts for an average of 21 disability days in 28, more than the amount reported in the present adult survey. Cognitive impairment mainly affected people aged 70 years and over, and most of these people reported coexisting chronic and disabling physical conditions. The SF12 mental health factor score was in the normal range (53.4) while the physical health factor score was low (39.7). No other mental disorder showed this factor reversal. Thus, cognitive impairment, in an otherwise well elderly person, is unlikely to account for a large number of disability days and the figure of 6.1 days is probably reasonable. Using the 21 day estimate for schizophrenia as an upper bound does not materially change the implications of the data in Table 3.2.

People with mental disorders reported 14 million disability days each month. These figures should be no surprise given that the Australian studies on burden of disease (Andrews, Mathers & Sanderson, 1998; Andrews, Sanderson & Beard, 1998) suggest that mental disorders account for some 40% of the years lived with a disability due to all diseases, and 20% of the total burden of disease. Expenditure on mental health is only 5% of the total health budget, not the 20% that one envisages should be spent if investing in health was determined only by burden of disease and unaffected by historical influences and treatment costs. Obviously one way of reducing the unmet need is to provide more money but, as Kessler points out (Chapter 5), one would have to specify which part of the health budget or other public endeavor this money should come from.

Within the mental disorders, half the disability associated with mental disorders is generated by two related disorders – the anxiety and affective disorders – and less than 10% by one disorder, schizophrenia. The present expenditure patterns in Australia are the converse, which may not be ideal, even though the need for emergency care for schizophrenia makes the cost per case much more expensive than treating a person with an anxiety or affective disorder (Andrews, 1997). However, the bottom line is really the efficiency of the interventions in reducing mortality and morbidity. Once we have such data then, instead of competing with our colleagues for a share of the mental health budget, we can compete for a share of the total health budget.

Consulting behavior

Some 40% who met criteria for an ICD-10 mental disorder some time during the 12 months obtained professional help, three-quarters from a general practitioner only, and one-quarter from a mental health specialist, usually a psychiatrist (Australian National Survey of Mental Health and Well-Being). If this is the met need, and this is a confident assumption that depends on the practitioners' making the right diagnosis and applying the correct treatment, then the unmet need is notionally 60%. Again this is an overestimate, for a substantial proportion of people who meet criteria for a disorder do not see themselves as having a need and will refuse any offer of treatment (Chapter 6; Brodaty & Andrews, 1983). We sometimes wrongly attribute our need to treat to our patients' apparent need for help. The 'met un-need' was also considerable – 35% of people who obtained help from a health professional for a mental problem (and 25% of people who saw a psychiatrist) did not meet criteria for a mental disorder covered by the survey during the year, presuming that diagnostic criteria are the arbiter of who should be treated.

In the Hulka et al. (1972) study people sought help when their symptoms were serious, chronic, disabling and when they thought that the doctor might help. In Chapter 12, Cooper makes it clear that many consult practitioners of complementary medicine when they do not think that their regular doctor can help. Jorm et al. (Chapter 28) show why many people might erroneously come to this conclusion – we have not taught people how to take care of their own mental health. Other people are quite correct when they decide that their doctor will not be able to help. The chapters by Hunt (Chapter 18) and Wittchen (Chapter 17) on anxiety disorders show that too many people find that 'treatment as usual' equals 'disease as usual', simply because their doctors persist in using treatments now known to be ineffective in the anxiety disorders despite the availability of very good treatments (Andrews, Crino, Hunt, Lampe & Page, 1994; Hunt & Andrews, 1998). The evidence-based medicine movement is preoccupied with developing clinical practice guidelines and encouraging doctors to adopt them. As mentioned previously, there is little discussion on how to get doctors to cease ineffective treatments which they persist in using for whatever reason, be it habit, ideology or income. Adopting new methods is always acceptable but discarding old treatments is hard, especially when it signifies a loss of clinical freedom (see Chapters 10 and 30; Andrews, in press).

Seeking help is therefore not the same as receiving appropriate treatment. Before discussing how to enlarge the scope and range of people receiving services one must ensure that all currently in treatment are receiving appropriate care. The current initiatives in clinical practice guidelines for psychiatrists, the collaboration between psychiatrists and general practitioners, and the educational programs for general practitioners are all steps in the right

Table 3.3. Rates of disability and consulting behavior among people with a current disorder in the month prior to the study

	Physical disorders	Mental disorders*
Disorders present this month	39%	12.8%
Disorder plus disability days this month	8%	4.5%
Disorder plus disability days and consulting this month	6%	2.1%
Percent of current cases disabled and consulting	15%	16%

*Excluding cognitive impairment and psychosis.

direction. Nevertheless, using consulting behavior as an indication of who warrants treatment is probably better than using perceived health needs. We know that, in the Australian environment where consulting at the primary care level is heavily subsidized, consulting is a behavior probably related to chronicity, disability, and the perception that something can be done.

The data from the survey are important in this respect. Whenever a person appeared likely to meet criteria for a mental or a physical disorder, we asked whether they had experienced one or more disability days or had consulted for that particular complaint, i.e., the disability and consulting were specific to the particular disorder and not affected by comorbidity. We were unable to ask these questions for schizophrenia or cognitive impairment. We used the physical disorders for comparison. Thirty-nine percent of respondents reported a current chronic physical disorder, and one in six (approximately 15%) of them reported both disability days and seeking help (Table 3.3). The determinants of consulting among people with mental disorders (neurasthenia, anxiety, affective disorder, substance use, or personality disorder) were similar, 12.8% of the population meet criteria for one of these diagnoses this month, 4.5% reported disability days and 2.1% of the population, one in six of those with current symptoms, reported both disability days and seeking medical help for these mental disorders in the past month, a rate comparable to that of people with physical disorders (Table 3.3). This is valuable information – again we demonstrate that people with mental disorders are not the worried well, they behave like all people who are sick and see a doctor when their disorder is chronic, disabling and when they perceive that the doctor could help. The second and very important corollary is that the number of people in the community who need help from the mental health services may be closer to the low 2.1% than estimates based on the annual prevalence figures of 24% or 28%.

As expected, disability and consulting were correlated. The probability of reporting disability days and of consulting is highest in neurasthenia and lowest in personality disorder (Table 3.4). Putting considerations of the

Table 3.4. Current mental disorder: disability days and consulting in the month prior to the study

Current disorder	1-month prevalence	% with disability days	% with disability days and consultations
Neurasthenia	1.2	72	41
Affective disorder	3.9	56	33
Anxiety disorder	6.5	37	17
Substance-use disorder	2.5	23	5
Personality disorder	5.0	15	8
Any of above disorders	12.8	35	16

appropriate level of consulting aside for the moment, one might conclude that the public's pattern of consulting is realistic, and that they choose to do so when disabled and when they perceive that the general practitioner might be useful. For example, personality or substance-use disorders do not frequently cause disability days and general practitioners usually have no simple remedies for these conditions.

Can the design of our health services be guided by data from the survey? I am still not sure whether it is sensible to respond to the claim that one in four or five of the population has a mental disorder that warrants treatment. Certainly they met criteria for a mental disorder sometime in 1998, but they are not sick in the sense that they are currently ill and disabled and would like treatment. It would be wiser to focus on the 14% of the population with a current disorder as the upper estimate of who should be treated. Unfortunately not everyone feels that less is more. The Survey showed that 41% of the population had significant mental symptoms sometime during the year even if only half met criteria for a diagnosis. Should treatment be offered to all such people? Even if we had the money and staff, some interventions can do more harm than good; for example, critical-incident, stress-debriefing of people recently exposed to trauma (Raphael, Meldrum & McFarlane, 1995). It is not a simple matter that more is better, as the McCord study (1978) so convincingly showed.

To return to the task of estimating the bottom line of who should be treated. Two percent of the population met criteria for a current mental disorder and reported that they had experienced disability days and had consulted. This figure does not include people with schizophrenia or cognitive impairment, or with other disorders not covered by the Survey. If these were added and the total came to 3% of the population, could they be seen by the resources currently available? I think that this is a manageable monthly workload for the specialist mental health and primary care physicians in Australia. Earlier I estimated that the private and public specialist services, general practitioners and the addiction services saw 1.34 million or 7.5% of the population for treatment of their mental disorders each year (Andrews, 1995). The current survey shows that 8.8% of the population consulted for a mental problem during the year. Given the ratio between one year and one month prevalences we seem to have sufficient services already in place to see the people with a current mental disorder who reported being disabled and seeking help, yet the level of dissatisfaction among consumers is high. People who are not in treatment cannot get appointments with someone expert in their disorder, people in treatment do not get better as quickly as one would expect from the efficacy literature. We need a better system than a health service that responds to demand. Clearly it is failing to satisfy the need, and people are either tolerating illness and not consulting, or turning to alternative services because of their frustration with the system.

In summary, the unmet need for direct treatment in most countries is considerable. Epidemiological studies show that half to three-quarters of people who meet criteria for a mental disorder do not seek, or cannot access, mental health services. In the four studies reviewed, a quarter to a half of all professional services are being delivered to people who do not meet criteria for a current mental disorder. Certainly if some of those met un-need services were redirected to people with mental disorders, the level of unmet need would fall, but still not to acceptable levels. The situation differs between countries but even in Australia, which has well organized public and private mental health sectors which are active in the community (Andrews & Issakidis, 1998), there is little information about whether the system is effective or efficient. It remains unclear whether there would still be a shortfall in services if we were to manage the services we do have efficiently, and not just attend to better ways of providing direct patient care to quieten the complaints of the consumers, carers and the concerned public. Somehow we need to shift the emphasis to the management of a disease, not just focus on the management of people with the disease.

The World Bank Burden of Disease project

Medicine in general, and mental health services in particular, have developed so many accepted methods of treatment that we have no possibility of being funded to do everything we might like to do, or our patients think we should do. We need intelligent ways to triage services, criteria that are independent of clinician whim and patient pressure, and criteria that will maximize the overall health gains. The World Bank Burden of Disease project has issued a final report which may be of value in informing such criteria.

The World Bank Burden of Disease project began in 1992, received initial exposure in the World Bank development report in 1993 (World Bank, 1993), and ends with ten source books, two of which were published in 1996 (*The Global Burden of Disease*, and *Global Health Statistics*) (Murray & Lopez, 1996a,b). The project had two major attributes, a worldwide scope that attempted to make all measures internally consistent; for instance, the total number of deaths attributed to the various causes could not be more than the total number of deaths known to occur. The second attribute was the use of the disability-adjusted life year (DALY) as the main unit of burden. Years of life lost through premature death are calculated as the difference between the actual age at death and the age to which a person could have been expected to live in an established market economy. The number of years of life lived with a disability is assessed in terms of expected duration weighted for severity, with death being regarded as total disability. The years of life lost from a disease and the weighted years lived with a disability due to that disease are summed as a measure of the burden due to that disease in DALYs lost, a measure that is age weighted and discounted for future costs.

The number of DALYs in an untreated population in any given year indicates the disease burden, while the DALYs currently averted by health interventions provide a measure of productivity or outcome. This composite DALY measure materially changes the ranking of health problems from that produced from mortality statistics alone. For example, for the world in 1990, the mental disorders studied (major depression, bipolar disorder, schizophrenia, alcohol and drug use, posttraumatic stress disorder (PTSD), OCD, panic disorder, dementia) accounted for only 0.4% of the years of life lost through early death, but accounted for 26% of all years lost through disability. Thus, when years lost through disability and death are combined, mental disorders account for 9.1% of the worldwide or global burden of disease. These same mental disorders account for 22.4% of the total burden of disease in established market economies, not because these countries are suffering an epidemic of mental disorder, but because the burden of other diseases has dropped, leaving the burden produced by mental disorders more prominent. In detail, the burdens attributed to the various mental disorders in established market economies by Murray & Lopez (1996a,b) were calculated to be as follows: unipolar depression 6.7%, bipolar disorder 1.7%, PTSD, OCD and panic disorder 2.4%, alcohol 4.7%, drugs 1.5%, schizophrenia 2.3%, dementia 2.9%, total 22.2% of the total burden of disease. Three common disorders that disable (See Table 3.2, and Andrews, Sanderson & Beard, 1998) – neurasthenia, social phobia and personality disorder – were not included in this tabulation and so the total DALYs due to mental disorders could be increased. The burden due to unipolar depression used a case history for the disability weighting procedure that was severe, not average, and no allowance was made for comorbidity between mental disorders. On both these grounds the burden attributable to mental disorders could be reduced. Nevertheless a preliminary estimate of the burden of disease in Australia that accommodates some of these changes (C. Mathers, personal communication, October 1997) shows the mental disorders to be, at 20%, the leading cause of burden when diseases are grouped by ICD-10 chapter.

While the relative importance may be different, the actual rates for the burden of mental disorder in DALYs in developed and developing countries are actually quite comparable. If this is true and not an artifact of ascertainment, it is an issue that needs thought, particularly as new data from developing countries suggest that rates of mental disorder are comparable with those in the developed world. Social advance and medical activity have, through prevention, risk factor reduction and direct treatment, reduced the burden of disease due to nonmental disorders in established market economies by some 60% over the rates observed in the rest of the world. This says something for the effect of public health and clinical medicine on the burden of physical illness. Strategies for prevention, risk factor reduction and effective treatment for people with mental disorders do exist, yet do not seem to have been effectively applied, at least as far as can be judged from the rates of DALYs associated with these disorders (established market economies 27.7/ 1000, rest of world 23.2/1000). Could this comparability of burden between the developed and developing worlds be evidence of the inefficiency of the mental health services in the developed world? The major question remains – why hasn't the provision of modern mental health services in developed countries resulted in a reduction of the burden of mental disorders of comparable extent to that which has occurred in the physical disorders.

What should be done? Cost minimization of personal care medicine seems the only strategy in use in most countries. A WHO Ad Hoc Committee addressed the problem of prioritizing investment in health research and development more creatively (Ad Hoc Committee on Health Research Relating to Future Intervention Options, 1996). They considered that the health sector should focus on quantitative measures of disease burden and the relative cost effectiveness of different interventions intended to reduce that burden. They recommended using a five-step method to determine priorities:

1. Calculate the burden of disease associated with the disorder, and favor disorders of large burden over those of small burden.
2. Identify the reasons why the disease burden persists, asking what proportion is currently being averted, what proportion could be averted with better use of existing resources (a health service delivery problem), what proportion could be averted if interventions were more cost-effective (a production problem), and presume that the remaining proportion cannot be averted with existing interventions (a research and development or R & D problem to discover new remedies or strategies for prevention).
3. Judge the adequacy of the existing knowledge base to overcome the barriers in health service delivery, production or discovery listed above.
4. Assess the promise of R & D effort in terms of the expected cost-effectiveness of any necessary new intervention and of the probability of successful development of it.
5. Assess the current level of R & D effort before costing the steps outlined above. Choose where to invest money in terms of the cost and likely benefit.

This Ad Hoc committee included representatives from industry. Presumably this is how successful industry operates – identify the major problem, look at the options available to solve it, and implement the preferred option. No such program has been implemented in mental health service provision. We seem preoccupied with meeting the demands of our patients, not in planning how to reduce the burden of mental disorders.

For example, panic disorder with or without agoraphobia had a point prevalence of 1.7% in the Australian Survey. The cases reported an average of 9.9 disability days per month or 2 million days in all. The burden is considerable. The American Psychiatric Association and the New Zealand Department of Health have both recently released guidelines for the treatment of people with panic disorder. These are good guidelines for how psychiatrists and primary care physicians should treat people with panic disorder using medication and cognitive behavior therapy. Despite the guidelines, the burden of disease appears to be unchanged. If one applied the five-step method a number of alternatives might be identified. Children at risk could be identified in school and taught by the education system how to manage anxiety more constructively (Roth & Dadds, 1999) so that panic never develops, cognitive therapy for panic could be developed and supplied by automated voice recognition technology over the phone line (c.f. Griest's COPE project for the cognitive therapy of Depression, Griest, 1998), and vicarious exposure for people with the agoraphobic complication could be supplied via the Internet (c.f. Newman C, New York University, personal communication, June 1998). Whether these ideas are practical is irrelevant, what is important is that all these alternatives exist outside the established health system and could be made commercially available. We have to implement whatever is necessary for disease management and not be bound by the need to see everything in terms of patient management.

Rationing of health care and caring for the chronically sick

It is one thing to argue for a five-step solution to guide investment in health research and development for disease management, and quite another to use a similar methodology to guide service delivery. Bobadilla, Cowley, Musgrove & Saxenian (1994) have used such a methodology, cost per DALYs averted, to rank services designed to meet the principal physical health problems of low- and middle-income countries. They argued that as no country in the world can provide health services to meet all the possible needs of the population, it is advisable to establish criteria for which services to provide. Oregon, in a similar initiative, made an attempt to have community groups develop a priority list of which treatments for which condition would be supplied under Medicare. Despite considerable difficulties, the endeavor has been seminal. Purchasers in high-income countries such as the USA, UK and Australia have begun to identify services for which they will not pay.

Rationing of health care is already a fait accompli (Klein, Day & Redmayne, 1996). Usually it is done by clinicians who privately decide who they will and will not treat, by administrators who decide what they will and will not fund, and by pressure groups who decide what they will and will not advocate. The reasons behind the rules as to who will be treated are never made public and can never be discussed, and often the rules themselves are never even clarified. It is a denial of natural justice that health, a public resource, is being secretly rationed. The World Bank Burden of Disease project, in terms of the calculations of DALYs lost due to a disease and likely to be gained from interventions, and the Ad Hoc Committee's strategies for investing in health, jointly provide a rational and transparent mechanism for prioritizing health expenditure.

What then are the barriers to the implementation of such a system? First, the calculation of the DALYs attributable to each disease or intervention will have to be recalculated by providers, payers and consumers using verified data to weight disability and techniques to adjust for comorbidity. Progress will only be possible when there is consensus among all stakeholders about the validity of the estimates. Second, providers, payers and advocates will have to be prepared to relinquish the power that presently goes with their ability to gainfully influence the deployment of resources. Neither of these steps will be easy.

One cannot over-emphasize the potential importance of the burden of disease estimates to psychiatry. In countries like the USA, the UK and Australia, mental disorders account for 22.4% of the burden of all disease. In these countries people with mental disorders commonly receive services that cost 5% to 10% of the health budget, instead of the 22.4% that would be their due if burden alone were the mechanism for funding. There is no doubt that such an increase in funding would reduce the need for hard decisions.

Within the constraints of the present mental health budget, the distribution of funds does not parallel burden or cost-efficiency. A large amount, more than half the budget in most countries, is spent on people with chronic psychoses, disorders which account for a minority of the mental disorder burden and for which interventions are not cost-effective. Too little is spent on people with depression and anxiety disorders, disorders which account for half of the burden and for which interventions are cost-effective. Mental health is not always, it seems, about prevention, cure, relief, and care. Certainly there is much to be done to put psychiatry's house in order before we start demanding a larger share of the health budget, but the World Bank Burden of Disease project has given us the tools to start on both tasks.

If we are to get the maximum health gain from the available funds, we do need to prioritize who we treat. This means that, in order to do the greatest good to the greatest number, we need to specify who we will exclude, and this is where most discussions of the problem end. Calman (1994) has argued that the UK National Health Service (NHS) budget could not meet all needs and would have to be prioritized, restricting specialist care to those services with the greatest cost-effectiveness, services that could still be afforded after the needs of the sick had been met for primary health care, emergency care, and shelter when ill. That is, while generalist mental health care would be a right, specialist mental health care would be rationed, and only provided to people for whom it was likely to be a cost-effective strategy.

It is instructive to examine how this model would affect current practice (Andrews, 1997). Australia spends about 5% of the health budget on people with mental disorders, approximately Aus$100 per capita per annum. The mental health component provided by general practitioners costs Aus$15, and the provision of emergency services, such as acute hospital admission and 24-hour crisis teams another Aus$50 per capita. One cannot easily triage either of these services and, under Calman's criteria that protect primary health care and emergency care, one would not. Access is the only criteria. Shelter when ill is presently undertaken in part by the emergency services and in part by other social agencies. Again no change in the status quo is envisaged. The remaining Aus$35 per capita is what is currently spent on specialist services, public and private, distributed on a historical basis. It could be apportioned among the specialist services according to burden and cost-effectiveness. A worked example for mental disorders has been published (Andrews, 1997), and while changes in the distribution of funds are significant, they are not radical, though they may become so as better data about burden and cost-effectiveness become available. Competition for this money by the specialists will hasten the process outlined by the Ad Hoc Committee, and see more people treated at a lower cost, simply because there is now an incentive to improve service delivery and to lower production costs by highlighting effective remedies (see Nathan & Gorman, 1998) and discarding the ineffective remedies. It should also facilitate the development of newer cost efficient remedies, particularly for the people who are presently excluded from specialist care. It is not often that one discovers a scenario where everybody wins, but prioritized health care based on burden and cost-effectiveness may be one such concept.

Conclusion

Defining the core business

If the results of the Australian survey apply to other countries then maybe many countries already have the staff to provide the services needed. Why doesn't it feel like that? It feels as though all mental health staff are overworked and lack the time to do many things properly. Perhaps it is because the core responsibilities are never defined. I have suggested that disability days are more important than symptoms in defining the relative burden of the mental disorders and that the practice of cost-effective treatments is to be preferred. The two pieces of information required by Bobadilla et al. (1994)

might well define the core responsibilities of the mental health services, for I am quite sure that the core business is to reduce the burden of mental disorders, that is, to attend to management of a disease and not just to the management of people with a disease.

There are two problems. There is community disquiet about the adequacy of mental health services. The community does not understand what mental disorders are, and often sees mental health services as resources that can help solve the causes of common human unhappiness, a task that is labor intensive and at which mental health services have never been shown to be more effective than other agencies, let alone cost-effective. We should carry out a community education program to demonstrate what mental health services can, and cannot do. The second problem is that, for historical and humane reasons, mental health services are seen to be responsible for maintaining public order challenged by people affected with psychoses and substance-use disorders. As there are reservations as to whether a period of compulsory hospitalization is beneficial in the long run for people with psychosis or substance-use disorders it may well be that the two roles, treatment of the severely disturbed and the maintenance of public order, should be separated. Monies for the maintenance of public order should not be a charge on the health budget. Acute inpatient units are costly to operate and seldom, for humane and risk management reasons, challenge the need for admission and continued hospitalization. There is no clear answer to this problem (see Treatment Protocol Project, 1999) but as half the mental health budget in Australia is spent on inpatient units, there should be.

Education

Many people who are disabled do not consult, either because they do not understand their illness or they do not believe their general practitioner can help. There are two steps needed to remedy this: general practitioners must be trained to be skillful with patients with the common mental disorders (see Andrews & Hunt, 1999, for a discussion of this issue). Then, once we have the resources in place, an education program about mental disorders should be a regular feature in press, radio, and television. It would be better if the profession, and not the proponents of complementary medicine, wrote self-help books for people who want to know about all the major mental disorders. Health department and University Internet home pages should carry such information. We must do more than only offer direct patient care. For an example directed at primary care but much used by patients, look at the anxiety disorders chapter from the Management of Mental Disorders (Treatment Protocol Project, 1997) at www.crufad.unsw.edu.au. In Australia the Heart Foundation endorses material that is consistent with established knowledge and this seal of approval is recognized. A similar seal of approval should exist in mental health. The consequence would be that more people would present for treatment informed as to why they have come. Provided that treatment is consistent with what they know to expect, they will persevere until they are cured or relieved. If the practitioner is perceived as competent, retention rates can be satisfactory whereas too often they are unacceptably low (Hunt & Andrews, 1992).

Prevention

Raphael (Chapter 9) reviews the evidence for primary prevention and finds good evidence for the effectiveness in anxiety/depression and in conduct disorder when used with at-risk children and adolescents. Other authors of this book also have seen the need to invest in primary prevention. Few health services put real effort into prevention. If prevention is effective it is hard for it not to be cost-effective, given the stream of direct and indirect costs that follow the development of a case. The problem is that the gains are long term and most administrators are simply trying to balance this year's budget, not looking for savings to accrue ten years hence. There is evidence that dropping out from high school, teenage pregnancy, being unemployable, and early drug use are risk factors for much adult psychopathology. There are programs to prevent or reduce these risk factors (Schorr, 1987), but there is no reason why they should be paid for from the health budget. Education, social welfare, housing, and the penal system all stand to benefit from changes to these behaviors.

Changing medical practice

Open-ended fee-for-service payments to private psychiatrists and hospitals, as used in Australia, can provide a perverse incentive that discourages efficient practice. It is not that fee-for-service is intrinsically inefficient, but it is when you pay for service not outcome, and it is when continuing sickness not increasing wellness is tacitly encouraged. The high burden of mental disorders in the developed world may well be due to the poor efficiency of current mental health practice. Seeing a psychiatrist or a general practitioner does not mean the patient will receive appropriate treatment (see Chapters 17 and 18). The compulsory continuing education programs at present in place now give credit for simply attending sessions. They will soon have to test knowledge and appropriateness of practice. It may also be that competent mental health practitioners cannot attain expected cures, simply because of the lack of time. Maybe the 5% of the health budget for people who represent 20% of the burden of disease is restricting the time needed to effect a cure, and only allowing time for practitioners to provide palliative relief and care. However it has come about, treatment as usual too often means disease as usual, an unfortunate outcome for the patient. The converse is also true, if doctors only have time for palliative care they will, unless very robust, lower their expectations further and become chronic doctors with chronic patients.

By encouraging clinicians to practice evidence-based medicine we hope to raise their efficiency to the point where more people are cured, no longer attend, and the onerous workloads become manageable. There is a large number of effective treatments in psychiatry, despite the caution of the Cochrane Collaboration reports (available at www.cochrane.co.uk). Nathan & Gorman (1998) organized a series of secondary analyses of randomized controlled trials and found substantive evidence for efficacy on 57 drug or psychological treatments for specific mental disorders. Their project was originally sponsored by the American Psychiatric and Psychological Associations but was disowned before publication, possibly because once one has identified the treatments that work one has to dissuade clinicians from practising those treatments for which there is no evidence of efficacy. Medical organizations are conservative and have suppressed unwelcome guideline information before (Andrews, in press; Deyo et al., 1997).

Setting priorities

In Australia we have sufficient clinicians to treat 3% of the population each month. If we educate the public about the treatment of mental disorders and educate primary care clinicians about appropriate treatment, some of the disabled who presently avoid treatment will come and the demand will rise. If we begin informed prevention programs for people at risk and self-treatment programs for people with milder disorders, the prevalence and latent demand will drop. If we train mental health clinicians to carry out treatments that work, and pay them accordingly, more people will be cured and the latent demand will drop (and the clinicians will find psychiatry a more exciting vocation). Bobadilla's challenge (Bobadilla et al., 1994) would allow us to set priorities based on the available evidence. This is something we should do.

Planning

Ministers of Health seek answers about planning for service delivery that are affordable and likely to benefit the electorate, or at least plans that will minimize complaints from consumers, carers, providers, and payers. Necessarily, such deliberations focus on the immediate future, and usually on the interface between the health services and the patients. The Ad Hoc Committee on Health Research Relating to Future Intervention Options (1996) took a longer view – calculate the burden of each disease and ask why that burden persists. If we already know enough to reduce the burden further then let us cost ways of doing so. If we lack the knowledge then let us cost the necessary research. Either way the focus should be on disease control, not on management of the consumers, carers, providers, and payers presently involved with the disease. The National Mental Health Strategy in Australia has expended significant money on a number of projects whose value was expected to be in the future. The Australian National Survey of Mental Health and Well-Being was one such project. Perhaps it is time to convene a multinational task force of clinicians, consumers, epidemiologists, economists, and lateral thinkers to prepare a plan for investing in mental health research and development so that we can indeed make sure that the burden does not unnecessarily persist and that the unmet need for effective treatment is, in the future, minimal. All nations face this problem – perhaps people from many nations can collaborate to solve it. The contributions in this book are a beginning.

References

Ad Hoc Committee on Health Research Relating to Future Intervention Options (1996). *Investing in Health Research and Development*. Geneva: World Health Organization.

Andrews, G. (1992). The prospect of cure: implications for mental health planning. *Behaviour Change*, **9**, 246–53.

Andrews, G. (1995). Workforce deployment: reconciling demands and resources. *Australian and New Zealand Journal of Psychiatry*, **29**, 394–402.

Andrews, G. (1996). Comorbidity and the general neurotic syndrome. *British Journal of Psychiatry*, **168** [Suppl. 30], 76–84.

Andrews, G. (1997). Managing scarcity: a worked example using burden and efficacy. *Australasian Psychiatry*, **5**, 225–8 (see also www.crufad.unsw.edu.au).

Andrews, G. (in press). Implementing evidence based medicine in psychiatry. *British Medical Journal*.

Andrews, G. & Hunt, C. (1999). The education of general practitioners in the management of mental disorders. In M. Tansella & G. Thornicroft (eds.), *Common Mental Disorders in Primary Care*. London: Routledge.

Andrews, G. & Issakidis, C. (1998). Mental health services in the city of Sydney, circa 1997. In D. Goldberg & G. Thornicroft (eds.), *Mental Health in our Future Cities*. London: Psychology Press.

Andrews, G., Anstey, K., Brodaty, H., Issakidis, C. & Luscombe, G. (in press). Recall of depressive episodes 25 years previously. *Psychological Medicine*.

Andrews, G., Crino, R., Hunt, C., Lampe, L. & Page, A. (1994). *The Treatment of Anxiety Disorders*. New York: Cambridge University Press.

Andrews, G., Mathers, C. & Sanderson, K. (1998). The burden of disease. *Medical Journal of Australia*, **169**, 156–8.

Andrews, G., Sanderson, K. & Beard, J. (1998). Burden of disease: methods of calculating the disability from mental disorder. *British Journal of Psychiatry*, **173**, 123–31.

Andrews, G., Slade, T.S. & Peters, L. (1999). Classification in psychiatry: ICD-10 versus DSM-IV. *British Journal of Psychiatry*, **174**, 1–3.

Australian Bureau of Statistics (1998). *Mental Health and Wellbeing. Profile of Adults, Australia, 1997*. Canberra: Australian Bureau of Statistics.

Bobadilla, J.-L., Cowley, P., Musgrove, P. & Saxenian, H. (1994). Design, content and financing of an essential national package of health services. In C.J.L. Murray & A.D. Lopez (eds.), *Global Comparative Assessments in the Health Sector. Disease Burden, Expenditures and Intervention Packages*. Geneva: World Health Organization.

Brodaty, H. & Andrews, G. (1983). Brief psychotherapy in family practice: a controlled prospective intervention trial. *British Journal of Psychiatry*, **143**, 11–19.

Calman, K.C. (1994). The ethics of allocation of scarce health resources: a view from the centre. *Journal of Medical Ethics*, **20**, 71–4.

Deyo, R.A., Psaty, B.M., Simon, G., Wagner E.H. & Omenn G.S. (1997). The messenger under attack: intimidation of researchers by special-interest groups. *New England Journal of Medicine*, **336**, 1176–80.

Griest (1998) *COPE, Self-Help Program for Depression*. Madison, WI: Healthcare Technology Systems.

Hulka, B.S., Kupper, L.L. & Cassel, J.C. (1972). Determinants of physician utilization: approach to a service-oriented classification of symptoms. *Medical Care*, **10**, 300–9.

Hunt, C. & Andrews, G. (1992). Dropout rate as a performance indicator in psychotherapy. *Acta Psychiatrica Scandinavica*, **85**, 275–8.

Hunt, C. & Andrews, G. (1998). Long-term outcome of panic disorder and social phobia. *Journal of Anxiety Disorders*, **12**, 395–406.

Jenkins, R., Bebbington, P., Brugha, T., Farrell, M., Gill, B., Lewis, G., Meltzer, H. & Petticrew, M. (1997). The national psychiatric morbidity surveys of Great Britain. *Psychological Medicine*, **27**, 765–74.

Kessler, R.C. & Frank, R.C. (1997) The impact of psychiatric disorders on work loss days. *Psychological Medicine*, **27**, 861–73.

Kessler, R.C., Frank, R.G., Edlund, M., Katz, S.J., Lin, E. & Leaf, P. (1997). Differences in the use of psychiatric outpatient services between the United States and Ontario. *New England Journal of Medicine*, **336**, 551–7.

Kessler, R.C., McGonagle, K.A., Zhao, S., Nelson, C.B., Hughes, M., Eshleman, S., Wittchen, H-U. & Kendler, K.S. (1994). Lifetime and twelve month prevalence of DSM-III-R psychiatric disorders in the United States. *Archives of General Psychiatry*, **51**, 8–19.

Klein, R., Day, P. & Redmayne, S. (1996). *Managing Scarcity: Priority Setting and Rationing in the National Health Service*. Buckingham: Open University Press.

Lin, E., Goering, P., Offord, D.R., Campbell, D. & Boyle, M.H. (1996). The use of mental health services in Ontario: epidemiological findings. *Canadian Journal of Psychiatry*, **41**, 572–7.

McCord, J. (1978). A thirty-year follow-up of treatment effects. *American Psychologist*, **33**, 284–9.

Murray, C.J.L. & Lopez, A.D. (eds.) (1996a). *The Global Burden of Disease: a Comprehensive Assessment of Mortality and Disability from Diseases, Injuries, and Risk Factors in 1990 and Projected to 2020*. Cambridge, MA: Harvard University Press.

Murray, C.J.L. & Lopez, A.D. (eds.) (1996b). *Global Health Statistics: a Compendium of Incidence, Prevalence and Mortality Estimates for over 200 Conditions.* Cambridge, MA: Harvard University Press.

Nathan, P.E. & Gorman, J.M. (eds.). (1998). *A Guide to Treatments that Work.* New York: Oxford University Press.

Raphael, B., Meldrum, L. & McFarlane, A.C. (1995). Does debriefing after psychological trauma work? *British Medical Journal,* **310,** 1479–80.

Regier, D.A., Narrow, W.E., Rae, D.S., Manderscheid, R.W., Locke, B.Z. & Goodwin, F.K. (1993). The de facto US Mental and Addictive Disorders System. *Archives of General Psychiatry,* **50,** 85–94.

Roth, J.H. & Dadds, M.R. (1999). Prevention and early intervention strategies for anxiety disorders. *Current Opinion in Psychiatry,* **12,** 169–74.

Schorr, L.B. (1987). *Within our Reach: Breaking the Cycle of Disadvantage.* New York: Doubleday.

Treatment Protocol Project. (1997). *Management of Mental Disorders* (2nd edition). Darlinghurst, NSW: World Health Organization Collaborating Centre for Mental Health and Substance Abuse.

Treatment Protocol Project. (1999). *Acute Psychiatric Inpatient Care: a Source Book.* Darlinghurst, NSW: World Health Organization Collaborating Centre for Mental Health and Substance Abuse.

United States Public Health Service (1995). *For a Health Nation: Returns on Investing in Public Health.* Washington, D.C.: US Government Printing Office 390–173 (20497).

Von Korff, M., Üstün, T.B. & Ormel, J. (1996). Self-report disability in an international primary care study of psychological illness. *Journal of Clinical Epidemiology,* **49,** 297–303.

Ware, J.E., Kosinski, M. & Keller, S.D. (1996). A 12-item short-form health survey: construction of scales and preliminary tests of reliability and validity. *Medical Care,* **34,** 220–33.

World Bank (1993). *World Development Report 1993: Investing in Health.* Oxford: Oxford University Press.

Unmet need: general problems and solutions

Introduction

Gavin Andrews

With the introductory chapters out of the way this book can settle to the serious work in hand. Chapter 4, by Regier et al., is an excellent start. It takes a 50-year perspective on the delivery of mental health services. It outlines the flurry of training that followed the Stirling County and Mid-Town Manhattan studies, the first studies that demonstrated the importance of non-psychotic mental disorders. Treatment capacity increased, but the proportion of cases in treatment did not, as revealed by the Epidemiologic Catchment Area (ECA) and the 1990 National Comorbidity Survey (NCS) studies. It notes the changes produced by legislation and the changes brought about by managed care. The message is of support for good data on which good service plans can be built. Kessler (Chapter 5) takes the argument one step further. He says that the problem of unmet need for people with mental disorders is part of the larger problem of resource allocation in health, and, if we are to succeed in reducing the unmet need, we will have to gather immaculate data to show that the health gains in psychiatry, in human capital terms, are sufficiently great to warrant increases in funding in competition with the costs and benefits of interventions in the physical diseases. The examples he finds as to how this could be done are quite exciting. Chapter 8, by Rupp and Lapsley, reinforces this perspective. If the range of possible interventions exceeds our ability to pay, then policy makers will be forced into ad hoc decisions unless provided with high quality data. For Rupp and Lapsley there is only one course of action – provide economic data to inform resource allocation or be ignored. Love and compassion are clearly no longer enough.

Bebbington (Chapter 6) looks at data from the overarching UK National Survey and from the very fine grained Camberwell Needs Survey and concludes that there is considerable unmet need for the treatment of depression and anxiety. Some of this is because the treatment was not and would not be sought, and some because it was not offered. That both are barriers to care means that the solution is not simple. Chapter 7, by Alegría et al., uses a revolutionary method to solve such problems – it combines health service data from a number of countries with different health delivery systems and discovers which elements of the systems produce the most equitable care.

Chapters 8–11 explore alternatives to routine mental health care. Pincus and Zarin (Chapter 10) discuss the gains that are possible from the implementation of evidence-based medicine and conclude that such quasi theoretical information has to be seen in relation to the realities of current practice. The American Psychiatric Association has developed a large practice research network that has the potential to inform in the same way that Alegría et al. (Chapter 7) can, by comparing the similarities and differences between countries on the one hand and practitioners on the other. Such lateral thinking has always been attractive. Raphael (Chapter 9) discusses prevention. Everyone provides lip service to prevention but few do it – the delights of the immediate improvement one sees in direct patient care outweigh the long haul needed before one can see benefit from prevention. Raphael shows that serious money should be invested in the prevention of anxiety/depression and in conduct/antisocial syndromes in children at risk. Given the heavy direct and indirect costs of illness, prevention has to be better at reducing need for treatment in economic terms, and, in pursuit of the main goal, saving children from a life of misery.

Readers of this book should remember that in most countries most treatment of people with mental disorders occurs in primary care. Üstün (Chapter 11) points out that there are now very good data indicating that some of the burden of mental disorders can be alleviated through an informed primary care sector. He sees the need for additional data and lists the specific items yet to be quantified. A most important chapter. Finally Cooper (Chapter 12) examines aspects of complementary or alternative medicine and notes that the unmet need of some patients is alleviated by such treatments. He discusses the ethos behind the treatments and regrets that orthodox medicine currently ignores the subject. He argues for collaborative investigations and for the inclusion of information about complementary treatments in the medical school curriculum.

4

The epidemiology of mental disorder treatment need: community estimates of 'medical necessity'

Darrel A. Regier, William E. Narrow, Agnes Rupp,
Donald S. Rae, and Charles T. Kaelber

A 50-year historical perspective is provided on US attempts to define and quantify the need for mental health services. Early epidemiological estimates of mental disorder prevalence were so far in excess of available treatment capacity that they supported initiation of major National Institute of Mental Health (NIMH) training programs to produce mental health specialists and to increase the supply of service center resources. Despite the increased treatment capacity demonstrated by the early 1980s, the Epidemiologic Catchment Area (ECA) study (Robins & Regier, 1991) indicated that of the 28% of the population that met annual diagnostic criteria for a mental or addictive disorder, over two-thirds received no treatment during the year – similar rates were demonstrated by the National Comorbidity Survey (NCS) in the 1990s (Kessler et al., 1994).

However, the 1990s brought a major change in the delivery of US mental health services. Managed behavioral health care resulted in marked decreases in definitions of need for inpatient mental health care, and greatly limited the indications of 'medical necessity' for outpatient treatment. Legislators have accelerated efforts to prioritize treatment need by specifying severe disorders (2.8% of the population) considered most in need of treatment and insurance coverage. Hence, the objectives of an epidemiological survey sensitive to the needs of patients, providers, managed care company guidelines, and policy planners in this context include the following: generate prevalence rates of disorders by disability levels; match these rates with need for specific treatment procedures; identify the unit and aggregate costs of treatment needed for the population in each category; and link such service costs to the benefits which would accrue for the health, social welfare, and productivity/ economy of the population.

This chapter will provide a developmental perspective on how the US mental health community has responded to periodic requests to define and quantify the need for mental health services in both public and private insurance sectors. It is now possible to look back over 40 years to when national planning for such mental health services took place in the mid1950s as part of the US Joint

Commission on Mental Illness and Health (Joint Commission on Mental Illness and Health, 1961) review process. Although community prevalence rates of mental disorders were more nonspecific at the time, available data from large epidemiological studies such as the Stirling County (Leighton, Harding, Macklin, Macmillian & Leighton, 1963) and Mid-Town Manhattan (Srole, Langer, Michael, Opler & Rennie, 1962) projects indicated a level of need which far surpassed available treatment resources.

Perhaps of even greater public policy consequence than the large community prevalence studies, at that time, were psychiatric-service-use findings from the study of social class and mental illness (Hollingshead & Redlich, 1958). This study demonstrated presumptive social inequities in that patients with lower socioeconomic status were more likely to be institutionalized and to receive severe mental illness diagnoses. It supported a strong hypothesis of that time that the stresses associated with poor living conditions could produce schizophrenia and other more severe forms of mental disorder. The rising patient populations and costs of state and county mental hospitals gave urgency to the Joint Commission on Mental Illness and Health for planning a new public mental health care system (Joint Commission on Mental Illness and Health, 1961). A Federally funded reform was endorsed by President Kennedy and implemented by President Johnson with the Community Mental Health Centers (CMHC) legislation. The service plans which ensued emphasized community-based alternatives for institutionalization, and prevention activities which often included community action and school consultation to improve community and individual living conditions.

In 1978, after 15 years of experience with the CMHC reforms, the President's Commission on Mental Health reviewed the impact of the CMHC system changes (The President's Commission on Mental Health, 1978). Although its recommendations for minor modifications in the Community Mental Health Systems Act were never implemented because of President Reagan's adoption of a block grant approach to the States, the Commission performed another valuable service. It documented our ability to describe the multiple components of the De Facto Mental Health Service System – with particular emphasis on the role of primary health care providers (Regier, Goldberg & Taube, 1978). The Commission also noted deficiencies in epidemiological information on the community prevalence of specific mental disorders, the degree to which they were treated or undertreated, and called for an improved database in order to plan for mental health services.

Over the past 20 years, with the impetus given by the President's Commission, we have been able to greatly increase the quantitative information on the contributions of various service system components, the level and cost of utilization, and the prevalence of mental and addictive disorders in the community. Major national level studies have included the ECA study (Robins & Regier, 1991) and the more recent NCS study (Kessler et al., 1994).

Radical changes in the organization and financing of mental health services in the USA have highlighted continued deficiencies in our ability to define adequate treatment for specific disorders and the level of need for care in the community. Although there is a well established distinction in public health and in health economics between the concepts of want, demand and need for medical services (Jeffers, Bognanno & Bartlett, 1971), the definition of need has generally been made by professionals and equated with a diagnosis. The equation of diagnosis with need for treatment has now been called into question – in particular by the managed behavioral health care industry which sees itself as being in the business of defining 'medical necessity' or need for treatment within its system (Regier et al., 1998).

Under traditional employer-based private insurance in the USA, physicians assigned a diagnosis and determined the need for treatment and the appropriate amount of care required in clinical settings. Such decisions were undoubtedly influenced by the patient's private insurance policy which provided specific limits and reimbursement rates for procedures. This provided the potential for excessive treatment if insurance coverage was available and 'undertreatment' if insurance coverage was limited. The cumulative effect of such financial incentives in the USA led to relatively rapid increases in the costs of treatments for mental health and substance-use disorders (Frank, McGuire, Regier, Mandersheid & Woodward, 1994). Under these circumstances, private health insurance companies and employers contracted with managed behavioral firms to change the utilization and cost patterns of care in two ways: they required more specific treatment objectives (with a focus on restoring function), and they required more objective evidence of a positive treatment outcome from the provider (Allo, Mintzes & Brook, 1988). Although the presence of managed care oversight theoretically offers greater flexibility than previous fixed benefits, determinations of medical necessity depend on the judgement of the care manager (an employee of the behavioral health care firm) and the judgement and reports of the treating clinician about the patient's status (Frank, McGuire, Bae & Rupp, 1997).

To plan for services in the current US context, it is necessary to extend beyond our knowledge of the prevalence of mental disorders or the implicit belief that all such disorders identified in community populations are clinically significant – meaning that they require professional treatment. With advances in epidemiological survey methods, we have been able to determine prevalence rates of DSM-III (American Psychiatric Association, 1980), subsequent DSM revisions, and ICD-10 (World Health Organization, 1993) syndromes in large community populations over multiple international settings. In virtually all of these studies, the prevalence of these syndromes far surpasses the perceived need for, demand for, and certainly the availability of professional treatment services. Policy makers and managed care actuaries can either despair of having useful epidemiological data for assessing and prioritizing service need, or more likely plan with different decision-making tools.

A useful illustration of the gap between community prevalence and treated prevalence was demonstrated by the ECA study in the USA which identified 28% of adults (age 18+) as having a mental or addictive disorder in one year (Regier et al., 1993). During that same time period 5.9% received services from mental health specialists, and an additional 5% received care only from general medical physicians in the health care system. The ECA recognized that many relevant services were also obtained from human service professionals outside the health care system. Approximately 3% of the population received some mental health services from human service professionals such as the clergy and social service workers, with a small percentage receiving intensive support from self-help groups as well as family and friends. Therefore, a total of slightly less than 15% used some mental health service in one year. When one attempts to compare those who received services with those who had disorders, we find that only 55% of the service recipients met diagnostic criteria. Perhaps of greater significance is the fact that only 28% of those with a mental or addictive disorder received any type of service in one year. These data are presented schematically in Figure 4.1.

The absence of precise information on who could benefit from care has very different consequences in the current managed care environment than it did in the previous mixed public care and private indemnity insurance system. The identification of large numbers of individuals with mental disorders in earlier population surveys (Leighton et al., 1963; Srole et al., 1962) and the demand for mental health treatment led to a major expansion in the supply of mental health facilities and providers. For example, in 1953 approximately 0.8% of the population of New Haven, Connecticut received any specialized mental health services (Hollingshead & Redlich, 1958). With the passage of the CMHC act, and a national commitment to training mental health specialists in psychiatry, psychology, social work, and nursing through NIMH-funded training grants, there was an explosion in the availability of outpatient services. Hence, by 1975, it was possible to document that 3.1% of the US population received specialized mental health services in one year (Regier et al., 1978). The logarithmic increase in access to specialty services continued between 1975 and 1983 to the point where the ECA documented the rate of specialty use in 5.9% of adults, as noted above (Regier et al., 1993). By the mid1980s, it appears that some leveling off of mental health service utilization had begun. In the 1992 NIMH-supported NCS, the rate of specialized mental health service use could be calculated from the reports as remaining at between 5% and 6% of the US population (Kessler et al., 1994, 1997).

Within the private sector, the revolution of managed behavioral health care (supported by a market economy response to employers' demands to

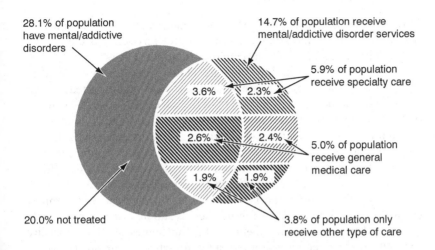

28.1% of population
have mental/addictive
disorders

14.7% of population receive
mental/addictive disorder services

5.9% of population
receive specialty care

3.6%   2.3%

2.6%   2.4%

5.0% of population
receive general
medical care

1.9%   1.9%

20.0% not treated

3.8% of population only
receive other type of care

Figure 4.1 The annual prevalence of mental/addictive disorders and services.

control costs) began to respond to the growth of specialized mental and addictive disorder treatment costs, costs that had mushroomed with the increased availability of private hospital and outpatient providers. Mental and addictive disorder treatment costs, which had reached as high as 10% of private indemnity plan benefit costs, were rapidly reduced through pre-admission screening, concurrent case-management review, and limitations on inpatient days and outpatient visits. The entire dynamic of fee-for-service medicine, in which it is to the providers' benefit to offer the best and most expensive forms of treatment, has been turned on its head. With prepaid, capitated, managed care, it is now in the providers' interest to limit care to that which is 'medically necessary' with savings redounding to the benefit of the employer (lower premiums), the managed care company (higher profits), and the provider (incentives to avoid specialty referrals or high-tech inter-ventions).

For epidemiological data to be useful for planning in the current managed care context, it must be closely linked to clearly defined indicators of treat-ment need – with equally well-defined cost implications of addressing differ-ent definitions of need. The concept of need has recently been linked more directly with treatment guidelines for specific disorders. However, despite the publication of detailed treatment guidelines for specific disorders by the American Psychiatric Association (1997) and the Agency for Health Care Policy Research (Depression Guideline Panel, 1993), the admission criteria and treatment guidelines of managed care companies (which focus on func-tional impairment, danger, and the availability of treatments to restore function) have much greater force in the current US environment. The treatment actually received, however, depends on the combination of the provider network structure, the providers' financial incentives, administrative mechanisms to monitor quality and use of services, and the general benefit limits negotiated with the employer (Frank et al., 1997).

Needs assessment research will require additional refinements in understanding the cost of appropriate treatments, given the expected clinical course and treatment effectiveness of these disorders. This expanded concept of 'medical necessity' will be linked with clinical service 'outcomes research', research in which the cost and consequences of undertreatment will be as visible to managed care company actuaries as the costs of inappropriate or excessive treatment are now (Steinwachs, Flynn, Norquist & Skinner, 1996). Although available empirical studies of the impact of managed behavioral health care consistently report substantial cost reductions and complex changes in service-utilization patterns, there is still little standardization of contractual arrangements and there are still only limited data on the quality and outcome of mental health and substance-abuse treatment (National Advisory Mental Health Council, 1998; Sturm, 1997). Of particular importance will be a definitive list of necessary services that will provide a publicly financed safety net for the severely ill, and serve as part of a comprehensive mental health service delivery system.

The remainder of this discussion will focus on a model of epidemiological data that will improve our ability to plan for mental health services. It reflects a research enterprise that is attuned to health policy service delivery innovations, service and economic research parameters, and treatment technologies involving both efficacy and effectiveness outcome measurement.

An epidemiology of clinically significant disorders

Criteria-based DSM and ICD-10 disorders

The first objective will be to improve our measurement of clinically significant mental and addictive disorders. Knowledge of the scope of mental illness in the US has increased greatly since the development of more explicit diagnostic criteria for mental disorders and the adoption of those criteria in the 1980 Diagnostic and Statistical Manual (DSM-III, American Psychiatric Association, 1980). Based on the first and second waves of the NIMH-sponsored ECA program, we now know that in one year, 28.1% of the US adult population (aged 18 and older) have symptoms of sufficient duration and severity to meet formal diagnostic criteria for a mental or addictive disorder. The more recently released data from the NCS for a younger population (ages 15–54) showed a similar one year prevalence of 29% (Kessler et al., 1994). The details for the prevalence of individual diagnoses are shown in Table 4.1.

Table 4.1. Twelve month prevalence of mental disorders

Disorder	NCS Data	ECA Data
Any affective disorder	11.3	9.5
Major depressive episode	10.3	5.0
Manic episode (bipolar)	1.3	1.2
Dysthymia	2.5	5.4
Any anxiety disorder	17.2	12.6
Panic disorder	2.3	1.3
Agoraphobia without panic	2.8	–
Social phobia	7.9	4.2
Simple phobia	8.8	9.1
Any phobia	–	10.9
Generalized anxiety disorder	3.1	–
Obsessive-compulsive disorder	–	2.1
Any substance-use disorder	11.3	9.5
Alcohol dependence or abuse	9.7	7.4
Drug dependence or abuse	3.6	3.1
Schizophrenia	0.5	1.0
Any mental disorder	29.5	28.1

NCS, National Comorbidity Survey; ECA, Epidemiologic Catchment Area Study.

Despite the apparent precision of these estimates for measuring the prevalence of adults meeting DSM-III/IV or ICD-10 diagnostic criteria, there has been considerable doubt about the clinical significance of these syndromes when found in community rather than clinical populations (Regier et al., 1998). Given the impossibility of providing specialized mental health services to 28% of the population, epidemiologists have begun to focus more carefully on the level of psychopathological impairment associated with these disorders.

Mental disorders classified by degree of impairment

The Marshfield study is one of the few such studies to present research, diagnosis and functional impairment criteria (Regier, Burke, Mandersheid & Burns, 1985). It found that approximately 30% of patients attending a primary care physician group practice in a three-month period had a Research Diagnostic Criteria (RDC) mental or addictive disorder. Most had no impairment, as determined by a global measure of functional impairment. Among the remainder, minimal impairment was most frequent (affecting 9%), while moderate and severe impairment were relatively infrequent (affecting 4% and 1.6%, respectively) (Regier et al., 1985). Equally interesting in the current climate, although unpublished, was the finding that about 5% of the population had a global assessment scale (GAS) score of less than 71 while

Table 4.2. Percentage of adults with severe mental disorders (Senate Committee definition)

Diagnosis	% of US adult population (age 18 and above)
Schizophrenia	1.5
Manic depressive (Bipolar)	1.0
Major depression	1.1
Panic	0.4
Obsessive-compulsive disorder	0.6
ANY OF ABOVE	2.8

having no mental disorder diagnosis. In this study, the GAS score was a more useful predictor of mental health service use than any RDC diagnosis or generalized health questionnaire (GHQ) symptom score.

Mental disorders classified by severity

In addition to examining prevalence rates qualified by disorder and functional impairment, legislators have requested epidemiological information that would clarify the implications of a health policy's granting differential insurance coverage for those with severe mental illness/disorders (National Advisory Mental Health Council, 1993). In what may prove to be a bellwether for psychiatric epidemiologists, the Senate Committee took the unusual step of defining the specific disorders that it considered were within the scope of severe disorders (see Table 4.2). Using specifications for severe mental disorders identified by the Senate Appropriations Committee, it was found that approximately 3% of the adult population has a *severe* mental disorder as defined above.

Combining criteria, impairment, and severity for children

Preliminary estimates from the four-site MECA study of about 1200 community residents suggest that a similar proportion of children aged 9–17 years have a severe mental disorder. The MECA assessment procedures permit estimates of six month prevalence based on symptom criteria only, and prevalence measures based on symptoms plus diagnosis-specific impairment criteria, and various global assessment of function levels, e.g., children's GAS (CGAS) <71 (22%), CGAS <61 (12%), CGAS <51 (5%), and, finally, the Senate definition of severe mental illness (SMI) (2.5%). The significance of these definitions for service use is shown in a somewhat complex figure (see Figure 4.2), in which health services, other human services (predominantly school based), and no service use are shown as a percentage of those with different functional impairment levels. For example, use of any mental health

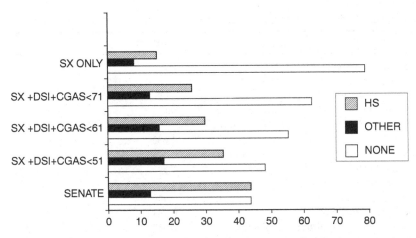

Figure 4.2 Percentage of children (aged 9–17) using services according to symptoms, diagnosis-specific impairment, and global impairment levels. SX, symptoms; DSI, diagnosis-specific impairment; CGAS, children's global assessment scale; HS, health services.

service increased from about 20% for those with diagnosis only, to 35% for those with diagnosis-specific impairment and a global impairment CGAS < 71, to 45% for those with a CGAS < 61, and to 50% for those with a CGAS < 51. The smaller group with the Senate definition of severe mental illness had a treatment rate of about 55%.

Disability and limited eligibility criteria

More limited definitions of severe mental disorder are also feasible – particularly when they are tailored to available eligibility requirements for specific types of welfare or clinical services. Table 4.3 illustrates the annual prevalence implications of different definitions of severe mental disorders: ranging from a high of 2.8% for those defined by the Senate as having severe mental disorders to a low of 0.05% for those requiring nursing home care or long-term hospitalization for mental disorders.

An epidemiology of mental disorder: course of illness

As helpful as the annual prevalence rates may be for focusing on the implications of different definitions of severity, they are insufficient to determine the clinical treatment needs or the related cost implications. Another relevant piece of information is the usual course of illnesses, as defined by various methods. As we can see from the longitudinal component of the ECA (see

Table 4.3. Definitions of severe mental disorder one-year prevalence by treatment

Definition	One-year prevalence
Senate Definition	
Prevalence (ECA)	2.8%
Receiving any services (ECA)	1.7%
Lasting > one year	0.8%
Marshfield Primary Care Study definition	
GAS < 50	1.6%
Social Security Administration definition	
SSI/SSDI Benefits	0.5%
Wisconsin/New Hampshire definitions	
Intermittent care	0.4%
Continuous care	0.1%
Nursing home/long-term hospitalization	0.05%

ECA, Epidemiologic Catchment Area Study; GAS, global assessment scale; SSI, Supplemental Security Income; SSDI, Social Security Disability Insurance.

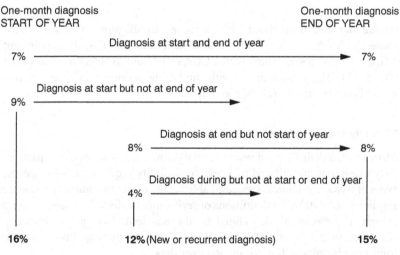

Figure 4.3 One-year prevalence of mental/addictive disorders: stability of diagnosis. The diagnosis at any time during the year: 7+9+8+4=28%. Note that the percentages are of the US adult population.

Figure 4.3), most episodes of mental illness are neither severe nor long-lasting. Although 28.1% of the US adult population have mental or addictive disorders during the course of a year, only 15.7% (rounded to 16%) of American adults have such a disorder at any one point in time. The two-wave longitudinal data from the ECA show that less than half of the one month prevalence group (7% of the population) will continue to have symptoms that fully meet diagnostic criteria during the year; the remainder will not.

Another 12% of the population who are not ill at the start of the year go on to develop a new or recurrent mental or addictive disorder. Hence, to determine treatment need, it is necessary to know which disorders are relatively brief and self-limiting (like a bad case of the 'flu), and which become chronic, disabling, and require long-term care (like a case of chronic obstructive pulmonary disease).

Disability-adjusted life years (DALYs)

Among the most interesting recent additions to the potential measures of need for treatment, few have generated as much interest as the recently defined disability-adjusted life years (DALYs) approach. The focus on a common metric for all physical and mental disorders, which combines prevalence, incidence, impairment/morbidity, course of illness, and mortality measures, offers new challenges to our field to produce empirical tests of the validity of the current estimates. In the meantime, the identification of mental disorders as resulting in 10.5% of all DALYs, with major depression resting in fourth place among all disorders at the present time, has been made possible because of the remarkable productivity of psychiatric epidemiologists worldwide (Murray & Lopez, 1996).

Use of the Diagnostic Interview Schedule (DIS) (Robins, Helzer, Croughan & Ratcliff, 1981) and the Composite International Diagnostic Interview (CIDI) (Robins et al., 1988) in studies around the world has facilitated secondary analyses and estimates of mental-disorder-related disability burdens in many different cultures. The validation of these estimates and public health efforts to organize health services to reduce such disability levels offers an organizing principle that can be appreciated by health service policy legislators and administrators.

An epidemiology of service use

Based on an epidemiological framework which differentiates those with severe mental disorders (SMI) from those with other mental disorders (nonSMI), as well as those with relatively brief versus those with a longer-term course, it will become increasingly useful to differentiate between those who access public and privately administered mental health services. This approach is intended to identify the prevalence of those who are treated and the locus of care for those with specific disorders that require specific types of treatment. Most American adults use some health care services in the course of a year. These service users include the 10.9% of the total adult population who use mental health or addictive disorder treatment services; virtually all of these use outpatient services, while only a small proportion of this group use some inpatient services (Manderscheid, Rae, Narrow, Locke & Regier, 1993; Regier et al., 1993).

More than half of those who suffer severe mental illness (53.1%) use mental health and substance-use services – particularly outpatient services – in the private sector during a year, while less than one-fifth use such services in the public sector. An evaluation of the future responsibilities of the public mental health system should begin with the fact that of the population that uses any public mental health services, about one-quarter have a severe mental disorder and the other three-quarters have other mental illnesses, which may be treatable within the private sector.

As past researchers attempted to predict the need for, and use of, mental health services, early studies demonstrated that diagnoses alone, as aggregated into diagnostic related groups (DRGs), were not a useful basis for such prediction (English, Sharfstein, Scherl, Astrachan & Muszynski, 1986; Taube, Lee & Forthofer, 1984). As a result, efforts have been made to combine diagnosis with various measures of disability (e.g., in work and school performance), comorbidity with other mental and addictive disorders, and need for social and economic supports – such as Supplemental Security Income, Social Security Disability Insurance, and Welfare – to estimate the type of service need (Regier, Shapiro, Kessler & Taube, 1984; Shapiro, Skinner, Kramer, Steinwachs & Regier, 1985). The massive gap between prevalence and service use required access to as many indicators as possible to explain this variance. Researchers have found that, in general, the need for, and use of, services can be more effectively predicted by the level of impairment, duration, comorbidity, and disability associated with symptoms or syndromes than by any specific diagnosis.

Consumer perceived need for care

More recent analyses of the NCS (Kessler et al., 1997) have also focused on the perceived need for treatment, which may be the product of supply-induced demand and subtle national expectations of entitlement to care that are independent of more objective indicators of need.

Linking the epidemiology of disorders, specific treatment needs, and predicted costs of care

With the advent of managed care, it may be useful to forge stronger links between the public health sciences of epidemiology and services research with the objective of matching specific treatments to patients – characterized by disorders, impairments, comorbidity, predicted clinical course, and cost of illness. With such a paradigm, it becomes important to assess the proportion of the population that needs a specific type of evaluation and treatment. A continuum of care can be conceptualized as follows:

1. Evaluation only
2. Short-term outpatient medication or psychotherapy < 10 visits/year
3. Medium-term outpatient medication management < 30 visits/year
4. Medium-term outpatient psychotherapy < 30 visits/year
5. Long-term outpatient psychotherapy > 30 visits/year
6. Brief (acute-care) hospitalization < 10 days/year
7. Medium-term hospitalization < 45 days/year
8. Long-term outpatient case-management/rehabilitation
9. Programs of assertive community treatment (PACT) – intensive
10. Long-term nursing home care
11. Long-term (chronic) hospitalization > 45 days/year

The dimensions of the above list include a progressive decrease in the treated prevalence and a progressive increase in the unit costs of care associated with each treatment procedure. The objectives of an epidemiological survey sensitive to the needs of mental health service providers and policy planners would be to identify the prevalence of disorders which would then be appropriately matched with each treatment procedure, the unit costs of treatment, the aggregate costs, and level of resources needed for the population in each category. A further objective would be to assess the health, social welfare, and productivity/economy benefits which would accrue to the treated population by providing such services.

Once the prevalence of treatment need is identified in this manner, the objective of a managed care company, or a public health entity contracting clinical services for this population, would be to develop an analysis similar to one developed for the State of New Hampshire for PACT low- to high-intensity type case management services, and for housing support for a designated severely mentally ill component of the population (G. Teague, personal communication). In this model, the number of clients served is given a treated prevalence population rate (0.4%), a total program cost for each type of service, a cost per user, and ultimately a cost per capita (see Table 4.4).

The science/political interface

Since 1993, a great deal of NIMH professional time has been focused on applying epidemiological data to health policy issues – first in the ill-fated

Table 4.4. Cost of case management services: New Hampshire, financial year 1993

	Users (no. of clients served)	Users per capita	Total program cost ($)	Cost per user ($)	Cost per capita ($)
Case management	3,939	0.3%	5,860,036	1,488	5.01
Continuous treatment team	753	0.065%	3,108,691	4,128	2.66
Housing support	707	0.06%	3,831,515	5,419	3.28
Combined	4,692	0.4%	12,800,242	2,728	10.95

Note: NH Total Population: 1,169,009.

President's Task Force on Health Care Reform (Frank et al., 1994), and more recently in assessing the costs of various legislative initiatives designed to produce parity of insurance coverage for mental and physical disorders (National Advisory Mental Health Council, 1993, 1998). It has become abundantly clear in our initial examinations of various State systems in which such legislation has been enacted, that managed care systems were either in place before the legislation was passed or put into service before the legislation was implemented.

Although most managed care systems have been in the private sector, public sector contracts for Medicaid and Medicare mental health services are rapidly growing. Information that will assist in the development of responsible contract bids, or in the monitoring of treatment adequacy in private and public systems, will require better measures of treatment need. One of the steps required to address these issues includes an improvement in the information gathered about the clinical significance of the prevalence rates of specific disorders – with specific attention given to functional status, course of illness, treatment matching, cost estimates, and quality or outcome of treatment analyses.

Planning challenge for determinations of need

It is worthwhile noting that many postwar social and political forces propelled early estimates of mental disorder prevalence and treatment need, such as the *Social Class and Mental Illness* (Hollingshead & Redlich, 1958), and the *Midtown Manhattan* (Srole et al., 1962) studies. Since that time, we have witnessed a major deinstitutionalization of the mentally ill, a major increase in mental health treatment capacity, increased demand and cost, and a pendulum swing to reduce demand while requiring more explicit indicators of treatment need priorities.

During the last few decades, psychiatric epidemiology has created better assessment instruments, utilized more sophisticated sampling designs, and generated better and more complex data sets concerning the need for mental health treatment in community populations. Further advances are likely to require consideration of the clinical, economic, health system management, and sociological variables that affect individual, community, and societal definitions of mental health service need in the private and public sectors of care.

The new social and economic forces driving our interest in meeting the unmet need are the managed care revolution in private insurance plans, the privatization of public mental health services, the search for social equity in insurance coverage for persons suffering from mental disorders, and the emergence of DALYs, which have integrated health and mental health issues in the health policy arena. In order for us to assist in formulating and monitoring public health policy, we will need to strengthen the link between epidemiology and the analysis of health economic and health services research. However, our credibility in the health policy arena will wither if we do not simultaneously attend to the uses of epidemiology other than community diagnosis and assessing the workings of the health care system as defined by Morris (Morris, 1964). More functional definitions of psychopathology in community studies will require further examination of the 'validity' of these syndromes in community populations by assessing clinical course, treatment outcome, genetic aggregation, and the other biological and environmental risk factors that will inform etiology and preventive strategies. The late Michael Shepherd referred to epidemiology as an integrating discipline for all of clinical medicine (Shepherd, 1978). To be most effective, the role of epidemiology must be inclusive enough to inform us about the unmet need for treatment in the community. Epidemiology in this broader context may serve as an integrating discipline for basic science, clinical medicine, public health and health policy.

References

Allo, C.D., Mintzes, B. & Brook, R.C. (1988). What purchasers of treatment services want from evaluation. *Alcohol Health and Research World*, 12, 162–7.

American Psychiatric Association (1980). *Diagnostic and Statistical Manual of Mental Disorders* (3rd edition). Washington, D.C.: American Psychiatric Association.

American Psychiatric Association (1997). Practice guideline for the treatment of patients with schizophrenia. *American Journal of Psychiatry*, 154 [Suppl. 4], 1–63.

Depression Guideline Panel (1993). *Depression in Primary Care. Clinical Practice Guideline, Number 5*. Rockville, MD: U.S. DHHS, PHS, Agency for Health Care Policy and Research.

English, J.T., Sharfstein, S.S., Scherl, D.J., Astrachan, B. & Muszynski, I.L. (1986). Diagnosis-related groups and general hospital psychiatry: the APA study. *American Journal of Psychiatry*, 143, 131–9.

Frank, R.G., McGuire, T.G., Bae, J.P. & Rupp, A. (1997). Solutions for adverse selection in behavioural health care. *Health Care Financing Review*, 18, 109–22.

Frank, R.G., McGuire, T.G., Regier, D.A., Manderscheid, R. & Woodward, A. (1994). Paying for mental health and substance abuse care. *Health Affairs*, 13, 337–42.

Hollingshead, A.B. & Redlich, F.C. (1958). *Social Class and Mental Illness*. New York: John Wiley & Sons.

Jeffers, J.R., Bognanno, M.F. & Bartlett, J.C. (1971). On the demand versus need for medical services and the concept of 'shortage'. *American Journal of Public Health*, 61, 46–63.

Joint Commission on Mental Illness and Health (1961). *Action for Mental Health: The Final Report of the Joint Commission on Mental Illness and Health*. New York: Basic

Books.

Kessler, R.C., Frank, R.G., Edlund, M., Katz, S.J., Lin, E. & Leaf, P. (1997). Differences in the use of psychiatric outpatient services between the United States and Ontario. *New England Journal of Medicine*, **336**, 551–7.

Kessler, R.C., McGonagle, K.A., Zhao, S., Nelson, C.B., Hughes, M., Eshleman, S., Wittchen, H.-U. & Kendler, K.S. (1994). Lifetime and twelve-month prevalence of DSM-III-R psychiatric disorders in the United States. *Archives of General Psychiatry*, **51**, 8–19.

Leighton, D.C., Harding, J.S., Macklin, D.B., Macmillan, A.M. & Leighton, A.H. (1963). *The Character of Danger*. New York: Basic Books.

Manderscheid, R.W., Rae, D.S., Narrow, W.E., Locke, B.Z. & Regier, D.A. (1993). Congruence of service utilization estimates from the Epidemiologic Catchment Area Project and other sources. *Archives of General Psychiatry*, **50**, 108–14.

Morris, J.N. (1964). *The Uses of Epidemiology* (2nd edition). Baltimore, MD: Williams & Wilkins.

Murray, C.J.L. & Lopez, A.D. (eds.) (1996). *The Global Burden of Disease: a Comprehensive Assessment of Mortality and Disability from Diseases, Injuries, and Risk Factors in 1990 and Projected to 2020*. Cambridge, MA: Harvard University Press.

National Advisory Mental Health Council (1993). Health care reform for Americans with severe mental illnesses: special report. *American Journal of Psychiatry*, **150**, 1447–65.

National Advisory Mental Health Council (1998). *Parity in Financing Mental Health Services: Managed Care Effects on Cost, Access, and Quality*. NIH Publication No. 98–4322. Rockville, MD: U.S. DHHS, NIH, National Institute of Mental Health.

Regier, D.A., Burke, J.D.J., Manderscheid, R.W. & Burns, B.J. (1985). The chronically mentally ill in primary care. *Psychological Medicine*, **15**, 265–73.

Regier, D.A., Goldberg, I.D. & Taube, C.A. (1978). The de facto US mental health services system: a public health perspective. *Archives of General Psychiatry*, **35**, 685–93.

Regier, D.A., Kaelber, C.T., Rae, D.S., Farmer, A., Knauper, B., Kessler, R.C. & Norquist, G.S. (1998). Limitations of diagnostic criteria and assessment instruments for mental disorders: implications for research and policy. *Archives of General Psychiatry*, **55**, 109–15.

Regier, D.A., Narrow, W.E., Rae, D.S., Manderscheid, R.W., Locke, B.Z. & Goodwin, F.K. (1993). The de facto US mental and addictive disorders service system. Epidemiologic catchment area prospective 1-year prevalence rates of disorders and services. *Archives of General Psychiatry*, **50**, 85–94.

Regier, D.A., Shapiro, S., Kessler, L.G. & Taube, C.A. (1984). Epidemiology and health service resource allocation policy for alcohol, drug abuse, and mental disorders. *Public Health Reports*, **99**, 483–92.

Robins, L.N. & Regier, D.A. (1991). *Psychiatric Disorders in America*. New York: The Free Press.

Robins, L.N., Helzer, J.E., Croughan, J. & Ratcliff, K.S. (1981). National Institute of Mental Health diagnostic interview schedule: its history, characteristics, and validity. *Archives of General Psychiatry*, **38**, 381–9.

Robins, L.N., Wing, J., Wittchen, H.U., Helzer, J.E., Babor, T.F., Burke, J., Farmer, A.,

Jablenski, A., Pickens, R. & Regier, D.A. (1988). The Composite International Diagnostic Interview. An epidemiologic instrument suitable for use in conjunction with different diagnostic systems and in different cultures. *Archives of General Psychiatry*, **45**, 1069–77.

Shapiro, S., Skinner, E.A., Kramer, M., Steinwachs, D.M. & Regier, D.A. (1985). Measuring need for mental health services in a general population. *Medical Care*, **23**, 1033–43.

Shepherd, M. (1978). Epidemiology and clinical psychiatry. *British Journal of Psychiatry*, **133**, 289–98.

Srole, L., Langer, T.S., Michael, S.T., Opler, M.K. & Rennie, T.A.C. (1962). *Mental Health in the Metropolis: The Midtown Manhattan Study*. New York: McGraw-Hill Book Co.

Steinwachs, D.M., Flynn, L.M., Norquist, G.S. & Skinner, E.A. (1996). *Using Client Outcomes Information to Improve Mental Health and Substance Abuse Treatment*. San Francisco, CA: Jossey–Bass.

Sturm, R. (1997). How expensive is unlimited health care coverage under managed care? *Journal of the American Medical Association*, **278**, 1533–7.

Taube, C., Lee, E.S. & Forthofer, R.N. (1984). DRGs in psychiatry. An empirical evaluation. *Medical Care*, **22**, 597–610.

The President's Commission on Mental Health (1978). The President's Commission on Mental Health: Report to the President from the President's Commission on Mental Health. Washington, D.C.

World Health Organization (1993). *The ICD-10 Classification of Mental and Behavioural Disorders. Diagnostic Criteria for Research*. Geneva: World Health Organization.

5

Some considerations in making resource allocation decisions for the treatment of psychiatric disorders

Ronald C. Kessler

Introduction

The key premise of the symposium on which this volume is based is that no society can afford to intervene to meet the needs of all the people found in psychiatric epidemiological surveys to have a clinically significant psychiatric disorder. Therefore, some triage rules are required to rationalize the allocation of limited resources. The assumption implied in the title of the symposium 'The Unmet Need for Treatment' is that differential need should be the main deciding factor from which these rules are developed. The challenge presented to speakers was to grapple with the complexities of operationalizing the concept of differential need for the purposes of developing such rules.

Health policy analysts have been concerned with the issue of resource allocation for quite some time (e.g., Bobadilla, Cowley, Musgrove & Saxenian, 1994; Patrick & Erickson, 1993; Wagstaff, 1991). The urgency of the issue as it concerns psychiatric disorders hit home in the mid1980s when the Epidemiologic Catchment Area (ECA) Study, the first general population survey of psychiatric disorders in the USA, documented that one out of every five people in the population meets criteria for a psychiatric disorder over a period of six months (Myers et al., 1984). President Clinton's proposal for national health reform further fuelled concerns about runaway health care costs. Cost containment for treating psychiatric disorders became a focal point of the ensuing health reform debate.

One response to these developments was to argue that many of the people reported to have a psychiatric disorder actually had relatively benign, self-limiting conditions of the sort that do not require treatment (Regier et al., 1998). The number of people with unmet need for treatment, according to this argument, is actually much smaller than the epidemiological data would seem to suggest. Consistent with this thinking, the National Advisory Mental Health Council of the US National Institute of Mental Health in 1993 called for a distinction between 'severe mental illness' (SMI) – which they defined as nonaffective psychosis, manic depressive disorder, autism, dementia, and severe forms of mood and anxiety disorders – and other less severe types of mental illness. The Council estimated that as few as 3% of the US population suffer from SMI in a given year compared to as many as 20% who meet criteria for some other mental disorder. The Council suggested that these two types of disorders should be treated differently in health care reform.

Shortly thereafter, the American Psychiatric Association (APA) published the fourth edition of its *Diagnostic and Statistical Manual of Mental Disorders* (DSM) and introduced for the first time an explicit requirement that 'the symptoms cause clinically significant distress or impairment' (American Psychiatric Association, 1994). This stipulation was included based on the assumption that the estimated prevalence of many disorders would decrease if significant distress or impairment was required.

About the same time, the US Congress, in Public Law (PL) 102-321, established a Block Grant for adults with 'serious mental illness' and children and adolescents with 'serious emotional disturbance.' A disorder was categorized as serious only if it substantially interfered with the patient's functioning in normal social roles. A subsequent attempt to operationalize the criteria stipulated in PL 102-321, using data from the ECA and National Comorbidity Survey (NCS), estimated that 5.4% of adults in the US population meet criteria for a serious mental illness in a given year (Kessler et al., 1996a). A parallel effort for youth estimated that between 4% and 8% of children and adolescents, depending on the definition of serious emotional disturbance (SED), meet criteria in a given year (Costello et al., 1997).

All of these efforts can be seen as ways to focus attention on the subset of psychiatric disorders that, in one way or another, are thought to be most in need of treatment. Need is implicitly defined in terms of impairment. This is an important focus, but it is inadequate for making decisions about the appropriateness of intervention. Instead, an intervention should be considered appropriate if, and only if, its expected benefits clearly exceed the sum of its direct costs and expected risks (Brook et al., 1986). There is no necessary relationship between level of need and appropriateness of intervention. Indeed, one could easily imagine a situation in which an effective intervention technology existed to prevent the progression from a mild to a severe form of a disorder but no effective method existed to treat the severe form, in which case it would be most appropriate to focus intervention on the nonsevere form.

It might be useful to ask ourselves why no society can afford to intervene with all people who have psychiatric disorders. After all, most societies have decided that they can afford to intervene with all the people who have some disorders. Virtually all societies, for example, provide universal treatment for tuberculosis. The same is true for a number of other diseases. Indeed, in some cases, the world health community not only offers treatment, but actively tracks down people with particular diseases and forces them to be treated.

Most of these cases involve rare diseases. The situation with psychiatric disorders is quite different. As many as one-third of the populations in some countries meet criteria for a psychiatric disorder in a given year. In the USA alone, there are over 50 million people with a psychiatric disorder (Kessler et al., 1994). Yet the decisions of some societies to offer universal intervention for certain illnesses are not confined to rare conditions. Nearly 250 million people in the USA, for example, have been vaccinated against polio and free polio vaccinations are available from public health departments throughout the USA for any and all. The same kind of universal intervention for a number of common disorders is found in many other countries around the world.

Why is it that so many countries have decided that they can afford to intervene in this way with hundreds of millions of people to address the problems of some physical illnesses, while they have decided that they cannot intervene with the smaller number of people who suffer from psychiatric disorders? The answer, I believe, involves the fact that the health conditions for which universal interventions are available are all generally recognized as costly conditions for which inexpensive and highly effective interventions exist. This means that the cost-benefit ratio is clearly in favor of intervening rather than not intervening.

Need is not the issue here, but rationality in calculating the costs of intervention relative to the costs of nonintervention. If we want to help rationalize social policy decisions about the allocation of scarce intervention resources among the large number of people with psychiatric disorders, we need to obtain data that can be used to make these calculations of cost ratios. A critical problem here is that we lack even the most basic understanding of the social costs of psychiatric disorders. Nor do we have a thorough understanding of the extent to which clinical or preventive interventions are capable of addressing these costs. As a result, the magnitude of the cost-benefit ratio of intervening versus not intervening is unclear.

It is much easier to make an exact calculation of the direct treatment costs of intervention than the often hidden indirect costs of nonintervention. When the former are low, it is sometimes not necessary to have a complete understanding of the latter. For example, the decisions to add fluoride to the drinking water or iodine to table salt were not based on detailed analyses of the societal costs of tooth decay or cretinism, but rather on a general appreciation of the low costs of these interventions in relation to their presumed positive effects on public health. The situation becomes more complex, though, when the costs of intervention are substantial, in which case social policy decisions require a clear reckoning of costs versus benefits. As evidence-based medicine has assumed increasing importance in clinical practice, the decision of whether to intervene or not has increasingly come to be based on careful cost-benefit analyses of this sort (e.g., Hillner & Smith,

1991; Pauker & Pauker, 1987). Rationality in making these decisions requires research aimed at addressing a number of questions, several of which psychiatric epidemiologists and services researchers are ideally suited to answer.

The prevalences of inappropriate treatment and nontreatment

Many instances of both inappropriate treatment and inappropriate nontreatment have been documented in numerous branches of medicine. An example of inappropriate treatment includes the finding that the majority of Medicaid patients in one state of the USA who were treated for a common cold, against which antibiotics are not effective, were nonetheless prescribed, and filed a prescription for, an antibiotic (Mainous, Hueston & Clark, 1996). Another example is the finding that nearly one-third of patients in The Netherlands who underwent angioplasty were subsequently determined not to be suitable for this procedure (Meijler et al., 1997). Examples of inappropriate nontreatment include the finding that more than one-fourth of 18-month-old children in the USA fail to receive all recommended vaccinations (Centers for Disease Control and Prevention, 1997), and that nearly half of pregnant women in the USA fail to receive the full set of prenatal tests and procedures specified in federal guidelines (Kogan, Alexander, Kotelchuck, Nagey & Jack, 1994).

It should not be surprising, in light of results such as these, that evidence for both inappropriate treatment and inappropriate nontreatment has also been found in psychiatry. For example, one study of patients in treatment for depression in the USA found that nearly one-third were inappropriately treated with tranquilizers (Wells, Katon, Rogers & Camp, 1994). Other studies have shown that only a minority of depressed people in the USA general population receive treatment in a given year (Regier et al., 1993) and that only a minority of those in treatment for depression receive therapies that meet federal practice guidelines (Katz, Kessler, Lin & Wells, 1998).

In the absence of such guidelines for the kinds of complex comorbid psychiatric conditions typically seen in clinical practice, there is no principled way to establish that care for psychiatric disorders has been either inappropriately provided or inappropriately withheld. As a result, we currently do not know what proportion of the people who receive psychiatric treatment should not have been treated. Nor do we know the proportion of nonpatients meeting criteria for a DSM or International Classification of Diseases (ICD) disorder in general population epidemiological surveys who are appropriate for treatment. Similarly, we have no way of determining the proportion of currently treated patients who would profit from appropriate treatment but are treated inappropriately.

Reducing inappropriate treatment and nontreatment

The first step in addressing the problems of inappropriate treatment and inappropriate nontreatment should be to document the prevalences and correlates of these problems. As guidelines become available for an increasing number of disorders, clinical epidemiological studies will be needed to investigate the prevalences and correlates of inappropriate treatment in representative patient samples. This will require collecting detailed data on the specifics of treatment. General population epidemiological studies will also be needed to investigate inappropriate nontreatment. This will require data to be collected on recent prevalences, symptom profiles, course, severity, and impairments in sufficient detail to distinguish untreated cases for which treatment would have been appropriate from untreated cases where treatment would not have been appropriate.

Procedures pioneered in other branches of medicine are available to encourage changes in clinical practice when a pattern of systematic inappropriate treatment is documented (Greco & Eisenberg, 1993). There is encouraging evidence to suggest that these approaches can be effective when clear guidelines are available, treatment processes are rigorously monitored in relation to these guidelines, relationships between these processes and outcomes are documented, and treatment providers are given incentives to participate in positive change efforts (Davis, Thomson, Oxman & Haynes, 1995; O'Connor et al., 1996; Pestotnik, Classen, Evans & Burke, 1996).

The problem of inadequate intervention resources

Even assuming that we could maximize appropriateness of treatment for psychiatric problems, we would still be confronted with the likelihood that the resources needed would far exceed the resources available. There are, logically, two approaches that could be used to address this problem. First, we could carry out a more serious evaluation than currently exists of the true indirect costs associated with failure to treat people with psychiatric disorders. If these costs are high, an increase in intervention resources might be seen as rational. Second, assuming that intervention resources are fixed, we could attempt to quantify the ratio of indirect cost reduction to direct intervention cost across a range of psychiatric conditions and treatment approaches in an effort to determine the most rational way of allocating limited resources so as to maximize benefits.

The indirect costs of psychiatric disorders

A rational evaluation of the pros and cons of intervention requires an initial investigation of the indirect costs of illness. The latter include the effects of the illness on well-being (e.g., pain, suffering, other aspects of quality of life, societal burden) as well as on longevity. These effects should ideally be considered not only for the ill person, but also for his or her family and friends, and for others whose lives are affected in some way by the illness. Some reorientation of thinking will be needed if psychiatric epidemiologists are to play a part in the rationalization of decision-making about the relative costs of intervention versus nonintervention for psychiatric disorders. This reorientation has already begun. In fact, research on the indirect costs of psychiatric disorders carried out by psychiatric epidemiologists has grown dramatically over the past decade. This has occurred in response to the rise of the managed care industry, and the increasing demands made in response to this development for evidence-based practice guidelines. This research has tended to focus on the short-term effects of psychiatric disorders on the role functioning of the ill person and to rely on the patients' self-reports as the main way of assessing functioning.

Some of these studies have been concerned with the effects of specific psychiatric disorders such as anxiety (Edlund, 1990), depression (Greenberg, Kessler, Nells, Finkelstein & Berndt, 1996), and schizophrenia (Wyatt & Clark, 1987). Other studies, in comparison, have been concerned with the effects of psychiatric disorders overall (Kouzis & Eaton, 1994; Rice, Kelman, Miller & Dunmeyer, 1990). In a few cases, the investigations have compared the costs of different psychiatric disorders (Kessler & Frank, 1997) or have compared the costs of a particular psychiatric disorder with the costs of specific physical disorders (Wells, Sturm, Sherbourne & Meredith, 1996).

My collaborators and I carried out a series of related studies as part of the NCS. One of these studies showed that employed people with psychiatric disorders in the USA have an average of nearly one and a half days of work loss or work cutback per month due to their disorders, accounting for a total of approximately one billion lost days of productivity per year in the civilian labor force (Kessler & Frank, 1997). Other NCS studies showed that people with psychiatric disorders have less supportive and more distant relationships than comparison subjects with their children, other family members, and friends (Mickelson, Kessler & Shaver, 1997), and that married people with psychiatric disorders are significantly more likely than other married people to experience marital violence.

These results suggest that psychiatric disorders are associated with impaired functioning in a variety of important social roles. It is noteworthy that these effects are not limited to the subset of disorders defined by the National Advisory Mental Health Council as 'severe mental illnesses.' However, this evidence is not definitive due to the fact that the functioning measures used in these studies relied on self-reports. We know that many people with psychiatric disorders, especially those with depression, have negative perceptual biases that lead them to overestimate the impairments caused by their disorders (Coyne & Gotlib, 1983). This can occur even in the assessment of such seemingly objective outcomes as work loss, because the vast majority of self-reported work loss due to psychiatric disorders is related to reduced performance on days at work rather than to sickness absence days (Kessler & Frank, 1997).

Concerns about biases in self-reported measures of role functioning have led to several recent research initiatives aimed at developing objective measures of functioning independent of self-report. One of the most practical and useful ways to obtain such measures is to study objective performance measures collected by employers to evaluate their workers. Berndt, Finkelstein, Greenberg, Keith & Bailit (1997) carried out a study of this sort that focused on biweekly productivity records collected over a period of several years in a large sample of insurance-claims processors. These performance records were combined with health insurance claims data over the same time period and analyzed to determine whether a drop in productivity occurred during illness episodes.

A substantial drop was documented in the six months prior to the onset of treated episodes of several disorders. Furthermore, a reversal of this drop was found for most, but not all, of these illnesses during treatment. One of the strongest patterns of this sort was associated with depression. Importantly, the indirect cost of the lost productivity associated with depression substantially exceeded the direct cost of treatment, suggesting that treatment of depression could prove to be a cost-saving measure if the treatment is effective in restoring the reduced productivity associated with this disorder.

Who bears the costs?

Rationality in allocating health care resources across interventions aimed at multiple risk factors and disorders requires decision rules to maximize benefits for a fixed investment. The development of these rules requires decisions about the relative values of morbidity compared to mortality, as well as about the relative values of one's life. These decisions vary depending on whose perspective is taken in evaluating costs and benefits. The cost-benefit ratio from the perspective of the employer of the ill person might be quite different from that of the patient, and the latter's might be different from that of the patient's family or members of the community in which the patient lives. Furthermore, two patients with identical objective impairments might make different evaluations of the importance of the limitations created by these impairments (Revicki, 1992).

Most social policy analysts have assumed that the perspective of the average person projected into the position of the patient should be the basis for evaluating benefits (Katz, 1987). The most commonly used metrics for this purpose have been averaged equivalence metrics such as time trade-offs (how many months or years of life one would be willing to give up if a treatment was available to cure the illness but with the side-effect of decreased longevity) or standard gambles (the risk, usually of death, one would be willing to take to cure the illness).

Any of several different commonly used equivalence metrics can be combined with treatment effectiveness data and survival data to compute a composite estimate of the number of adjusted lost life years associated with each disease, where the estimate is the sum of actual lost years of life and years of morbidity weighted by the equivalence metric. For example, a disease that typically shortens life by five years and is associated with a decade of morbidity prior to death would be defined as leading to $5 + 10e$ lost quality-adjusted life years (QALYs), where e = the estimated loss in time-equivalent quality of life (Torrence & Feeny, 1989). This metric, in turn, can be compared across different medical conditions to evaluate the relative benefits of different interventions per unit of direct cost.

There are many other ways to study benefit maximization in the allocation of health care resources. These various approaches differ in their assumptions about the costs and benefits of illness and treatment as well as in the perspective used to make the valuation (e.g., the perspective of the patient, of the general public, or of the health care professional). Two of these approaches have been especially important in research on resource allocation in the treatment of psychiatric disorders: the cost offset approach and the workplace cost approach. These two approaches differ from the social policy approach in that they evaluate the indirect versus direct costs from the perspective of the health care provider or the workplace rather than from the perspective of the patient.

The cost offset approach begins with the observation that many of the patients who are heavy general medical service utilizers have emotional problems rather than, or in addition to, physical problems (Russo et al., 1997). These patients create management problems for general practitioners because they often present vaguely defined physical complaints that are difficult to treat and have high demands for services. They create financial problems for managed care plans because primary care providers often respond to their demands by ordering unnecessary and expensive medical tests. In light of these high costs to providers, health services researchers have speculated that psychiatric treatment of these patients might actually reduce overall medical costs by decreasing inappropriate and inefficient primary care costs, more than offsetting the direct costs of psychiatric treatment. If so, there would be a benefit to managed care plans of offering psychiatric treatment to such patients even if the benefit to the patients themselves would not justify the direct costs of such treatment.

Definitive data on this speculation are scant. One experimental trial carried out to evaluate whether a program aimed at detecting and treating primary care patients with depression might have an offset effect of this sort failed to find evidence of direct cost savings (Simon et al., 1996). However, nonexperimental evidence suggests that there might be more powerful offset effects associated with adjunctive psychiatric treatment in samples of patients with chronic physical conditions (Stoudemire, 1995). Controlled studies are needed to evaluate these effects more rigorously (e.g., Roose & Glassman, 1994).

The workplace cost approach begins with the observation that untreated psychiatric disorders are highly prevalent in the labor force (Eaton, Anthony, Mandel & Garrison, 1990; Kouzis & Eaton, 1994), and that these disorders are associated with substantial lost productivity (Kessler & Frank, 1997). If treatment could be shown to be successful in restoring this lost productivity, and there is good reason to believe it could for certain disorders (Berndt et al., 1997; Judd, Paulus, Wells & Rapaport, 1996; Mintz, Mintz, Arruda & Hwang, 1992), then aggressive outreach and treatment of workers with these disorders would represent an investment opportunity for employers rather than a health care cost, irrespective of the benefit to the patients themselves.

Two large field trials are currently underway to evaluate whether aggressive screening and treatment of major depression, the most common impairing psychiatric disorder among workers, has a performance-enhancement effect of this sort and, if so, whether the magnitude of this effect in terms of increased value to the employer offsets the direct costs of treatment. One of these trials is being carried out by Roger Kathol and his colleagues at the University of Iowa in the entire workforce of a single large corporation. The other trial is being carried out by a group of researchers from Harvard Medical School (Richard Frank and Ronald Kessler) and the John D. and Catherine T. MacArthur Foundation (Robert Rose), studying a sample of workers from a number of different large corporations. Both trials are attempting to arrive at an objective assessment of the decreased performance associated with major depression, to calculate the financial costs to employers of this decreased performance, and to determine experimentally how much of this decreased performance can be recovered by aggressive outreach and treatment.

The comprehensive comparative assessment of indirect costs

Neither the cost offset approach nor the workplace cost approach attempts to develop a comprehensive assessment of all the societal costs of psychiatric disorders. Instead, these approaches focus on the indirect costs of psychiatric disorders from the perspective of an organization – either the managed care organization or the employer organization. They then attempt to determine whether these indirect costs are large enough that their reduction would justify the increased direct costs associated with treating currently untreated psychiatric disorders from the perspective of that organization (i.e., taking into consideration only the indirect costs to the organization and ignoring any positive effects of treatment from the perspective of the patient). If so, then no broader considerations of other indirect costs are needed.

Cases of this sort clearly exist, as witnessed by the aggressive screening and treatment for substance-use disorders carried out by employers of workers in safety-sensitive jobs (e.g., truck drivers, oil refinery workers). Some researchers and policy analysts believe that this scenario will turn out to be true in many more cases than we currently realize, especially with regard to workplace costs, once a complete indirect cost accounting of the sort promised by studies like the Iowa and Harvard field trials is carried out. Indeed, studies such as these might show that certain types of aggressive outreach and treatment efforts should be conceptualized as corporate investment opportunities to enhance competitive advantage rather than workplace costs.

Rigorous field trials of this sort are able to assess cost–benefit ratios by limiting the analysis of indirect costs to a single set of these costs (e.g., reduction in workplace performance due to the disorder) associated with a single disease. From a narrow point of view, rational treatment decisions can be based on data of this sort. That is, it is rational in a narrow sense for a company to invest in the treatment of a particular disease if the direct costs of treatment are less than the indirect cost savings in improved productivity associated with treatment.

However, the broader question of whether the same direct cost investment would have yielded a higher return if it had been used to intervene in another way (e.g., to fire all the workers with the disease and use the money that would otherwise have gone to treatment to pay for hiring and training of new employees) is much more difficult to answer. This difficulty is multiplied when we move from a narrow focus on only one disorder and one set of indirect costs to the much broader perspective of a society aiming to maximize the quality of life of its citizens.

Societal decisions about health care resource allocations across a wide range of risk factors and disorders require nothing less than a comprehensive comparative assessment of the epidemiology and burden of all major diseases. The World Health Organization has accepted the challenge of carrying out such an assessment in its Global Burden of Disease (GBD) Study (Murray & Lopez, 1994, 1996). The GBD Study is an attempt to quantify the burden of disease and injury in an objective fashion that combines epidemiological information on the morbidity and mortality of specific diseases. The goal is to develop a reproducible set of assessment procedures to arrive at a single measure of burden for each disease that can be used in cost-effectiveness analysis.

This is a daunting task. As in most other attempts to combine information about morbidity and mortality into a single metric (e.g., Patrick & Erickson, 1993), a time-based approach is used by the GBD investigators. That is, epidemiological information about years of lost life is combined with weighted information about years of morbidity to arrive at a single estimate of the burden of each disease under study (Murray, 1994). However, the GBD investigators have departed from the conventional use of survey-based equivalence metrics linked to quality of life perceptions to generate the morbidity weight. Instead, they have attempted to base their evaluations on actual observations of disease burden whenever possible and to make this information available to an expert panel of raters in each major region of the world to generate ratings of perceived disease burden. A standardized protocol has been developed for this purpose in which the raters are required to deliberate about the implications of their initial decisions and to revise ratings for a series of sentinel diseases iteratively until they reach consensus.

The GBD project is still in process. Although initial estimates of the burden associated with each of many different diseases have been made, the GBD investigators are well aware that these estimates are based on incomplete information and imperfect methods of synthesizing the available information (Murray, 1994). Future research by psychiatric epidemiologists could help inform this process in a number of ways. One of the most useful types of these would be to carry out studies that provide more objective information than currently exists about the indirect costs of psychiatric disorders. This information could be used to help validate the estimates of burden developed in the GBD Study and provide a gold standard to be used by subsequent generations of GBD expert panels to revise their evaluations of disease burden.

My collaborators and I have carried out a series of preliminary studies that illustrate this type of work by focusing on the associations between psychiatric disorders and subsequent major life course transitions in the domains of education, parenting, marriage, and employment. We studied the effects of prior psychiatric disorders in predicting these transitions in a series of analyses that combined retrospectively reported information on age of onset of psychiatric disorders collected in the NCS with information about the timing of role transitions to construct synthetic data files of implied temporal orderings between disorder onsets and role transitions.

These files were analyzed using the method of discrete-time survival analysis (Efron, 1988), with the disorders treated as time-varying covariates to predict subsequent role transitions. A detailed description of this analysis method can be found in Kessler, Magee & Nelson (1996b). The results document powerful associations between psychiatric disorders and virtually all of these outcomes. In particular, people with a history of early-onset psychiatric disorders were found to be at elevated risk compared to controls of truncated educational attainment (Kessler, Foster, Saunders & Stang,

1995), teenage childbearing (Kessler et al., 1997a), marital instability (Kessler & Forthofer, 1999), and poor labor market outcomes (Ettner, Frank & Kessler, 1997; Jayakody, Danziger & Kessler, 1998).

In addition to providing input to future GBD evaluations, increased knowledge about the indirect costs of psychiatric disorders has the potential to increase the constituents for aggressive outreach and treatment of these disorders based on more narrow considerations of indirect costs. For example, while only 16% of births in the USA are to teenage mothers, over 50% of the federal budget to Aid for Families with Dependent Children (AFDC) goes to families started by teenage mothers (Moore & Burt, 1982). This has led critics of AFDC to make reduction of teenage pregnancy a central goal in the welfare debate (Maynard, 1996). While the methods for doing this remain a major point of contention in the debate, the documentation that early-onset psychiatric disorders are powerful risk factors for teenage child-bearing has led to a new enthusiasm for developing targeted interventions to treat early-onset psychiatric problems on the part of welfare reformers, based on the hope that these interventions might help prevent teenage pregnancy.

Preventive interventions

It is important to include preventive interventions in the pool of interventions considered in comparisons of cost-effectiveness. A recent report from the Institute of Medicine noted that prevention of mental disorders has a low priority in the health care agendas of most countries (Institute of Medicine, 1994). This is in sharp contrast to the situation with physical disorders. Public health efforts to reduce the proportion of people who smoke and to increase the use of seat belts have saved literally hundreds of thousands of lives each year in the USA alone through the prevention of physical illness and fatal injuries. Clinical efforts to intervene with high-risk patients defined in terms of having elevated blood pressure, being overweight, and having other known risk factors for serious physical illness are now a routine part of general medical practice. Yet no comparable efforts exist to prevent the onset of psychiatric disorders.

Preventive interventions might make even more sense for psychiatric than physical disorders because of the comparatively early age of onset of many psychiatric disorders, the high rates of chronicity of many early-onset psychiatric disorders, their substantial effects on the subsequent emotional and social development of the people who suffer from them, and the availability of new intervention models that may prevent specific early-onset psychiatric disorders. It is noteworthy that the reversibility of the indirect costs of psychiatric disorders is likely to be quite different depending on the timing of the intervention. This means that cost-effectiveness calculations for early preventive interventions might show greater effects than clinical interventions if long-term effects on role functioning are considered. This issue has not yet been thoroughly integrated into the GBD framework, although initial steps have been made along these lines.

The Institute of Medicine report suggested that the time is now right for a new emphasis on prevention of mental disorders. Several factors came together to lead the authors of the report to this conclusion. Among the most important of these factors were the dramatic growth of knowledge about both environmental and genetic risk factors for psychiatric disorders in the 1980s and 1990s, and the availability of a number of very promising models for early intervention (see reviews in Dryfoos, 1990; Hamburg, 1992; Institute of Medicine, 1994).

It is important to realize, though, that there are formidable barriers to the success of preventive interventions. Even interventions that are fairly inexpensive on an individual basis become very expensive overall when they have to be delivered to a large part of the population. Rigorous cost-effectiveness analyses often show that seemingly inexpensive preventive interventions for physical disorders are actually very expensive per unit of saved QALY or DALY when we consider the fact that only a small minority of the people exposed are affected by low-dose preventive interventions, that the people affected are often those with only a moderate risk of the illness outcome, and that the risk factors targeted in the interventions are only some of the many factors contributing to the outcome (e.g. Pharoah & Hollingsworth, 1996; Shepherd et al., 1995).

As one illustration, Robertson (1996) calculated that the preventive use of pharmacotherapy for patients with moderately elevated cholesterol in a general medical practice in Great Britain would require a 50% increase in the total medication budget for the practice and would save only one life every 7.5 years out of the average of 2000 patients seen by the typical general practitioner. This would clearly not be cost-effective since the same resources could be allocated more productively to alternative interventions. On the other hand, some preventive interventions are cost-effective. For example, Tosteson et al. (1997) showed that inexpensive public education efforts to reduce cholesterol have an estimated total cost of only $3200 per year of life saved.

Rigorous cost-effectiveness studies are needed to evaluate the likely effects of preventive interventions for mental disorders. There will be formidable logistic complications here. For example, currently available preventive interventions for mental disorders generally target the reduction of risk factors and the enhancement of protective factors that have been implicated in a number of different mental disorders (e.g., Beardslee et al., 1992; Johnson, 1990). This means that it will be very difficult to rigorously trace out the reductions in morbidity associated with these interventions.

Another complexity is that many of these interventions occur a number of years prior to the time the disorders would have been expected to occur. This means that long-term follow-up is needed to evaluate the effectiveness of the interventions. However, these complexities are not unique to preventive interventions or to mental disorders. Similar difficulties arise in evaluating the effects of clinical interventions aimed at increasing both quality of life and longevity. We simply have to do the best we can to combine thoughtful long-term tracking with extrapolation and adjustment for the inevitable loss to follow-up of some patients, and the necessity of making interim policy recommendations prior to completing a full long-term follow-up period.

One issue of special importance in preventive interventions for mental disorders is that a very large proportion of young people can be considered at risk for clinically significant psychiatric problems. A family history of psychiatric disorder, parental divorce, family adversity, and other risk factors for childhood- and adolescent-onset psychiatric disorders are highly prevalent in the general population (Kessler, Davis & Kendler, 1997c). Furthermore, a very high proportion of youngsters have problems with mood regulation that involve either acting out, depression, anxiety, or some combination of these symptoms (Cohen et al., 1993; Costello et al., 1997; Reinherz, Giaconia, Lefkowitz, Pakiz & Frost, 1993). Although many of these problems resolve spontaneously in the course of development, others progress into full-blown psychiatric disorders.

It is not clear how to target interventions in a situation of this sort. One strategy for targeting preventive interventions that is fairly unique to psychiatric disorders builds on the fact that the majority of patients with psychiatric disorders carry more than one diagnosis (Wolf et al., 1988). Similar patterns are found in general population samples (Kessler, 1997). The NCS identified more than 80% of all severe current psychiatric disorders in the USA among the 13% of the population who have a lifetime history of three or more disorders (Kessler et al., 1994). These results suggest that the prevention of comorbidity (i.e., the prevention of the first onset of a second disorder) might reduce a substantial proportion of all lifetime psychiatric disorders, and possibly an even greater proportion of ongoing disorders. If so, then it might be useful to consider developing interventions aimed at the primary prevention of secondary psychiatric disorders in the sector of the population who already suffer from an initial psychiatric disorder.

There would be several practical advantages of conducting preventive interventions in populations at risk for comorbid disorders (Kessler & Price, 1993). For one, the ease and reliability of targeting respondents are greater when they already meet criteria for a primary disorder. In addition, already diagnosed groups are at very high risk of developing secondary disorders, which increases the efficiency and power of preventive interventions. Furthermore, primary prevention of secondary disorders may allow prevention researchers to include current treatment technologies, including pharmacological and cognitive-behavioral interventions, in their preventive intervention strategies. The experience gained from using and developing these interventions to treat psychiatric disorders may enable some of them to be used in prevention.

There is considerable stigma associated with psychiatric disorders. Therefore, preventive trials with diagnosed clinical populations at risk of developing secondary disorders might increase the social justification for preventive intervention. In particular, various community and professional groups may be more ready to acknowledge that it is appropriate to intervene when a person is already suffering from a disorder. Furthermore, the recipients of the interventions might already be experiencing sufficient distress to make the intervention more acceptable. This is an especially important issue since preventive interventions are often compromised by the fact that many recipients refuse to participate because they are not suffering enough.

Despite these advantages, it is not clear whether primary preventive interventions for psychiatric disorders are feasible. A number of practical problems need to be considered. For example, it is likely that more intensive effort is needed to prevent secondary disorders, because the primary disorders will complicate prevention efforts in the same way they complicate treatment efforts. Furthermore, if we rely on existing diagnoses to identify individuals with a primary disorder, we will restrict the interventions to people who are already in the health care system. Yet if we go beyond treatment samples to make diagnoses in the general population, we risk stigmatization. It might also be that it is more difficult to prevent the onset of secondary disorders than to prevent the onset of primary disorders for reasons that involve differences in the causal processes underlying these different kinds of onset. These are complex issues that need to be addressed before we can seriously consider launching interventions for the primary prevention of secondary disorders.

One example of this approach that has been of special interest to my research group over the past few years involves the primary prevention of substance abuse occurring as an unintended consequence of self-medicating a primary mental disorder. The NCS data show that this is a very common type of comorbidity that is usually associated with childhood- and adolescent-onset anxiety and mood disorders, leading to the development of substance-use problems during the teenage years and early twenties (Kessler et al., 1996a, 1997b). Simulations of NCS data suggest that successfully intervening, and severing the link between these temporally primary anxiety and mood disorders among adolescents and the subsequent onset of substance-use disorders would prevent as much as one-third of all alcohol and drug dependence in the USA.

A research team headed by Kathleen Merikangas, David Kupfer, and myself is currently involved in developing an intervention to prevent the onset of substance-use disorders that occur secondary to preexisting adolescent-onset anxiety and mood disorders. Targeting for the intervention uses school-based screening for anxiety and mood disorders among adolescents, while the intervention itself involves a combination of cognitive-behavioral therapy and pharmacotherapy aimed at treating the primary disorders, and social skills training. This training aims to provide the patients with strategies for coping with their dysphoria in ways that avoid secondary substance-use problems from developing. The intervention is currently being piloted in a series of secondary schools in three parts of the USA (in collaboration with Greg Clarke in Oregon, Mary Ann Albano in Kentucky, and Rick Heimberg and Phil Kendall in Pennsylvania), in preparation for a full field trial in 1999. Consistent with the ideas earlier in this chapter, we are designing the evaluation of this trial so that it will provide information about not only treatment-effectiveness but also cost-effectiveness that can be interpreted in terms of prevention of indirect costs based on QALYs and DALYs.

Using research to establish standards for quality assurance

A validated mechanism to monitor the quality of intervention delivery is needed if the results of research into intervention and its effectiveness are to be put into practice. This is crucial because the concerns that benefits managers in a managed care environment have about quality assurance are a critical barrier to their adoption of innovative psychiatric treatments. Although this is currently an issue of greatest concern in the USA, it will surface elsewhere as evidence-based medicine makes greater inroads into delivery systems throughout the world. Currently in the USA, the majority of people with health insurance obtain their coverage through their employer. This means that benefits managers are critically important in determining the types of services available through health insurance plans. These managers are particularly concerned about mental health benefits, because they believe that they have poorer ways of monitoring the quality of treatment for psychiatric disorders than for many physical disorders.

Many benefits managers have dealt with this uncertainty by imposing more extreme limits on the treatment of mental than physical disorders, and by casting an especially critical eye on the mental health benefits in their contracts. These managers are unwilling to increase mental health coverage because they have no way of measuring quality of care. Therefore, if cost-effectiveness research is to be successful, it needs not only to demonstrate that mental health interventions delivered in the context of a controlled trial are appropriate and cost-effective, but also to provide tools for quality assurance once expanded services are made available.

A number of systems are already in use in the USA to monitor quality of medical care. Some of these are broad-based systems that sample a small number of indicators of quality in an effort to globally evaluate the quality of entire health care organizations (e.g., Felt-Link & St. Peter, 1997; Jencks, 1995; National Committee for Quality Assurance, 1997). However, most of these systems include only fairly superficial evaluations of the quality of mental health care (National Committee for Quality Assurance, 1997).

As a result, it would be valuable to have focused systems available to monitor quality of care for specific commonly treated psychiatric syndromes. A number of such systems currently exist for specific physical conditions and medical procedures (e.g., Chassin, Hannan & DeBuono, 1996; Schneider & Epstein, 1996). There is good evidence that some of these systems have led to improvements in quality of care (e.g., Hannan, Kilburn, Racz, Shields & Chassin, 1994; Korn, Casey-Paal, Lazovich, Ball & Slater, 1997). There is no reason to believe that the same would not be true of systems focused on the treatment of psychiatric disorders.

Three approaches are available to evaluate quality of care (Donabedian, 1980). These three focus either on measures of structure (e.g., percent of providers in a system who are board certified), process (e.g., percent of medications prescribed at recommended doses), or outcomes (e.g., mortality rates at a specified time after discharge). There is considerable controversy about which of these approaches is to be preferred (Brook, McGlynn & Cleary, 1996; Ellwood, 1988). All of them are limited in one way or another.

Structural standards have long been the mainstay of system-accreditation processes. Minimum structural requirements are, of course, necessary to ensure adequate care; or they should be, but most research has failed to find strong effects of structural variations on either quality process or outcome measures (Brook et al., 1996).

Process standards are useful in that they serve an educational function that helps guarantee a minimal level of care for all patients. This might be especially true for the treatment of psychiatric problems, as much of this treatment is provided in the general medical sector by providers who have little expertise in treating this class of disorders. However, there are difficulties associated with process standards in that they may reduce the flexibility and efficiency of providers who are skilled at treating psychiatric problems. As it is impossible to specify all the details of clinical interventions for psychiatric disorders, creating process standards might focus attention on the minimally acceptable procedures rather than on excellence, and reduce the providers' responsibility for successful outcomes.

Outcome standards would resolve the concerns about the impossibility of specifying process standards in enough detail to guarantee high-quality and cost-effective treatment. However, appropriate expectations for outcome vary enormously depending on a great many factors that are beyond the control of the treating physician. Included here are such things as genetic predisposition, environmental factors that might either facilitate or impede treatment, and variation in patient compliance with treatment regimens. Service providers are, understandably, hesitant to accept outcome standards as the basis for evaluating the quality of their work when they have no control over so many critical factors. Furthermore, adverse outcomes are often rare and take a great deal of time to emerge, which means that quality evaluations that rely largely on outcome measures may be insensitive.

All these considerations have led to a growing consensus that a rich and evolving assessment of process measures should be the core of most disorder-specific systems that assess quality of care (Brook et al., 1996). However, there are exceptions. For example, outcome assessment focusing on 30-day mortality has been used to good effect in the evaluation of coronary artery bypass graft surgery (O'Connor et al., 1996). This has been possible because mortality is not a rare outcome for this procedure and usually occurs rather quickly after the procedure has been completed. Furthermore, it is possible to obtain good clinical information prior to the procedure that can be used to adjust for between-patient variation in risk in order to adjust for between-doctor and between-organization case mix.

There is a much greater array of appropriate treatments and types of providers (psychiatrists, nonspecialist physicians, psychologists, psychiatric nurses, psychiatric social workers) available to treat psychiatric disorders compared with most physical disorders. Therefore, there are likely to be special challenges in developing quality of care assessment systems for psychiatric disorders that rely exclusively on process measures. This is especially true for psychotherapies. At the same time, there are two special features of psychiatric disorders that might make them especially appropriate for outcomes assessment. The first is that, unlike the situation for many physical disorders, excellent treatment outcome measures for psychiatric disorders can be obtained during the course of treatment and shortly after it ends, based entirely on patients' self-reports. The second is that a great deal is known from epidemiological research about the risk and protective factors for psychiatric disorders. This information could be measured in a systematic and comparable way when patients first access services from a sample of providers and treatment organizations. These data could then be used to develop powerful risk-adjustment equations for use in comparing outcomes across providers and organizations in outcomes-based quality-assessment systems.

It is important to be aware of the two major risks associated with a system that focuses on outcomes rather than process evaluation. One is that it might be difficult to find differences in outcome even when they exist because of low statistical power in the face of rare adverse outcomes. However, given that the results of psychiatric treatment can be assessed not only in terms of rare, sharply defined outcomes (e.g., suicide, long-term disability, hospitalization after outpatient treatment) but also in terms of well-distributed continuous outcomes (e.g., frequency/intensity of residual symptoms, impairment in role functioning), this is unlikely to be a problem when assessing treatment outcomes for most psychiatric disorders. The second problem is that risk adjustment may be inadequate to remove case mix bias, in which case some providers or service delivery organizations will be incorrectly classified as having unacceptable outcomes when, in fact, they actually treated more intractable cases. However, this will not be a long-term problem if outcome assessment is used as part of continuous quality improvement (Berwick, 1991; Blumenthal, 1993), and if process assessment is used in conjunction with outcomes assessment in order to discriminate between providers and organizations whose seemingly poor performance can be explained in terms of inappropriate processes and those whose process measures appear to be good despite poor outcomes.

Overview

I began this chapter by provisionally accepting the main premise of the symposium on which this volume is based, that no society can afford to intervene to meet the needs of all the people found in psychiatric epidemiological surveys to have a clinically significant psychiatric disorder. However, I challenged the secondary premise, that need (i.e., severity, chronicity, impairment) should be the main deciding factor on the basis of which triage rules are developed. I suggested, instead, that appropriateness of treatment should be determined, based on the extent to which the benefits of treatment clearly exceed the sum of its direct costs and expected risks.

Cost-effectiveness studies that explicitly compare benefits in relation to costs and risks in other areas of medicine were reviewed. These studies show that it is possible to improve quality of care both in terms of reducing inappropriate treatment and increasing appropriate treatment when clear guidelines for appropriateness are available, treatment processes are rigorously monitored in relation to these guidelines, relationships between these processes and outcomes are documented, and treatment providers are given incentives to participate in positive change efforts. There is every reason to believe that similar effects may be achieved in rationalizing the allocation of intervention resources to psychiatric problems. However, I noted that there are practical impediments to moving forward in this agenda. Treatment guidelines are not available for most psychiatric disorders, making it impossible to rigorously study process measures that would provide needed information about the prevalences of inappropriate treatment and inappropriate nontreatment. Furthermore, we lack persuasive knowledge about either the indirect costs of psychiatric disorders or about the extent to which intervention can reverse these costs.

I reviewed a number of research initiatives currently underway to study the indirect costs of psychiatric disorders and the extent to which these costs can be reversed with intervention. I also located these studies in the larger literature on the burden of disease. I suggested that it is critical for cost-effectiveness studies of psychiatric interventions to be presented in ways that can be compared with the broader literature on the cost-effectiveness of medical interventions. This is true because the ultimate social-policy decisions regarding resource allocation to interventions for psychiatric disorders will hinge on evidence regarding the relative impact of these interventions compared to interventions for other classes of disease on the populations' disability and quality of life.

Finally, I cautioned that mechanisms to assure the quality of interventions have to be developed as part of cost-effectiveness studies if we hope to persuade policy makers to increase the allocation of health care resources to psychiatric disorders. I argued that while process assessments have to play a prominent role in any plan for the quality assurance of psychiatric interventions, special features of psychiatric disorders make them especially appropriate for outcomes assessment. It is important to be aware of the risks associated with a system that focuses on outcomes rather than process evaluation, but I discussed why these risks are likely to be lower in the evaluation of psychiatric interventions than interventions for other classes of disorders. I also argued that process assessment should be used in conjunction with outcomes assessment in order to guard against these risks.

The set of considerations discussed here might seem to have moved considerably away from the initial question posed by the conference convenors. However, I believe that these are the key considerations we need to grapple with if we are serious about confronting the problem of unmet need. This problem is, at its heart, part of the larger problem of resource allocation faced by the entire health care field. If we believe that psychiatric disorders are a major factor in disease burden and reduced quality of life in the population, and if we believe that interventions to address these problems either by prevention or treatment are effective, then we have to follow the lead of other specialty areas. We have to objectively document disease burden, rigorously demonstrate that this burden can be prevented or reversed with intervention, quantify the cost-benefit ratios using metrics that can be compared with other interventions for other diseases, and develop quality assurance mechanisms. I have tried throughout the chapter to call attention to areas where epidemiological and services researchers have a role to play in moving this agenda forward. It is an ambitious agenda, but one that we are capable of carrying out if we embrace it and keep the larger aims in mind as each of us works on our separate research components.

References

American Psychiatric Association (1994). *Diagnostic and Statistical Manual of Mental Disorders* (4th edition) Washington, D.C.: American Psychiatric Association.

Beardslee, W.R., Hoke, L., Wheeler, I., Rothberg, P.C., van de Velde, P. & Swatling, S. (1992). Preventive intervention for families with parental affective disorders: initial findings. *American Journal of Psychiatry*, **149**, 1335–40.

Berndt, E.R., Finkelstein, S.N., Greenberg, P.E., Keith, A. & Bailit, H. (1997). *Illness and Productivity: Objective Workplace Evidence.* (Working Paper 42-97.) MIT Program on the Pharmaceutical Industry.

Berwick, D.M. (1991). Controlling variation in health care: a consultation from Walter Shewhart. *Medical Care*, **29**, 1212–25.

Blumenthal, D. (1993). Total quality management and physicians' clinical decisions. *Journal of the American Medical Association*, **269**, 2775–8.

Bobadilla, J.L., Cowley, P., Musgrove, P. & Saxenian, H. (1994). Design, content, and financing of an essential national package of health services. *Bulletin of the World Health Organization*, **72**, 653–62.

Brook, R.H., Chassin, M.R., Fink, A., Solomon, D.H., Kosecoff, J. & Park R.E. (1986). A method for detailed assessment of the appropriateness of medical technologies. *International Journal of Technology Assessment in Health Care*, **2**, 53–63.

Brook, R.H., McGlynn, E.A. & Cleary, P.D. (1996). Quality of health care. Part 2: Measuring quality of care. *New England Journal of Medicine*, **335**, 966–70.

Centers for Disease Control and Prevention (1997). National, state, and urban area vaccination coverage levels among children aged 19–35 months – United States, January–December 1995. *Morbidity and Mortality Weekly Reports*, **46**, 176–83.

Chassin, M.R., Hannan, E.L. & DeBuono, B.A. (1996). Benefits and hazards of reporting medical outcomes publicly. *New England Journal of Medicine*, **334**, 394–8.

Cohen, P., Cohen, J., Kasen, S., Velez, C.N., Hartmark, C., Johnson, J., Rojas, M., Brook, J. & Streuning, E.L. (1993). An epidemiological study of disorders in late childhood and adolescence. 1: Age- and gender-specific prevalence. *Journal of Child Psychology and Psychiatry*, **34**, 851–67.

Costello, E.J., Angold, A., Burns, B.J., Erkanli, A., Stangl, D.K. & Tweed, D.L. (1997). The Great Smoky Mountains study of youth: functional impairment and serious emotional disturbance. *Archives of General Psychiatry*, **53**, 1137–43.

Coyne, J.C. & Gotlib, I.H. (1983). The role of cognition in depression: a critical appraisal. *Psychological Bulletin*, **94**, 472–505.

Davis, D.A., Thomson, M.A., Oxman, A.D. & Haynes, R.B. (1995). Changing physician performance: A systematic review of the effect of continuing medical education strategies. *Journal of the American Medical Association*, **274**, 700–5.

Donabedian, A. (1980). *Explorations in Quality Assessment and Monitoring.* Volume 1. *The Definition of Quality and Approaches to its Assessment.* Ann Arbor, MI: Health Administration Press.

Dryfoos, J.G. (1990). *Adolescents at Risk: Prevalence and Prevention.* New York: Oxford University Press.

Eaton, V.W., Anthony, J.C., Mandel, W. & Garrison, R. (1990). Occupation and the prevalence of major depressive disorder. *Journal of Occupational Medicine*, **32**,

1079–87.

Edlund, M.J. (1990). The economics of anxiety. *Psychiatric Medicine*, 8, 15–26.

Efron, B. (1988). Logistic regression, survival analysis, and the Kaplan–Meier curve. *Journal of the American Sociological Association*, 83, 414–25.

Ellwood, P.M. (1988). Outcomes management: a technology of patient experience. *New England Journal of Medicine*, 318, 149–56.

Ettner, S.L., Frank R.G. & Kessler, R.C. (1997). The impact of psychiatric disorders on labour market outcomes. *Industrial and Labour Relations Review*, 51, 64–81.

Felt-Link, S. & St. Peter, R. (1997). Quality assurance for Medicaid managed care. *Health Affairs*, 16, 248–52.

Greco, P.J. & Eisenberg, J.M. (1993). Changing physicians' practices. *New England Journal of Medicine*, 330, 435–6.

Greenberg, P.E., Kessler R.C., Nells, T.L., Finkelstein S.N. & Berndt E.R. (1996). Depression in the workplace: an economic perspective. In J.P. Feighner & W.F. Boyer (eds.), *Selective Serotonin Re-Uptake Inhibitors: Advances in Basic Research and Clinical Practice*, pp. 327–63. New York: John Wiley & Sons.

Hamburg, D.A. (1992). *Today's Children: Creating a Future for a Generation in Crisis*. New York: Times Books.

Hannan, E.L., Kilburn, H. Jr., Racz, M., Shields, E. & Chassin, M.R. (1994). Improving the outcomes of coronary artery bypass surgery in New York state. *Journal of the American Medical Association*, 271, 761–6.

Hillner, B.E. & Smith, T.J. (1991). Efficacy and cost-effectiveness of adjuvant chemotherapy in women with node-negative breast cancer. *New England Journal of Medicine*, 324, 160–8.

Institute of Medicine (1994). *Reducing Risks for Mental Disorders: Frontiers for Preventive Intervention Research*. Washington, D.C.: National Academy Press.

Jayakody, R., Danziger, S. & Kessler, R.C. (1998). Psychiatric disorders and male socio-economic status. *Social Science Research*, 27, 371–87.

Jencks, S. (1995). Changing health care practices in Medicare's health care quality improvement program. *Joint Commission Journal on Quality Improvement*, 21, 343–7.

Johnson, D.L. (1990). The Houston parent-child development center project: disseminating a viable program for enhancing at-risk families. *Prevention in Human Services*, 7, 89–108.

Judd, L.L., Paulus, M.P., Wells, K.B. & Rapaport, M.H. (1996). Socioeconomic burden of subsyndromal depressive symptoms and major depression in a sample of the general population. *American Journal of Psychiatry*, 153, 1411–17.

Katz, S. (ed.) (1987). The Portugal Conference: measuring quality of life and functional status in clinical and epidemiological research. *Journal of Chronic Disease*, 40, 459–650.

Katz, S.J., Kessler, R.C., Lin, E. & Wells, K.B. (1998). Appropriate medication management of depression in the United States and Ontario. *Journal of General Internal Medicine*, 13, 17–85.

Kessler, R.C. (1997). The prevalence of psychiatric comorbidity. In S. Wetzler & W.C. Sanderson (eds.), *Treatment Strategies for Patients with Psychiatric Comorbidity*, pp. 23–48. New York: John Wiley and Sons.

Kessler, R.C. & Forthofer, M.S. (1999). The effects of psychiatric disorders on family formation and stability. In J. Brooks-Gunn & M. Cox (eds.), *Family Risk and Resilience: The Roles of Conflict and Cohesion*, pp. 301–20. New York: Cambridge University Press.

Kessler, R.C. & Frank, R.G. (1997). The impact of psychiatric disorders on work loss days. *Psychological Medicine*, **27**, 861–73.

Kessler, R.C. & Price, R.H. (1993). Primary prevention of secondary disorders: a proposal and agenda. *American Journal of Community Psychology*, **21**, 607–33.

Kessler, R.C., Berglund, P.A., Foster, C.L., Saunders, W.B., Stang, P.E. & Walters, E.E. (1997*a*). The social consequences of psychiatric disorders. II: Teenage parenthood. *American Journal of Psychiatry*, **154**, 1405–11.

Kessler, R.C., Berglund, P.A., Zhao, S., Leaf, P.J., Kouzis, A.C., Bruce, M.L., Friedman, R.M., Grosser, R.C., Kennedy, C., Kuehnel, C., Laska, T.G., Manderscheid, E.M., Narrow, R.W, Rosenbeck, R.A., Santoni, T.W., Schneier, M. (1996*a*). The 12-month prevalence and correlates of Serious Mental Illness (SMI). In R.W. Manderscheid & M.A. Sonnenschein (eds.), *Mental Health, United States, 1996*, pp. 59–70. Washington, D.C.: U.S. Government Printing Office.

Kessler, R.C., Crum, R.M., Warner, L.A., Nelson, C.B., Schulenberg, J. & Anthony J.C. (1997*b*). The lifetime co-occurrence of DSM-III-R alcohol abuse and dependence with other psychiatric disorders in the National Comorbidity Survey. *Archives of General Psychiatry*, **54**, 313–21.

Kessler, R.C., Davis, C.G. & Kendler, K.S. (1997*c*). Childhood adversity and adult psychiatric disorder in the US National Comorbidity Survey. *Psychological Medicine*, **27**, 1101–19.

Kessler, R.C., Foster, C.L., Saunders, W.B. & Stang, P.E. (1995). The social consequences of psychiatric disorders. I: Educational attainment. *American Journal of Psychiatry*, **152**, 1026–32.

Kessler, R.C., Magee, W.J. & Nelson, C.B. (1996*b*). Analysis of psychosocial stress. In H.B. Kaplan (ed.), *Psychosocial Stress: Perspectives on Structure, Theory, Lifecourse, and Methods*, pp. 333–66. Orlando, FL: Academic Press.

Kessler, R.C., McGonagle, K.A., Zhao, S., Nelson, C.B., Hughes, M., Eshleman, S., Wittchen, H.-U. & Kendler, K.S. (1994). Lifetime and 12-month prevalence of DSM-III-R psychiatric disorders in the United States: results from the National Comorbidity Survey. *Archives of General Psychiatry*, **51**, 8–19.

Kogan, M.D., Alexander, G.R., Kotelchuck, M., Nagey, D.A. & Jack, B.W. (1994). Comparing mothers' reports on the content of prenatal care received with recommended national guidelines for care. (*Public Health Reports, 109*, 637-646). Hyattsville, MD: National Center for Health Statistics.

Korn, J.E., Casey-Paal, A., Lazovich, D., Ball, J. & Slater, J.S. (1997). Impact of the Mammography Quality Standards Act on access in Minnesota (*Public Health Reports, 112*, 142-145). Minneapolis, MN: Minnesota Department of Health.

Kouzis, A.C. & Eaton, V.W. (1994). Emotional disability days: prevalence and predictors. *American Journal of Public Health*, **84**, 1304–7.

Mainous, A.G. III, Hueston, W.J. & Clark, J.R. (1996). Antibiotics and upper respiratory infection: do some folks think there is a cure for the common cold? *The Journal of Family Practice*, **42**, 357–61.

Maynard, R.A. (ed.) (1996). *Kids Having Kids: Economic Costs and Social Consequences of Teen Pregnancy.* Washington, D.C.: Urban Institute Press.

Meijler, A.P., Rigter, H., Berstein, S.J., Scholma, J.K., McDonnell, J., Breeman, A., Kosecoff, J.B. & Brook, R.H. (1997). The appropriateness of intention to treat decisions for invasive therapy in coronary artery disease in the Netherlands. *Heart,* **77,** 219–24.

Mickelson, K.D., Kessler, R.C. & Shaver, P.R. (1997). Adult attachment in a nationally representative sample. *Journal of Personality and Social Psychology,* **73,** 1092–106.

Mintz, J., Mintz, L.I., Arruda, M.J. & Hwang, S.S. (1992). Treatments of depression and the functional capacity to work. *Archives of General Psychiatry,* **49,** 761–8.

Moore, K.A. & Burt, M.R. (1982). *Private Crisis, Public Cost: Policy Perspectives on Teenage Childbearing.* Washington, D.C.: Urban Institute Press.

Murray, C.J.L. (1994). Quantifying the burden of disease: the technical basis for DALYs. *Bulletin of the World Health Organization,* **72,** 429–45.

Murray, C.J.L. & Lopez, A.D. (eds.) (1994). *Global Comparative Assessments in the Health Sector.* Geneva: World Health Organization.

Murray, C.J.L. & Lopez, A.D. (eds.) (1996). *The Global Burden of Disease: A Comprehensive Assessment of Mortality and Disability from Diseases, Injuries, and Risk Factors in 1990 and Projected to 2020.* Cambridge, MA: Harvard University Press.

Myers, J.K., Weissman, M.M., Tischler, G.I., Holzer, C.E., Leaf, P.J., Ovaschel, H., Anthony, J.C., Boyd, J.H., Burke, J.D., Kramer, M. & Stoltzman, R. (1984). Six-month prevalence of psychiatric disorders in three communities. *Archives of General Psychiatry,* **41,** 959–67.

National Advisory Mental Health Council (1993). Health care reform for Americans with severe mental illnesses. *American Journal of Psychiatry,* **150,** 1447–65.

National Committee for Quality Assurance (1997). *HEDIS 3.0: Narrative: What's in it and why it matters.* Washington, D.C.: National Committee for Quality Assurance.

O'Connor, G.T., Plume, S.K., Olmstead, E.M., Morton, J.R., Maloney, C.T., Nugent, W.C., Hernandez, F. Jr., Clough, R., Leavitt, B.J., Coffin, L.H., Marrin, C.A.S., Wennberg, D., Birkmeyer, J.D., Charlesworth, D.C., Malenka, D.J., Quinton, H.B. & Kasper, J.F. (1996). A regional intervention to improve the hospital mortality associated with coronary artery bypass graft surgery. *Journal of the American Medical Association,* **275,** 841–6.

Patrick, D.L. & Erickson, P. (1993). *Health Status and Health Policy: Quality of Life in Health Care Evaluation and Resource Allocation.* New York: Oxford University Press.

Pauker, S.P. & Pauker, S.G. (1987). The amniocentesis decision: ten years of decision analytic experience. *Birth Defects,* **23,** 151–69.

Pestotnik, S.I., Classen, D.C., Evans, R.S. & Burke, I.P. (1996). Implementing antibiotic practice guidelines through computer-assisted decision support: clinical outcomes and financial outcomes. *Annals of Internal Medicine,* **124,** 884–90.

Pharoah, P.D. & Hollingsworth, W. (1996). Cost effectiveness of lowering cholesterol concentration with statins in patients with and without pre-existing coronary heart disease: a life table method applied to health authority population. *British Medical Journal,* **312,** 1443–8.

Regier, D.A., Kaelber, C.T., Rae, D.S., Farmer, M.E., Knauper, B., Kessler, R.C. &

Norquist, G.S. (1998). Limitations of diagnostic criteria and assessment instruments for mental disorders: implications for research and policy. *Archives of General Psychiatry*, **55**, 109–15.

Regier, D.A., Narrow, W.E., Rae, D.S., Manderscheid, R.W., Locke, B.Z. & Goodwin, F.K. (1993). The de facto US mental and addictive disorders service system: epidemiologic catchment area prospective 1-year prevalence rates of disorders and services. *Archives of General Psychiatry*, **50**, 85–94.

Reinherz, H.Z., Giaconia, R.M., Lefkowitz, E.S., Pakiz, B. & Frost, A.K. (1993). Prevalence of psychiatric disorders in a community population of older adolescents. *Journal of the American Academy of Child and Adolescent Psychiatry*, **32**, 369–77.

Revicki, D.A. (1992). Relationship between health utility and psychometric health status measures. *Medical Care*, **30**, 274–82.

Rice, D.P., Kelman, S., Miller, L.S. & Dunmeyer, S. (1990). *The Economic Costs of Alcohol and Drug Abuse and Mental Illness: 1985*. Rockville, MD: Alcohol, Drug Abuse, and Mental Health Service Administration.

Robertson, M. (1996). Cost effectiveness of lowering cholesterol: costs in general practice. *British Medical Journal*, **313**, 1143–4.

Roose, S.P. & Glassman, A.H. (1994). Antidepressant choice in the patient with cardiac disease: lessons from the Cardiac Arrhythmia Suppression Trial (CAST) studies. *Journal of Clinical Psychiatry*, **55** [Suppl. A], 83–7.

Russo, J., Katon, W., Lin, E., VonKorff, M., Bush, T., Simon, G. & Walker, E. (1997). Neuroticism and extraversion as predictors of health outcomes in depressed primary care patients. *Psychosomatics*, **38**, 339–48.

Schneider, E. & Epstein, A. (1996). Influence of cardiac-surgery performance reports on referral practices and access to care: a survey of cardiovascular specialists. *New England Journal of Medicine*, **335**, 251–6.

Shepherd, J., Cobbe, S.M., Ford, I., Isles, C.G., Lorimer, A.R., MacFarlane, P.W., McKillop, J.H. & Packard, C.J. (1995). Prevention of coronary heart disease with pravastatin in men with hypercholesterolemia: West of Scotland Coronary Prevention Study Group. *New England Journal of Medicine*, **333**, 1301–7.

Simon, G.E., VonKorff, M., Heiligenstein, J.H., Revicki, D.A., Grothaus, L., Katon, W. & Wagner, E.H. (1996). Initial antidepressant choice in primary care: effectiveness and cost of fluoxetine vs tricyclic antidepressants. *Journal of the American Medical Association*, **275**, 1897–902.

Stoudemire, A. (1995). *Psychological Factors Affecting Medical Conditions*. Washington, D.C.: American Psychiatric Press.

Torrence, G.W. & Feeny, D. (1989). Utilities and quality-adjusted life years. *International Journal of Technology Assessment in Health Care*, **5**, 559–75.

Tosteson, A.N., Weinstein, M.C., Hunink, M.G., Mittleman, M.A., Williams, C.W., Goldman, P.A. & Goldman, L. (1997). Cost effectiveness of population-wide educational approaches to reduce serum cholesterol level. *Circulation*, **95**, 24–30.

Wagstaff, A. (1991). QUALYs and the equity-efficiency trade-off. *Journal of Health Economics*, **10**, 21–41.

Wells, K.B., Katon, W., Rogers, B. & Camp, P. (1994). Use of minor tranquilizers and antidepressant medications by depressed outpatients: results from the medical outcomes study. *American Journal of Psychiatry*, **151**, 694–700.

Wells, K.B., Sturm, R., Sherbourne, C.D. & Meredith, L.S. (1996). *Caring for Depression*. Cambridge MA: Harvard University Press.

Wolf, A.W., Schubert, D.S.P., Patterson, M.B., Marion, B., Grande, T.P., Brocco, K.J. & Pendleton, L. (1988). Associations among major psychiatric disorders. *Journal of Consulting and Clinical Psychology*, **56**, 292–4.

Wyatt, R.J. & Clark, K. (1987). Calculating the cost of schizophrenia. *Psychiatric Annals*, **17**, 586–91.

6

The need for psychiatric treatment in the general population

Paul Bebbington

Defining the need for psychiatric care is essentially the province of experts, and the concept of need thus differs from the empirically related concepts of demand and utilization. Despite the importance of assessing population levels of need for treatment, this has almost invariably been done by indirect methods based on consideration of prevalence, disability, and utilization. Such data do have some use, and I use the results of the household component of the British National Survey of Psychiatric Morbidity to demonstrate that there must be a considerable, if imprecisely defined, shortfall in treatment for depression and anxiety in the British population. In the Camberwell Needs for Care Survey (Bebbington et al., 1997), we adapted the Needs for Care Assessment for use in the community in an attempt to provide a detailed account of the treatment needed by individuals, whether it was provided, and if not, why. This allows statements of aggregate levels of need and its fulfillment. The results of these two studies cohere in identifying considerable unmet need for treatment of depression and anxiety. Some of this arises because treatment was not and would not be sought, some because it was not offered. The problems of remedying this situation are complex.

Need, demand and utilization

The performance of organizations and agencies responsible for delivering psychiatric care can be assessed in relation to what care is delivered, to whom, and with what effect. This is set against the background of the moral imperative of health economics: that resources should not be used in one way, if using them differently would increase the overall health benefit. The relationship between the provision of health care and the needs of its consumers can be examined by looking at the three areas of demand, utilization, and need.

Demand is the overall requirement that members of a population have for given treatments and services. This is the result of individuals' perception of distress and disability, and what they regard as effective and desirable treatment. Both of these perceptions may differ from those of the professionals to whom they turn.

Utilization is relatively straightforward, indicating the take-up of treatment and services by individuals. Some of this utilization will be seen as appropriate by professionals and some will not. Thus, many people whom professionals would like to treat may not present themselves, and many for whom no treatment is available, or suitable, may nevertheless make contact with medical services. Moreover, in psychiatry, the existence of compulsory treatment legislation is a clear indication that utilization and demand may not coincide at all.

The word 'need', in our view, is best kept to refer to expert-defined, or normative, need (Bradshaw, 1972). Demand is sometimes referred to as 'perceived need', but we think the conceptual distinction should be maintained. The whole idea of professional expertise is predicated on the belief that, in certain arenas, people are not necessarily the best judge of what is good for them. This distinguishes the functions of professionals such as physicians and lawyers from those of grocers and butchers. This may sound condescending, but in medicine it refers to the simple fact that lay people may not be in a position to judge the empirical effectiveness of treatment. However, there is a dynamic tension between perceived need and expert-defined need. People present problems to consultants, who then proceed to suggest solutions. However, the consulting person may, in the light of the proposed solutions, reframe the problems or negotiate about the solution. Nevertheless, it is the professional's expertise that drives the interaction.

Strategies for identifying need, met and unmet, at the population level

Until recently, epidemiological studies in psychiatry produced two sorts of data relevant to these issues: the prevalence of various mental disorders and the extent to which people utilize services. Prevalence was seen as a proxy for need. However, this presupposes that clinicians judge the need for treatment solely on the basis of the process of diagnosis. This involves allocating the attributes of individuals to diagnostic classes. The diagnostic classes are essentially set up for theoretical purposes. However, they are useful for several different theoretical concerns, and are therefore unlikely to serve any one of them perfectly. Thus, a major preoccupation of those setting up diagnostic classifications is etiology, and consequently diagnostic classes correspond only approximately to treatment classes. For this reason, the prevalence of a disorder is only an approximation of the need for treatment at the community level, and may indeed be a rather poor approximation. Thus, diagnosis is merely suggestive of treatment, not prescriptive. Treating clinicians are also likely to consider the course of the disorder, the level of distress, and disability, and the likely outcome without treatment. Attempts to get closer to need by combining case identification with utilization or disability data have been made (Lehtinen et al., 1990; Shapiro, Skinner, Kramer, Steinwachs & Regier, 1985). However, there is a very strong argument for attempting to assess need for treatment in populations directly. Our own community psychiatric survey in Camberwell appears to be the first to attempt to do this (Bebbington, Marsden & Brewin, 1997; Bebbington, Marsden, Brewin & Lesage, 1996).

Utilization data from the British National Survey of Psychiatric Morbidity

The combination of prevalence and utilization data does at least give a feel for the extent to which treatment needs go unmet. We will, therefore, first describe data from the British National Survey of Psychiatric Morbidity. These data are presented more extensively elsewhere (Meltzer, Gill, Petticrew & Hinds, 1995). The methods used have been described by Jenkins et al. (1997a, b). The survey was of a stratified random sample of the whole population of Great Britain. Response rates were good and we were able to interview around 10,000 individuals. Neurotic psychiatric disorders were assessed using the Revised Clinical Interview Schedule (CIS-R) (Lewis, Pelosi, Araya & Dunn, 1992). This provides prevalences relating to a one-week period. Symptom data can be subjected to a computer algorithm providing ICD-10 diagnoses. In addition, those scoring above 12 on the overall summed score, who were not allocated to specific ICD-10 categories, were classed as suffering from mixed anxiety depressive disorder.

Some information about consultation with general practitioners was asked of all respondents, with more detail being requested of those with neurotic disorders. People with such disorders were also asked about their contact with secondary care services. Detailed information was collected on medication and other forms of treatment. This included data about two broad categories of medication: antidepressants, and hypnotics and anxiolytics. Information on two other forms of treatment, psychotherapy and counseling, was also sought.

In Table 6.1 we present the sorts of treatment given to people with neurotic disorders. There are two striking features of this table. First, very few people who were diagnosed as having a neurotic disorder were actually in receipt of treatment. There was a rough correspondence to the likely severity of the disorder and disability associated with it. However, even for depressive disorder, 75% of cases were not in receipt of treatment. The prescription of antidepressants was most frequent for depressive disorder, and there is therefore some evidence of specificity. However, appreciable proportions of people with other disorders were also being given antidepressants. The prescription of anxiolytics and hypnotics was almost as prevalent as that of

Table 6.1. Type of treatment by type of neurotic disorder in the British National Survey of Psychiatric Morbidity

Type of treatment	Mixed anxiety & depressive disorder, % (n=750)	GAD, % (n=439)	Depressive episode, % (n=220)	Phobia, % (n=180)	OCD, % (n=157)	Panic, % (n=93)
Any medication	6	12	21	21	16	13
Antidepressants	3	8	16	15	12	11
Anxiolytics and hypnotics	2	7	10	11	9	3
Any counselling or therapy	4	7	11	14	9	6
Any treatment	9	16	25	28	19	15

Source: Meltzer, Gill, Petticrew & Hinds, 1995.
GAD, generalized anxiety disorder; OCD, obsessive-compulsive disorder.

Table 6.2. Type of treatment by number of neurotic disorder in the British National Survey of Psychiatric Morbidity

Type of treatment	One neurotic disorder, % (*n*=1348)	Two or more neurotic disorders, % (*n*=209)
Any medication	6	25
Antidepressants	4	18
Anxiolytics and hypnotics	3	12
Any counseling or therapy	5	12
Any treatment	10	30

Source: Meltzer, Gill, Petticrew & Hinds, 1995.

antidepressants, even in the category of depressive episode. Even if some people identified as having neurotic disorder did not require treatment, these data strongly suggest that many needs were not being met.

There was some evidence that severity had an effect. Thus, in Table 6.2, treatment is more likely in cases where more than one category of neurosis had been identified. Nevertheless, 70% of people with two or more neurotic disorders were still not receiving treatment.

The Camberwell Needs for Care Survey and the Needs for Care Assessment

In the second part of this chapter, we are able to evaluate more specifically the extent to which needs for psychiatric treatment are being met in the general population. This comes from the Camberwell Needs for Care Survey (Bebbington et al., 1996, 1997). This was based in the catchment area of the Bethlem/Maudsley Hospital, a socioeconomically deprived area of inner south London. The sample was randomly selected from the electoral roll.

The survey was carried out in two stages. In stage one, respondents were asked to fill in the generalized health questionnaire GHQ-28 (Goldberg & Hillier, 1979) and to provide basic sociodemographic information. All people above the standard cut-off, and a proportion of those below, were invited for a second interview. Our data can thus be weighted back to the original sample. At stage two, people were assessed using *SCAN Schedules for Clinical Assessment in Neuropsychiatry* (World Health Organization, 1992), the Medical Research Council (MRC) Social Role Performance Schedule (Hurry & Sturt, 1981), the Life Events and Difficulties Schedule (Brown & Harris, 1978), and a treatment inventory specially developed for the study. Seven hundred and sixty people were assessed at stage one, and 408 were successfully interviewed at stage two.

The information obtained from the various assessment instruments was then used as a basis for rating needs for care. In order to do this, we developed a community version of the MRC Needs for Care Assessment (NFCAS) (Brewin, Wing, Mangen, Brugha & MacCarthy, 1987; Brewin et al., 1988). While the community version retains the philosophy of the original, it is a very different instrument (Brewin, Bebbington & Lesage, 1994). Its psychometric properties have been established by Lesage et al. (1996). The instrument has seven clinical domains: psychosis, depression, anxiety, alcohol abuse, drug abuse, eating disorders, and adjustment disorders. The actual items of treatment provided are compared with an explicit model of care based on current clinical consensus and the literature on treatment effectiveness. Each item of care is rated according to whether it is provided, and whether it is appropriate and effective in the context of a given level of disability. The ratings allow the establishment of a primary need status falling in the potential categories: met need, unmet need, no need, and no meetable need.

There is also a facility for rating over-provision (described elsewhere in this book as met un-need). There is an elaborate rating for each individual actual or potential item of care for a given clinical domain. It should be noted that the convention of the assessment is to record 'no need' where there is no effective treatment available, even if there is a clear disability. In other words, needs are recorded only when there is a practical treatment. The ratings were made by a psychologist and psychiatrist following presentations of case vignettes describing disabilities, symptoms, and treatments.

Need for treatment in the general population: depression and anxiety

In Table 6.3 we present a summary of the weighted prevalence from the Camberwell Needs for Care Survey. While the prevalence of meetable need for treatment was very similar to the prevalence of all ICD-10 disorders, the people with needs for treatment did not wholly overlap with diagnosed cases. The identified needs for treatment in Camberwell are broken down further in Table 6.4. It can be seen that unmet needs outnumbered met needs. Unmeetable needs comprised an appreciable minority of all needs.

There is obviously considerable clinical interest in looking in more detail at the items of care that were assessed. In this chapter we will focus on depressive and anxiety disorders, since these were the commonest groups. Individuals were rated in relation to 'care episodes'. Up to two of these were rated in the year prior to assessment. If people had symptoms in more than one clinical domain and these required treating in their own right, they could have had simultaneous care episodes for different conditions. Thus there are two separate reasons for there to be more care episodes than individuals. In

Table 6.3. Camberwell Needs for Care Survey: weighted prevalence

	1-month prevalence, %	1-year prevalence, %
All ICD-10 disorders	9.8	12.3
Depressive disorders	3.1	5.3
Anxiety states	2.8	2.8
Meetable needs for treatment	9.5	10.4

Source: Bebbington et al., 1997.

Table 6.4. Identified needs for treatment in Camberwell: unweighted numbers; weighted percentages

	Care episodes		People needing treatment	
Need status	Current	Whole year	1 month	1 year
Met	19 (4%)	29 (6.1%)	17 (3.6%)	18 (3.7%)
Unmet	41 (6.8%)	49 (8.2%)	34 (5.9%)	37 (6.7%)
Unmeetable	9 (1.5%)	13 (2.3%)	8 (1.3%)	10 (1.6%)

Source: Bebbington et al., 1997.

Table 6.5. Treatment needs and provision: anxiety and depression

	Total care episodes	
Need status	Depression	Anxiety
Met	8 (1.2%)	2 (0.3%)
Unmet	21 (4.0%)	13 (2.5%)
Unmeetable	4 (0.8%)	1 (0.1%)

Source: Bebbington et al., 1997.

Table 6.5, we present the needs status in relation to all the care episodes rated for depression and anxiety. Note that in the NFCAS depression is distinguished from adjustment reaction on clinical grounds. The ratio of unmet/met need was high in depression (3.3 to 1), and it was very high indeed in anxiety disorders (8.3 to 1).

Altogether 30 respondents were assessed in the depression section. For 21 of these, the provision of antidepressant medication was evaluated in relation to 26 care periods. In only six instances (23%) was effective medication provided, while in a further case it was provided but not regarded as being fully effective. Many respondents did not like to medicalize their low mood, and this is reflected in 12 instances (46%) where the whole idea of medical

Table 6.6. Items of care for depression (n=30)

	Medication	Support	Psychotherapy	Cognitive therapy	Other
Needed/ effective	6	4	–	–	–
Needed/part-effective	–	1	–	–	1
Noncompliant	1	–	–	–	–
Rejection of treatment	12	3	2	2	–
Needed/not given	6	12	3	10	–

treatment was rejected. There were, however, six cases (23%) where medication would have been acceptable but had not been prescribed. Of these, two had seen their general practitioner for 'nerves'. Most respondents would have welcomed some professional support, but in most instances this had not been provided (see Table 6.6). Interestingly, in two cases where psychotherapy was thought appropriate, it was rejected by the individual. In three others, there was felt to be an unmet need for psychotherapy, cases in which the depressive condition emerged from a long-standing depressive personality and a history of early adversity.

In the view of the assessment team, 12 respondents (40% of the total individuals assessed for depression) would have benefited from cognitive therapy because of persistent problems with self-esteem and recurrent depressed mood. In most cases, this was rated as an unmet need. No person was actually receiving this form of treatment for depression, and the need was rated as unmet in over 80%. Two rejected the whole idea of treatment and would not consider cognitive therapy.

In Table 6.7, we record information on 17 persons who were assessed as having anxiety symptoms or treatment for them. Again, many care episodes (13/24) were characterized by an unmet need for treatment. In general, we were reluctant to consider medication for such conditions, unless they were likely to be of short duration, and pharmacotherapy would serve a useful function in the short-term. In two individuals we identified an unmet need for medication, and in four others medication that had been prescribed was seen as appropriate and fully or partly effective. There was an interesting contrast to those with depression: those with anxiety were unlikely to reject the idea of treatment (only 2 of the 17 did so). Unmet needs for cognitive therapy were identified in eight individuals, and three (25% of the 12 in which it was regarded as appropriate) were actually receiving treatment of this type.

Table 6.7. Items of care for anxiety ($n=17$)

	Medication	Support	Assessment	Cognitive therapy	Other
Needed/effective	2	1	–	1	–
Needed/part-effective	2	–	–	2	–
Noncompliant	–	–	–	–	1
Rejection of treatment	–	1	–	1	–
Needed/not given	2	1	2	8	–

The bottom line so far

The two surveys used in this chapter to illustrate needs for psychiatric treatment complement each other. In the smaller, more intensive study, needs were assessed directly using a newly developed standardized technique. This revealed that many needs for treatment were not being met in the community, and that this applied to the two commonest groups of disorder, depression and anxiety. In the large British National Survey of Psychiatric Morbidity, needs were not measured directly. However, it is reasonable to assume that an appreciable proportion, particularly of the more severe disorders such as depressive episode, would have been judged in need of treatment. This can then be set against the utilization of services and the provision of treatment, and the findings relating to this are so striking that one is left with the inevitable inference that only a minority are getting the treatment they need.

Thus in the Needs for Care Survey, the proportion of meetable needs for the treatment of depression that were actually met was less than a quarter, and for anxiety it was not much more than 10%. This tallies quite well with the National Survey data, in which 75% of cases of depressive episode were completely untreated, and even more for other neurosis diagnoses. It is of particular interest that antidepressant medication was given infrequently, and that this often came about because the respondents themselves were very wary of it. They were less wary of psychological treatment but this was rarely available.

The research context

The results presented here are very consistent with others in the literature. A high frequency of unmet need was reported from Epidemiologic Catchment Area (ECA) data by Shapiro and his colleagues (1984, 1985) and a more elaborate study from Finland gave similar findings (Lehtinen et al., 1990) –

4% of respondents were receiving appropriate and adequate treatment, while 14% showed an unmet need.

There is evidence from elsewhere that people with anxiety disorders are often not treated, and when they are they do not get the right treatment (Chapter 18), despite the cost-effectiveness of cognitive behavior therapy. The problem of antitreatment attitudes has also been identified by others. Wilhelm and Lin (Chapter 15) showed that much undertreated depression comes about because of the antitreatment attitudes of those who suffer from it. A large survey in Australia confirms that members of the general public have a low opinion of the effectiveness and appropriateness of antidepressants as a treatment for depression (Chapter 28), and similar findings were obtained in Germany (Matschinger & Angermeyer, 1996).

Finally, the effect of severity, as reflected in comorbidity, in increasing the likelihood that treatment is provided has also been noted in the Munich Prospective Community Survey. The number of comorbid anxiety disorders predicted utilization (Chapter 17).

Conclusion

The issue of severity illuminates the moral dilemma posed by these results. More severe cases are more likely to get treatment, and in a cash-limited service one might be inclined to approve of this trend, feeling that the service has at least some claims to be a just one. However, some severe disorders are nevertheless untreated, and it may yet be very cost-effective to treat milder conditions, partly because it may preempt deterioration, and partly because even these disorders impose a burden of disability and cost. There exists a major problem in designing services that are capable of delivering treatments known from specific studies to be effective, and this problem includes the financing of the service in a way that is free from perverse incentives. The main benefit of focusing on needs for treatment is that it initiates debate on how these problems might be overcome.

References

Bebbington, P.E., Marsden, L. & Brewin, C.R. (1997). The treatment of psychiatric disorder in the community: report from the Camberwell Needs for Care Survey. *Psychological Medicine*, 27, 821–34.

Bebbington, P.E., Marsden, L. Brewin, C. & Lesage, A. (1996). Measuring the need for psychiatric treatment in the general population: the community version of the MRC Needs for Care Assessment. *Psychological Medicine*, 26, 229–36.

Bradshaw, J. (1972). A taxonomy of social need. In G. McLaclan (ed.). *Problems and Progress in Medical Care, Seventh Series.* London: Oxford University Press.

Brewin, C.R., Bebbington, P.E. & Lesage, A.D. (1994). *The MRC Needs for Care Assessment Community Version Instruction Manual* (version 3.0 June 1994). London: MRC Social Psychiatry Unit, Institute of Psychiatry.

Brewin, C.R., Wing, J.K., Mangen, S.P., Brugha, T.S. & MacCarthy, B. (1987). Principles and practice of measuring need in the long term mentally ill: the MRC Needs for Care Assessment. *Psychological Medicine,* 17, 971–81.

Brewin, C.R., Wing, J.K., Mangen, S.P., Brugha, T.S., MacCarthy, B. & Lesage, A. (1988). Needs for care among the long-term mentally ill: a report from the Camberwell high contact survey. *Psychological Medicine,* 18, 457–68.

Brown, G.W. & Harris, T. (1978). *Social Origins of Depression: A Study of Psychiatric Disorders in Women.* London: Tavistock.

Goldberg, D.P. & Hillier, V.F. (1979). A scaled version of the General Health Questionnaire. *Psychological Medicine,* 9, 139–45.

Hurry, J. & Sturt, E. (1981). Social performance in a population sample: relation to psychiatric symptoms. In J. Wing, P. Bebbington, & L. Robins (eds.), *What is a Case? The Problem of Definition in Psychiatric Community Surveys,* pp. 202–13. London: Grant MacIntyre.

Jenkins, R., Bebbington, P.E., Brugha, T., Farrell M., Gill, B., Lewis, G., Meltzer, H. & Petticrew, M. (1997a). The National Psychiatric Morbidity Surveys of Great Britain. I: Strategy and methods. *Psychological Medicine,* 27, 765–74.

Jenkins, R., Lewis, G., Bebbington, P.E., Brugha, T., Farrell, M., Gill, B. & Meltzer, H. (1997b). The National Psychiatric Morbidity Surveys of Great Britain. II: The Household Survey. *Psychological Medicine,* 27, 775–89.

Lehtinen, V., Joukamaa, M., Jyrkinen, E., Lahtela, K., Raitasalo, R., Maatela, J. & Aromaa, A. (1990). Need for mental health services of the adult population in Finland: results from the Mini Finland Health Survey. *Acta Psychiatrica Scandinavica,* 81, 426–31.

Lesage, A., Fournier, L., Cyr, M., Toupin, J., Fabian, J., Gaudette, G., Vanier, C., Bebbington, P.E. & Brewin, C. (1996). The reliability of the community version of the needs for care assessment. *Psychological Medicine,* 26, 237–43.

Lewis, G., Pelosi, A.J., Araya, R.C. & Dunn, G. (1992). Measuring psychiatric disorder in the community: a standardized assessment for use by lay interviewers. *Psychological Medicine,* 22, 465–86.

Matschinger, H. & Angermeyer, M.C. (1996). Lay beliefs about the causes of mental disorders: a new methodological approach. *Social Psychiatry and Psychiatric Epidemiology,* 31, 309–15.

Meltzer, H., Gill, B., Petticrew, M. & Hinds, K. (1995). *OPCS Surveys of Psychiatric Morbidity In Great Britain. Report No. 2. Physical Illness, Service Use and Treatment of Adults with Psychiatric Disorders.* London: OPCS.

Shapiro, S., Skinner, E.A., Kessler, L.G., Von Korff, M., German, P.S., Tischler, G.L., Leaf, P., Benham, L., Cottler, L. & Regier, D.A. (1984). Utilisation of health and mental health services: three epidemiologic catchment area sites. *Archives of General Psychiatry,* 41, 971–8.

Shapiro, S., Skinner, E.A., Kramer, M., Steinwachs, D.M. & Regier, D.A. (1985). Measuring need for mental health services in a general population. *Medical Care*, **23**, 1033–43.

World Health Organization (1992). *SCAN Schedules for Clinical Assessment in Neuropsychiatry*. Geneva: World Health Organization.

7

Comparing data on mental health service use between countries

Margarita Alegría, Ronald C. Kessler, Rob Bijl, Elizabeth Lin, Steven G. Heeringa, David T. Takeuchi, and Bodhan Kolody

The International Consortium of Psychiatric Epidemiology (ICPE) has brought together mental health researchers from around the world to compare the prevalence of mental health disorders and the utilization of mental health services in a variety of settings. The analyses compare results on patterns of service utilization in four of the ICPE study sites: USA, Ontario, The Netherlands, and Puerto Rico. The goals of this chapter are the following: to present data on past-year mental health service use, and to discuss the practical and methodological issues to be considered when developing a core set of questions about people's use of psychiatric services for use in psychiatric epidemiological surveys.

Formal mental health care was significantly higher for The Netherlands (13.4%), similar for Puerto Rico and the USA (8.3% and 8.1%, respectively) and lowest for Ontario (6.6%). A cross-national comparison examining differences in level of need in relation to use of mental health services showed that the number of psychiatric disorders was a major determinant of the individual's interaction with the formal mental health care system in all four sites. Observed differences in the use of mental health services could be attributed to differences in individual factors, in provider characteristics and in health care systems between the countries. By combining data from several countries, the ICPE provides an analytical base for monitoring the equity of service systems for people with mental illness. This chapter is only the beginning of our efforts to understand cross-national differences in patterns of care.

This is the first report of the mental health services work group of the ICPE. The ICPE is a World Health Organization (WHO) and National Institute of Mental Health (NIMH) collaborative effort to bring together researchers from a number of countries to foster cross-national comparative research on psychiatric disorders and mental health service use. (See Acknowledgement for address of the ICPE home page and more detailed information on the Consortium.) The mental health services work group of the ICPE has two mandates. The first is to catalogue all data on mental health services collected in completed ICPE surveys and coordinate comparative analyses of these data. The second mandate is to design a standardized set of questions on mental health services that can be used in future ICPE surveys in an effort to expand the comparative data available on this topic.

Preliminary results of work on both these mandates are presented in this chapter. In the first section, we present preliminary data on mental health service use from the first four countries that have contributed data on this topic to the ICPE master data bank. The last section discusses some of the methodological and substantive issues confronted in designing a standardized series of questions about service use that can be employed in future surveys carried out across the world.

General overview of cross-national comparisons

The usefulness of field surveys in psychiatric epidemiology would be enhanced considerably if, in addition to assessing morbidity, they examined the relationship between the individual with a psychiatric disorder and the health care system. Adding service-use data to psychiatric epidemiology studies may also increase our capacity to assess how well countries allocate resources to meet mental health care needs (Burke & Jack, 1995).

At present we are a long way from meeting these ambitious goals. Most data on service use, if collected at all in epidemiological surveys, are collected for understanding specific issues within countries, and are not intended for international comparisons. In the USA, very recent large-scale surveys (Kessler et al., 1994; Regier et al., 1993) asked some questions about service use, but these were limited in scope and the question format tended to vary between the sites. In other countries, collection of data on service use is even less regular (Gater & Goldberg, 1991). In spite of these limitations, our efforts are geared towards improving the capacity to compare service-use data across countries.

Methods

Survey information

The ICPE has brought together mental health researchers from several countries to conduct cross-national analyses of the prevalence and patterns of mental health disorders and the utilization of mental health services in a variety of different social, cultural, and political settings. The analyses presented in this chapter compare results on mental health utilization rates and patterns of service use in four of the ICPE study sites: the 1990 National Comorbidity Survey (NCS) of the US household population; the 1990

Mental Health Supplement (the Supplement) to the Ontario (Canada) Health Survey; the 1996 Netherlands Mental Health Survey and Incidence Study (NEMESIS); and the 1992 Puerto Rico Mental Health Care Utilization (MHCU) Project.

In this chapter, we illustrate the use of the multiple data sources by comparing use of any services for mental health problems in the 12 months prior to the survey. Three of these surveys (NCS, the Supplement and NEMESIS) interviewed a probability sample of the general population and obtained information on the past-year prevalence of psychiatric disorders based on the WHO's Composite International Diagnostic Interview (CIDI; Wittchen, 1994; Wittchen, Kessler, Zhao & Abelson, 1995; World Health Organization, 1990) and information about formal and informal care for psychiatric problems during that same time period. The MHCU interviewed a probability sample of adults residing in poor neighborhoods of the island. These data make it possible to compare rates of past-year service use across subsamples defined in terms of their need for services. For some analyses, need for services is defined as the number of past-year CIDI/DSM-III-R disorders. For other analysis, need is equated with specific CIDI diagnoses. The sample design for each of the four studies is based on a multistage area probability sample of the respective survey population. Although the age range for each sample varied by country, all the analyses presented in this chapter are restricted to respondents 18–54 years of age.

Contextual information about the four ICPE sites

It is important to note that the mental health service systems in these four countries are quite different. The Netherlands has universal health coverage available to all residents of the country. Most outpatient and inpatient mental health care is financed through social health insurance. Most providers are paid on a fee-for-service basis subject to tariff regulations under social health insurance. About 4% of service costs are paid by individual patients, either through out-of-pocket expenses or with supplemental health insurance. Although the general practitioner is supposed to act as the gatekeeper to the mental health care system, about 40% of those who receive outpatient mental health care do so without being referred by the general practitioner.

Ontario also has universal insurance coverage open to all legal residents of the province (Freeman, 1994; Ontario Ministry of Health, 1993; Roche-fort, 1992). Mental and physical health are both covered, with no limits on the number of visits for mental health problems. Physician services are billed primarily to the provincial health plan on a fee-for-service basis. Other mental health care is paid for by the Ministry of Health through the salaries of professionals such as psychologists, nurses, and other mental health specialists who work in hospitals or health care agencies.

In the USA, services are offered by a public and private system of care. About 60% of the population is covered through private insurance, often made available through employment. Some mental health coverage is available through virtually all these private insurance plans, although most often the coverage is subject to special limits or is under capitation funding; that is, programs receive a fixed payment per client (Lehman, 1987). Public financing systems of Medicare and Medicaid pay for mental health care for the elderly and poor. Coverage of mental health in these plans is generous. About 15% of the USA population has no form of third-party payment and must rely on state-financed mental health systems, which vary in the quality of, and access to, care.

In Puerto Rico, mental health services are provided in both the private and public sector (Health Department of the Commonwealth of Puerto Rico, 1989). Since 1993, the government has acted both as payer and provider of mental health services, subsidized in part by federal Medicaid funds. Under a Medicaid waiver, Puerto Rico does not use income thresholds to define eligibility for the public health system. Anyone who needs health or mental health care automatically qualifies for free health and mental health care from public facilities. Users of the public system cannot choose the provider, but there are no restrictions on the number of visits to mental health services. Demand for specialty services in the public system of health is controlled by limiting the supply of mental health specialty providers in community mental health settings. The private sector offers mental health care through various institutions, providers, and hospitals without a clearly delineated structure of care delivery. Mental health providers operate as an informal network on a fee-for-service model. Consumers have access to private specialty services as long as they can afford the fees or the co-payments required by their insurance, which is typically 20% of the contracted fee. Most private insurance will not pay for more than 10 or 12 ambulatory visits to the specialty sector.

One might imagine from this variation in service systems that availability of mental health providers would be quite different across these countries. However, as shown in Table 7.1, there is striking similarity in the number of psychiatrists per capita in the four countries – between 0.09 and 0.13 per 1000 population. Consistent with the fact that specialty inpatient treatment is more prominent in The Netherlands than in the other three countries, we find that the number of psychiatric hospital beds per capita is higher in The Netherlands (1.83 per 1000 population) than in Ontario (0.52 per 1000), USA (0.40 per 1000) or Puerto Rico (0.41 per 1000). The number of general practitioners per capita, in comparison, is considerably lower in The Netherlands (0.46 per 1000) than in the other countries (0.77–0.80 per 1000). Wide variation in psychiatrist-to-population ratios within countries are well known.

Table 7.1. Characteristics of the service system in four selected International Consortium of Psychiatric Epdemiology (ICPE) sites

	Psychiatrists (/1000 population)	Psychiatric hospital beds (/1000 population)	General practitioners (/1000 population)
Ontario	0.13	0.52	0.78
The Netherlands	0.11	1.83	0.46
United States of America	0.09	0.40	0.77
Puerto Rico	0.13	0.41	0.80

Measures

The first challenge in conducting cross-national comparisons in the ICPE surveys was that the CIDI does not include a core of questions on service use (WHO, 1990). When our group initiated its work, 12 ICPE surveys that contained some data on mental health services were available for analysis (see Table 7.2). However, as shown in Table 7.3, there were discrepancies in the type of providers assessed in the questions about service use. As shown in Table 7.4, there was also considerable variation in the time frame assessed. Annual use of mental health services was the most common time frame; therefore, the rate contrasted across countries. Furthermore, studies differed significantly on whether information was obtained about the number of visits made, the reasons for stopping treatment, use of medications, and other important service-use questions.

We have dealt with this variability for the purposes of the present chapter by focusing the analyses on those service-use questions included in more than one survey. The areas assessed in the surveys discussed are:

Formal care (divided into specialty and general medical care) – this includes visits to any general medical or mental health specialty provider as defined below.

Specialty care – this corresponds to visits to a psychiatrist, psychologist, hospital psychiatric emergency room, psychiatric outpatient clinic, mental health center, drug or alcohol outpatient clinic or inpatient drug clinic.

General medical care – this represents discussion of a mental health problem with a general practitioner; family physician; company doctor; cardiologist; gynecologist; or other physician; nurse; occupational therapist; or other health professional who is not a social worker or counselor.

Human services care – this includes mental health care provided by a social

Table 7.2. Description of the International Consortium of Psychiatric Epidemiology (ICPE) surveys with mental health service utilization information

Country	Name of survey	Type of survey	Target population	Sample size
Canada	Ontario Health Survey	Regional	15 or over	9953
Canada	Toronto Study	Regional	18–55	1393
Chile	Concepcion & Santiago National Study	Regional	15 or over	2136
Mexico	Psychiatric Morbidity in Mexico City	Regional	18–64	1734
Mexico	Tialpan & Xochilmilco	Regional	15–80	1482
The Netherlands	NEMESIS	National	18–64	7000
Puerto Rico	Mental Health Service utilization among Puerto Ricans	National	18–64	wave I: 3504; wave II: 3263
Turkey	Mental Health Profile of Turkey	National	18 or over	6095
USA	American Indian Veterans	Regional	men, Vietnam era	621
USA	Chinese–American Psychiatric Epidemiological Study	Regional	18–64	wave I: 1747; wave II: 1503
USA	Fresno	Regional	18–59	4000
USA	National Comorbidity Study	National	15–54	8098

NEMESIS, The 1996 Netherlands Mental Health Survey and Incidence Survey.

Table 7.3. Provider alternatives included across 12 sites/countries

Type of provider or care sector	Number of sites with provider option
General medical	
General practitioner, family physician	9
Private office of general doctor (nonpsychiatrist)	6
Cardiologist, gynecologist, or other physician	5
Nurse, occupational therapist, other health professional	7
Hospital medical emergency room	6
General hospital	1
Company doctor	1
Specialty mental health sector	
Psychiatrist	9
Psychologist	8
Private office – psychiatrist, psychologist	3
Psychiatric outpatient clinic	7
Drug or alcohol outpatient clinic	7
Mental health center	3
Hospital psychiatric emergency room	1
Inpatient drug or alcohol treatment center	1

worker or counselor in a social or government agency; in a private
office; or health care setting.

Informal care – this includes mental health care given by a minister, priest,
rabbi, or other religious representative; self-help group; telephone
hotline; spiritualist; herbalist; natural healer/therapist; folk healer;
'santero'; astrologist; 'sobador'; psychic; medium.

Findings

In this chapter, we present several cross-national comparisons. They are
illustrations of how these data viewed as a whole, rather than separately by
each country, can be an important clue for understanding and evaluating
which health systems facilitate mental health services. Comparative analysis
of service-use data may point to solutions for improving services at the
structural level of organizations and systems as well as the consumer, family
and provider level.

Use of different sectors of care for mental health problems

It is important to examine the utilization rates for mental health services

Table 7.4. Time frame of questions on mental health service utilization by 12 ICPE surveys

Survey	Past month/ current	Past 6 months	Past 12 months	Ever/ lifetime
Ontario Health Survey, Canada	+	+	+	+
Toronto Study, Canada			+	
Concepcion & Santiago National Study, Chile		+		
Psychiatric Morbidity in Mexico City, Mexico	+	+	+	+
Tialpan & Xochilmilco, Mexico		+	+	
NEMESIS, The Netherlands	+	+	+	+
Mental Health Service utilization among Puerto Ricans, Puerto Rico		+	+	
Mental Health Profile of Turkey			+	
American Indian Veterans, USA		+	+	
Chinese–American Psychiatric Epidemiological Study, USA		+	+	
Fresno, USA	+	+	+	+
National Comorbidity Study, USA	+	+	+	+
Total	5	10	10	6

Note: + Survey includes this time frame in their service utilization questions.

across countries, adjusting for the presence of disorders. Before adjustments (see Table 7.5), the percentage of the population receiving mental health services was significantly higher for The Netherlands (13.4%), similar for Puerto Rico and the USA (8.3% and 8.1%, respectively), and lowest for Ontario (6.6%). Differences in the rates of receiving any formal mental health care between countries are significant ($p < 0.05$), except for those between the USA and Puerto Rico ($Z = -0.28$, $p = 0.39$).

When one focuses on a particular sector of mental health care, it appears that The Netherlands, even though it has fewer general practitioners than the other sites, has at least double the rate of general medical sector care for mental health services (10%) than the other countries (3.7–4.6%). Some other important differences are noted in Table 7.5. In The Netherlands and Ontario, the unadjusted rates of receiving mental health care from a general medical provider are higher than those for receiving care from a specialty provider. The opposite was observed for the USA and Puerto Rico.

Several intriguing patterns related to the sector of care for mental health problems can also be seen in Table 7.5. Only in the USA does the human services sector provide a considerable amount of mental health care. People in The Netherlands appear more ready to use most of the service sectors (i.e.,

Table 7.5. Unadjusted estimated percentages of mental health services in the last 12 months for four selected ICPE sites

	Type of service				
	Any formal care % (SE)	General medical % (SE)	Specialty % (SE)	Human services % (SE)	Informal care % (SE)
Ontario	6.6 (0.4)	4.6 (0.4)	3.5 (0.2)	1.3 (0.2)	2.3 (0.2)
The Netherlands	13.4 (0.5)	10.0 (0.5)	6.5 (0.3)	2.3 (0.2)	4.8 (0.3)
United States of America	8.1 (0.5)	3.7 (0.4)	5.5 (0.4)	4.3 (0.3)	3.2 (0.3)
Puerto Rico	8.3 (0.5)	4.2 (0.4)	5.4 (0.4)	1.3 (0.3)	3.2 (0.4)

general medical, specialty and informal), apart from the human services, compared with those in the three other countries.

Psychiatric need and service use

A second cross-national comparison examined how differences in the level of need, as measured by the number of CIDI/DSM-III-R psychiatric diagnoses, are related to variations in the rates of mental health service use (see Table 7.6). It should be noted that the number of disorders assessed by the different studies varied greatly (four in Puerto Rico versus 17 in the USA). These data compare rates of past-year formal mental health care treatment across sub-samples in the four ICPE sites, controlling for level of need. We present these descriptive data not as evidence on which to base conclusive statements, but to suggest interesting cross-national hypotheses for future work. Based on the number of past-year CIDI/DSM-III-R disorders, several patterns appear uniform across the four countries. There is a strong positive linear relationship between the number of diagnoses and the probability of receiving any formal mental health care in all four countries. For example, the rates of receiving formal mental health care are less than 8% of the general population in all countries for individuals with no CIDI/DSM-III-R diagnosis in the previous year. For all sites included, the number of psychiatric disorders is a major determinant of the individual's interaction with formal mental health care services.

This partitioning of mental health service use along a gradient of need can clarify many of the previously described similarities and differences between countries. The Netherlands appears to provide higher rates of any formal care for those with and without psychiatric disorders. Ontario reflects a completely different picture, whereby only 3.2% of those with no psychiatric disorder use any formal mental health care.

Table 7.6. Comparison of any formal use of mental health services for respondents defined in need on the basis of the number of past year CIDI/DSM-III-R disorders

	No past 12-month diagnosis % (SE)	One past 12-month diagnosis % (SE)	More than one past 12-month diagnosis % (SE)
Ontario	3.2 (0.4)	13.6 (2.0)	36.7 (2.9)
The Netherlands	7.7 (0.4)	21.0 (1.4)	51.9 (2.7)
United States of America	4.0 (0.5)	12.4 (1.4)	24.2 (1.7)
Puerto Rico	5.6 (0.5)	24.2 (2.9)	39.9 (6.5)

Table 7.7. Comparison of specialty and general medical use of mental health services for respondents defined in need on the basis of the number of past year CIDI/DSM-III-R disorders

	No past 12-month diagnosis		1 past 12-month diagnosis		More than 1 past 12-month diagnosis	
	Specialty % (SE)	General % (SE)	Specialty % (SE)	General % (SE)	Specialty % (SE)	General % (SE)
Ontario	1.6 (0.2)	2.3 (0.3)	6.0 (1.1)	10.2 (1.7)	23.8 (3.7)	24.7 (2.9)
The Netherlands	3.4 (0.2)	5.2 (0.4)	8.7 (0.9)	16.0 (1.2)	31.1 (2.1)	41.8 (2.5)
United States of America	2.5 (0.3)	1.9 (0.4)	7.5 (0.9)	6.2 (1.2)	18.8 (1.1)	18.8 (2.5)
Puerto Rico	3.4 (0.4)	2.7 (0.4)	18.4 (2.9)	12.7 (2.1)	26.2 (5.8)	24.3 (5.8)

There are also between-country differences in the prevalence of any formal use of mental health services among people with more than one last-year CIDI diagnosis (see Table 7.6). One in every two people with more than one last-year CIDI diagnosis receives formal care in The Netherlands in contrast to one in every four in the USA.

When we focus on specialty care for people who were classified as having one disorder in the past 12 months, we see remarkable differences between countries in the proportions who use specialized mental health care (see Table 7.7). In Puerto Rico, 1 out of every 5 respondents with one disorder used specialty services compared to 1 out of 11 in The Netherlands, 1 out of 13 in the USA, and 1 out of 17 in Ontario. For respondents with more than one psychiatric disorder, the proportion of specialty use in The Netherlands was 1:3 in contrast to 1:4 in Ontario and Puerto Rico, and 1:5.5 in the USA. This seems to suggest a higher proportion of specialty use in The Netherlands and Puerto Rico as compared to Ontario and the USA.

Table 7.7 also presents information on the relationship between the num-

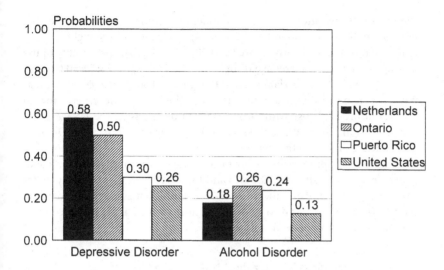

Figure 7.1 Probability of any formal use of mental health services in the previous year among those with a depressive disorder and among those with an alcohol-abuse/ dependence disorder by site (weighted analysis). Covariates are fixed at: each country's average for sex, age, education, marital status, employment status, income and chronic physical illnesses.

ber of psychiatric disorders and the probability of receiving specialty treatment. In The Netherlands, Ontario and Puerto Rico, those with more than one past-year CIDI/DSM-III-R diagnosis are more likely to receive specialty treatment as compared to those in the USA. It is also interesting that mental health services in three of the four sites are just as likely to be provided in the specialty sector as in the general medical sector for those with two or more psychiatric disorders. Roughly half the people with two or more psychiatric disorders in Ontario, the USA and Puerto Rico are provided with services from the general medical sector and the other half from the specialty sector, recognizing that some receive services from both.

Type of disorder and mental health service use

Another example of cross-country comparison is shown in Figure 7.1. We estimated the probability of any formal use of mental health services among two groups for each site: those complying with criteria for a past-year depressive disorder (includes a diagnosis of major depression or dysthymia), and those with alcohol abuse/dependence. To compare the treatment rates for a standard population group, the estimated probabilities were calculated while fixing the covariates at the country's average. For example, the probability of seeking formal care was calculated, where the average income over the site was substituted for each respondent's income. Among those with a depressive disorder, respondents in The Netherlands had the highest probability of receiving any formal care (p=0.58, SE=0.04). The probability of use among those with a depressive disorder in the USA (p=0.26; SE=0.02) was half that for The Netherlands and Ontario (p=0.50; SE=0.05). A similar pattern can be observed among those meeting diagnostic criteria for an alcohol disorder. Those with alcohol-related disorders in the USA are less likely to use the mental health services than their counterparts in Ontario, Puerto Rico, or The Netherlands.

Relative to the probability of any formal care for respondents with alcohol abuse/dependence disorder, Ontario and Puerto Rico do considerably better than The Netherlands or the USA. These findings suggest the need to tie service use to particular disorders in an effort to conduct between-country comparisons of unmet need and patterns of care.

Demographic variations in mental health service use

For an additional illustration of cross-national comparisons, we focused on the characteristics related to help-seeking among a particular group of individuals – those who met criteria for depression in the previous 12 months. Two patterns emerged when the gender, education, and marital status of depressed respondents who had sought formal services in the previous 12 months were compared with those who did not. First, despite differences in the culture and health system between the four sites, there are some consistent trends between those with treated and untreated depression. Those seeking formal care are more likely to be female (in all sites except Puerto Rico), to be high-school graduates (except in The Netherlands), and to be in a disrupted marital status (all sites). The second pattern is that these differences, while consistent, are slight. The only statistically significant odds ratio is the 'high-school graduate' for The Netherlands. These results suggest that there are minor sociodemographic differences between those depressed individuals who seek care and those who do not, an essential step in uncovering the selection biases that operate in help-seeking beyond the current clinical status (Dew, Dunn, Bromet & Schulberg, 1988).

Discussion

Our cross-national comparisons offer a reasonable basis from which to generate hypotheses about what accounts for similarities and differences in the rates of mental health service use between countries. One possible explanation for the elevated rates of any formal care for mental health problems in The Netherlands as compared to the other three sites is that it is the only country where screening for mental health conditions is included in the clinical prevention guidelines designed for the primary care sector. This may account for the finding that those with and without psychiatric disorders are more likely to report discussing mental health problems with their general practitioner in The Netherlands than in any of the other three sites. Training of general practitioners in the screening of psychiatric morbidity and the enforcement of clinical guidelines to appropriately identify and treat psychiatric disorders may account for the large proportion of patients treated by mental health services in general medical care settings in The Netherlands.

In addition, most general practitioners in The Netherlands remain in the same setting, organized in small professional groups (*maatschappen*), working in only one hospital over their lifetime (Maarse, Mur-Veeman & Spreeuwenberg, 1997). Having the same provider evaluate the patient over several years may foster a greater therapeutic alliance, which could make it easier to detect mental illness and other social conditions that may impinge upon the patient's well-being. Always having the same doctor may improve the patients' trust in and relationship with health care services, which can increase their receptivity and willingness to discuss mental health problems.

Also, the higher education in The Netherlands may result in there being less stigma associated with discussing and seeking treatment for mental health problems. There may be more resources in The Netherlands for providing information on how to deal with mental health problems, the nature of psychiatric symptoms, and the location of their nearest provider. Alternatively, the larger proportion of those affected being treated may simply result from the more positive attitudes towards formal and informal interventions for emotional conditions in The Netherlands than in Ontario, the USA and Puerto Rico. These findings suggest several mechanisms that may maximize entrance into mental health treatment: screening for mental conditions by general practitioners; the possible benefits of having provider continuity in detecting mental health problems; and consumer education as a way to lessen stigma and promote more positive attitudes towards mental health care.

The general practitioners' gate-keeping role in The Netherlands may explain why general medicine provides such a large amount of the care for mental health conditions in this country. If the health care system requires that people with mental health problems see a general practitioner first, as in The Netherlands, their likelihood of receiving specialty care may be minimized when the general practitioner is capable of treating the most common mental disorders, such as anxiety and depression. This may be particularly true when general practitioners use treatment guidelines for mental disorders, as in The Netherlands, and believe that mental health care is also their responsibility.

The data in Table 7.5 compare use of the human services sector for mental health problems in the USA, Ontario, The Netherlands, and Puerto Rico. Excluding counselors and social workers from the definition of formal care may partly explain why the health services were used less in the USA than in the other three sites. Care provided by the human services sector was not included as a component of any formal care sector because of the dissimilarities in training and education of counselors, social workers and other professionals who provide mental health service to patients across the ICPE sites. Counselors and social workers appear to represent a low-cost option for public health facilities to provide mental health care to the poor in the USA. The cost-effectiveness of this provider option for treating mental illness is an area for future assessment; particularly in countries with a low psychiatrist-to-population ratio.

The increase in the prevalence of service use as the level of need increases (as measured by the number of CIDI/DSM-III-R psychiatric diagnoses) implies that there is a certain measure of rationality in the help-seeking process and in the allocation of resources to people with different levels of need in all four sites (Table 7.6). Mental health services research assumes that, given limited resources, services should be targeted to those with greater need. However, others may argue that services should be directed to those who will benefit most, or to those who, if not treated, will financially burden the society. This may well be an area for future empirical work by the ICPE.

When considering the high rates of use of formal services by people who do not have CIDI disorders in The Netherlands and Puerto Rico, we have no way of knowing whether those people have other disorders not presently assessed or whether they are simply seeking treatment for distress or life problems that are not associated with a psychiatric diagnosis (Greenley, 1984). It is worth remembering that the set of diagnoses included in the CIDI instrument is limited. The CIDI does not include an assessment of all Axis I disorders or an assessment of the Axis II personality disorders. Furthermore, the CIDI does not evaluate more culture-bound syndromes that might be the basis of help-seeking in some countries, such as 'ataque de nervios' in Puerto Rico (Guarnaccia, Rubio-Stipec & Canino, 1989).

Differences in access to care may result in varied rates of treatment for the more mentally ill between countries. For example, Ontario, Puerto Rico, and the USA treat a lower proportion of those with a chronic mental illness than is the case in The Netherlands, which appears to have better outreach services. A second possible explanation for the differences between countries in their rates of any formal care for those with more than one past-year CIDI/DSM-III-R diagnosis is that there are cultural differences in the expectations of treatment effectiveness. At present, the collected ICPE data provide no information on whether these lower rates of formal care in the USA reflect pessimism about the therapeutic effects of formal treatment. Thus, consumers' expectations of treatment effectiveness need to be assessed in surveys if we are to understand the differences in help-seeking behavior between countries.

In addition, the observation that, in the USA, those with most need (two or more CIDI/DSM-III-R diagnoses) have a low probability of receiving specialty care may emphasize problems in the referral pathways of the more seriously ill into the specialty sector (Lincoln & McGorry, 1995). More empirical studies are needed to identify efficient ways to reduce the extensive delays in gaining access to specialty treatment (Johnstone, Crow, Johnson & MacMillian, 1986) as well as how to prevent further problems from developing. Clearly, this is a critical issue for any system.

Consumers' inability to discriminate between treatments offered by providers (i.e., psychiatrists, psychologists, general medical providers, social workers, and counselors) may also help to explain why consumers are just as likely to choose general practitioners as specialty providers, even at the highest level of need in three of the four sites. Recent studies suggest that general medical providers are the most likely to treat substance-use and adjustment disorders, while psychiatrists provide a high proportion of the services to patients with depression, bipolar disorder, and schizophrenia (Olfson & Pincus, 1996). Symptomatology appears to influence the selection of providers. The consumers' ambiguous presentation of physical and psychiatric symptoms when they first discuss their complaint with their service provider and family members may also deter appropriate referral to specialty care (Beiser, Erickson, Fleming & Iacono, 1993; Helgason, 1990). We need to analyze more closely how providers and consumers weight different decision factors in this sorting process and how they choose the specialty sector of care in different countries (Table 7.7).

While the structure and financing of the service system have an impact on the provision of mental health care for those in need, they are only two of several factors affecting why people reach for, remain in, and benefit from, mental health treatment. We badly need a better grasp of what influences patients' readiness to engage in treatment, their expectations about the effectiveness of treatment, and the role of social networks in resistance and referral to treatment. We must also evaluate any coexisting stressful circumstances that can disrupt the patient's family or social life and may trigger the early detection and treatment of mental illness (Monroe, Simons & Thase, 1991; Phillips & Murrell, 1994). Attitudes at the community and country level that stereotype 'mental illness' and the 'benefits' of discussing mental health problems with informal and formal providers may also explain the observed differences in the patterns of care. Future studies should assess the therapeutic alliance between the client and the clinician, and compare their goals (see also Chapter 13).

Please note that although these data reveal that mental health services are more readily used in one country than in another, they shed no light on the quality of that care. The data of the ICPE surveys are constrained by the lack of information on the content and quality of the treatment offered. In this respect, future work by the ICPE services work group should assess not only utilization rates but the treatments offered, and this might lead us to better understand the differences or similarities in treatment outcomes across countries.

Issues to be considered when designing a core bank of questions on service use

Before designing a core bank of questions on service use, we should be clear why we are trying to find out this information. Questions for clinical populations on their use of mental health services tend to have a different focus compared with those aimed at providing information for the planning and allocation of services for the community. Clinical samples can better address issues of treatment pathways, description of services provided, factors influencing continuation and cessation of services, performance indicators of the mental health care system, and treatment match with patients' needs. Community samples can be more informative about referral pathways, how symptoms are discussed and conceptualized by informal sources (i.e., family, friends, co-workers) and lay providers (i.e., ministers, hot-lines, self-help groups), and the provider's response to the patient's consultation for a mental health problem. Thus, it is essential to identify what you need to know rather than simply ask questions on the data available.

We emphasize the importance of departing from questionnaires focused on a service model. When designing a core bank of questions about service use, one must consider more than just a description of service utilization. In the past, most epidemiological surveys in psychiatry have been simply a description of need, where need is defined by measures of symptoms, distress, symptom severity or diagnosis; or by measures of impairment or complications, e.g., suicide attempts or ideation. Later a description of service use was deemed necessary to describe the unmet need – had the person received help from the informal sector only, or from the specialty mental health sector, the general medical sector or from other human services agencies? Some studies noted the costs of treatment, others the person's usual source of care. This focus has recently been extended to describe the help-seeking process (Dew et al., 1988; Gallo, Marino, Ford & Anthony, 1995; Lin, Inui, Kleinman & Womack, 1982) and the pathways to care and continuity of services (Alegría, Pescosolido, Santos & Vera, 1997). Topics to be measured include how the problem is recognized as one needing treatment, the pathways to care and the factors (personal, community and service behaviors) that determine whether a person seeks and complies with treatment. Future developments should also encompass the patient, provider and system characteristics that are associated with a successful outcome (Chamberlain & Rapp, 1991; Leff, Mulkern, Lieberman & Raab, 1994). These might include evaluating the mental health status and level of functioning given the intervention; the clients' satisfaction with treatment and their perception of the effectiveness of care; and the outcome in terms of quality of life and the reduction in family burden. Depending on the study objectives, one has to choose the variables that will be measured to assess the need, service use, help-seeking behavior, and outcome of care to guide the instrument design.

Given the limited time available for asking questions (10 minutes versus 45 minutes), and the need to obtain specific information, it is important to select and prioritize the topics for assessment. There is no consensus on how best to define need, nor any established definitions of service sectors or an identified core set of concepts pertinent to help-seeking. The topics to be covered need to be reviewed for their relevance in all countries. Some areas in understanding help-seeking behavior are of common interest in many of these countries: the high rates of unmet need, attitudes that delay people from seeking help, and treatment pathways into specialty care.

A uniform phenomenon across countries is the high rate of unmet need. Some of the questions that need to be posed are: what types of psychiatric conditions are more likely to be identified and labeled by the person and his/her significant others as 'mental health problems'? How do people conceptualize their mental health problems and how distant are these conceptualizations from their psychiatric diagnoses? How are symptoms discussed within the context of lay and informal networks? How do these informal and lay networks delay or precipitate care being sought? What types of referral pathways sort persons with mental health illnesses into the different sectors of care – specialty, general medical, human services or informal?

Another topic of interest is the individual and family attitudes that operate as barriers to formal care. Frequently the reason for not seeking care among those that recognize a mental health problem is the decision to deal with the problem themselves – what can be called a self-reliant attitude. What characterizes people who are likely to present a self-reliant attitude when dealing with mental health problems? What strategies do self-reliant people use to successfully deal with their mental health problems? At what threshold does a self-reliant person, or their family, seek formal mental health care? What personal and community attitudes influence help-seeking behavior and the choice of providers of mental health care? What individual and family factors influence the entry into, and maintenance of, treatment?

Pathways into formal care are also of interest in most countries. What are the typical pathways for those who never reach specialty care? Does strong family support restrain people with mental illness from seeking care until it becomes an unbearable burden? What attracts consumers to lay networks for mental health services?

Relative to outcomes, some areas that need to be addressed are: personal and psychosocial factors that influence positive outcomes for mental health treatment; provider and system characteristics that reduce relapse; and family and social network determinants that promote and sustain patient recovery. These are only a few of the topics that future cross-national comparative pilot studies can flesh out.

The third issue is the type of questions, the format, and the optimal placement of the service-use questions in the survey. Greater attention should be paid to how best to obtain the information needed, taking as reference what respondents can answer. Sorting out what information is needed and whether the question will elicit it requires careful analysis. Mechanic (1992) contends that the ECA Studies overestimated the number of people in treatment for emotional problems with a primary care doctor. The ECA asked people, 'Did you tell a doctor about . . . emotional problems?'. Mechanic's (1992) argument is that many people mention to a doctor that they have been a little stressed out lately during their visit for a physical examination, and the doctor usually dismisses the comment without follow-up, treatment, or referral. If the 'yes' response to this question defines 'getting treatment', use of formal mental health services might be overestimated.

On the other hand, the 1990 NCS Study asked people, 'Did you go to a doctor for help with . . . emotional problems?'. Other researchers argued, correctly, that this might underestimate service use. Some people presumably end up getting treatment for emotional problems after going to a physician for some other reason (e.g., headaches). If this is the case, those respondents will not be counted. Based on this argument, some sustain that the NCS Study underestimates the number of people being treated by a family doctor for emotional problems.

Neither the ECA nor the NCS study questions ask anything about how the doctor responds. In both surveys we might learn that the person made four visits to a family doctor for emotional problems, but, for all we know, the patient could have gone to four different doctors and all four could have ignored the patient's complaint. Or maybe, all four told the patient to wait a while and see if the problem would go away on its own. In other words, we know about help-seeking behavior but not about treatment. It would be very useful to have a set of questions about the latter.

The placement of the service-use section within the complete questionnaire also demands serious attention. Respondents may be less willing to endorse service use after undergoing an hour of diagnostic assessment. The alternative of placing a service screener early in the questionnaire might maximize the opportunities for identifying service users. After the battery of diagnostic questions, a more detailed assessment of service and treatment could be collected for those who, either in the service screener or in the diagnostic battery, are identified as service users.

Attention to these three issues – the objectives and overall service model of each survey, the specific content or topics to be elucidated, and methodological issues such as question format and placement – is, in our judgement, critical to the development of international services research. We should also comment on two additional topics that are relevant to this field. First, it would be worthwhile to develop a common set of covariates (to be either measured directly or controlled for in the sample design) to allow greater cross-site comparability. The most obvious candidates are sociodemographic characteristics such as age, gender, and socioeconomic status, but there may well be others that are particularly relevant to services research. Second, the assessment of alternative services (e.g., nonwestern medicine) is a neglected area, but one which we feel is a necessary component of any core battery of service use designed for international comparisons. This is true for both developed and developing countries since there is abundant evidence that even in industrialized nations (Eisenberg et al., 1993), many people use these types of treatment either alone or as a supplement to Western medical services. Inclusion of questions about use of alternative services would create a more all-purpose battery and allow some potentially interesting comparisons; for example, between the outcomes of alternative versus formal health care.

The ICPE work group is currently developing a service module. We expect to design a series of questions to generate cross-national information that can elicit recommendations to facilitate treatment seeking and better treatment outcomes for people who need mental health services.

Organizational and market changes are generating unprecedented alterations in the delivery of health services not only in the USA but in many other countries (Kemper et al., 1996). International comparisons could play a central role in policy making by providing meaningful information about how system changes, such as managed care or universal access, impact service delivery for those in need. Health care delivery differs between countries because of availability of resources, culture, policy, history, and values in health and health promotion. Cross-national information about use of mental health services may assist the understanding of how the individual, his or her family, the social structure, and the context of the system impacts upon access, treatment and, ultimately, the outcomes of care (Jenkins, 1990). In addition, cross-national comparisons can highlight factors affecting access and potential outcomes that operate regardless of the country or type of health care system. Such findings can suggest areas that need more detailed research, as well as populations in greater need of outreach services and targeting.

By combining data on mental disorders and service utilization in several countries with diverse systems of care, the ICPE may be able to provide information and an analytical base to monitor the equity of service systems across countries for people with mental illness. Therefore, information at the cross-national level can enable comparisons of met and unmet need. Future comparisons could eventually elucidate how to improve outcomes of treatment from the mental health services, and how best to organize the service system to accomplish these outcomes.

Acknowledgements

This chapter was prepared with support from the International Consortium of Psychiatric Epidemiology (ICPE). The ICPE is a consortium sponsored by the World Health Organization (WHO), designed to foster cross-national comparative research on psychiatric disorders by bringing together researchers from around the world who have carried out general population surveys using the WHO Composite International Diagnostic Interview (CIDI). Information about participating ICPE sites and investigators and a bibliography of ICPE publications can be obtained from the ICPE home page at http://www.hcp.med.harvard.edu/icpe. Four surveys are used in the current report, the National Comorbidity Survey (NCS) (Ronald C. Kessler, Ph.D., principal investigator), the Puerto Rico Mental Health Utilisation (PRMHU) Project (Margarita Alegría, Ph.D., principal investigator), the Mental Health Supplement of the Ontario (Canada) Health Survey (David R. Offord, Ph.D., principal investigator) and The Netherlands Mental Health Survey and Incidence Study (NEMESIS) (Rob Bijl, Ph.D., principal investigator). Support for the NCS came from the US National Institute of Mental Health (Grants MH46376, MH52861, and MH49098) with supplemental support from the National Institute of Drug Abuse (through a supplement to MH46376) and the W.T. Grant Foundation (Grant 90135190). The Puerto Rico Mental Health Utilisation Project is supported by the US National Institute of Mental Health (Grant R01-MH42655). The Mental Health Supplement to the Ontario Health Survey is supported by the Ontario Ministries of Health and Community and Social Services through the Ontario Mental Health Foundation. The Netherlands Mental Health Survey and Incidence Study (NEMESIS) is being conducted by The Netherlands Institute of Mental Health and Addiction (Trimbos-Instituut) in Utrecht, and financially supported by The Netherlands Ministry of Health, Welfare and Sport (VWS), The National Institute of Public Health and Environment (RIVM), and The Medical Sciences Department of The Netherlands Organization for Scientific Research (NWO).

References

Alegría, M., Pescosolido, B.A., Santos, D. & Vera, M. (1997). Can we conceptualize and measure continuity of care in individual episodes? The case of mental health services in Puerto Rico. *Sociological Focus*, **30**, 113–29.

Beiser, M., Erickson, D., Fleming, J.A. & Iacono, W.G. (1993). Establishing the onset of psychotic illness. *American Journal of Psychiatry*, **150**, 1349–54.

Burke, J. & Jack, D. (1995). Mental health services research. In M.T. Tsuang, M. Tohen, & G.E.P. Zahner (eds.), *Textbook in Psychiatric Epidemiology*, pp. 199–209. New York: John Wiley and Sons.

Chamberlain, C. & Rapp, C.A. (1991). A decade of case management: a methodological review of outcome research. *Community Mental Health Journal*, **27**, 171–88.

Dew, M.A., Dunn, L.O., Bromet, E.J. & Schulberg, H.C. (1988). Factors affecting help-seeking during depression in a community sample. *Journal of Affective Disorders*, **14**, 223–34.

Eisenberg, D.M., Kessler, R.C., Roster, C., Norlock, F.E., Calkins, D.R. & Deleanco, T.L. (1993). Unconventional medicine in the United States. *New England Journal of Medicine*, **328**, 246–52.

Freeman, S.J.J. (1994). An overview of Canada's mental health system. In L.L. Bachrach, P. Goering, & D. Wasylenki (eds.), *Mental Health Care in Canada*. San Francisco: Josey-Bass.

Gallo, J.J., Marino, S., Ford, D. & Anthony, J.C. (1995). Filters on the pathway to mental health care. II: Sociodemographic factors. *Psychological Medicine*, **25**, 1149–60.

Gater, R. & Goldberg, D. (1991). Pathways to psychiatric care in South Manchester. *British Journal of Psychiatry*, **159**, 90–6.

Greenley, J.R. (1984). Social factors, mental illness, and psychiatric care: recent advances from a sociological perspective. *Hospital and Community Psychiatry*, **35**, 813–20.

Guarnaccia, P.J., Rubio-Stipec, M. & Canino, G. (1989). Ataques de nervios in the Puerto Rico Diagnostic Interview Schedule: the impact of cultural categories on psychiatric epidemiology. *Culture, Medicine & Psychiatry*, **13**, 275–95.

Health Department of the Commonwealth of Puerto Rico (1989). Manual de Estructura y Organización del Departamento de Salud. In *Health Department Structure and Organization Manual*, pp. 51-63. San Juan: Departamento de Salud.

Helgason, L. (1990). Twenty years' follow-up of first psychiatric presentation for schizophrenia: what could have been prevented? *Acta Psychiatrica Scandinavica*, **81**, 231–5.

Jenkins, R. (1990). Towards a system of outcome indicators for mental health care. *British Journal of Psychiatry*, **157**, 500–14.

Johnstone, E.C., Crow, T.J., Johnson, A.L. & MacMillan, J.F. (1986). The Northwick study of first episodes of schizophrenia. I: Presentation of the illness and problems relating to admission. *British Journal of Psychiatry*, **148**, 115–20.

Kemper, P., Blumenthal, D., Corrigan, J.M., Cunningham, P.J., Felt, S.M., Grossman, J.M., Kohn, L.T., Metcalf, C.E., St. Peter, R.F., Strouse, R.C. & Ginsburg, P.B. (1996). The design of the community tracking study: a longitudinal study of health system change and its effects on people. *Inquiry*, 33, 195–206.

Kessler, R.C., McGonagle, K.A., Zhao, S., Nelson, C.B., Hughes, M., Eshleman, S., Wittchen, H-U. & Kendler, K.S. (1994). Lifetime and twelve month prevalence of DSM-III-R psychiatric disorders in the United States. *Archives of General Psychiatry*, 51, 8–19.

Leff, H.S., Mulkern, V.M., Lieberman, M. & Raab, B. (1994). A model guided approach to measuring access, adequacy, and appropriateness in mental health programs. *Administration and Policy in Mental Health*, 21, 141–60.

Lehman, A. (1987). Capitation payment and mental health care: a review of the opportunities and risks. *Hospital and Community Psychiatry*, 38, 31–3.

Lin, K.M., Inui, T.S., Kleinman, A.M. & Womack, W.M. (1982). Sociocultural determinants of the help-seeking behavior of patients with mental illness. *Journal of Nervous and Mental Disease*, 170, 79–85.

Lincoln, C.V. & McGorry, P. (1995). Who cares? Pathways to psychiatric care for young people experiencing a first episode of psychosis. *Psychiatric Services*, 46, 1166–71.

Maarse, H., Mur-Veeman, I. & Spreeuwenberg, C. (1997). The reform of hospital care in the Netherlands. *Medical Care*, 35, OS26–OS39.

Mechanic, D. (1992). Treating mental illness: generalist versus specialist. *Health Affairs*, 9, 61–75.

Monroe, S.M., Simons, A.D. & Thase, M.E. (1991). Onset of depression and time to treatment entry: roles of life stress. *Journal of Consulting and Clinical Psychology*, 59, 566–73.

Olfson, M. & Pincus, H.A. (1996). Outpatient mental health care in nonhospital settings: distribution of patients across provider groups. *American Journal of Psychiatry*, 153, 1353–6.

Ontario Ministry of Health (1993). *Putting people first: the reform of mental health services in Ontario*. Toronto: Queen's Printer for Ontario.

Phillips, M.A. & Murrell, S.A. (1994). Impact of psychological and physical health, stressful events, and social support on subsequent mental health help seeking among older adults. *Journal of Consulting and Clinical Psychology*, 62, 270–5.

Regier, D.A., Narrow, W.E., Rae, D.S., Manderscheid, R.W., Locke, R.Z. & Goodwin, F.K. (1993). The de facto US mental and addictive disorders service system: epidemiologic catchment area prospective 1-year prevalence rates of disorders and services. *Archives of General Psychiatry*, 50, 85–94.

Rochefort, D.A. (1992). More lessons, of a different kind: Canadian mental health policy in comparative perspective. *Hospital and Community Psychiatry*, 43, 1083–90.

Wittchen, H.-U. (1994). Reliability and validity studies of the WHO-Composite International Diagnostic Interview (CIDI): a critical review. *Journal of Psychiatric Research*, 28, 57–84.

Wittchen, H.-U., Kessler, R.C., Zhao, S. & Abelson, J. (1995). Reliability and clinical validity of UM-CIDI DSM-III-R generalized anxiety disorder. *Journal of Psychiatric Research*, 29, 95–110.

World Health Organization (1990). *Composite International Diagnostic Interview* (CIDI Version 1.0). Geneva, Switzerland: World Health Organization.

8

The challenges of meeting the unmet need for treatment: economic perspectives

Agnes Rupp and Helen Lapsley

Introduction

One of the greatest challenges facing mental health care today is its financing. With increasing emphasis being placed on controlling costs in both publicly and privately financed health insurance systems, mental health providers need to develop informed policy on priority setting for financing mental health care and research. Research on the management of mental and addictive disorders to date has been conducted separately in various scientific disciplines such as epidemiology, clinical sciences, economics, and public health. There is a need to integrate these different research areas and, although this chapter is focused on economic perspectives, it also tries to demonstrate how researchers from different disciplines can work together to assist decision makers to formulate mental health policy. The central task for researchers who deal with the unmet need for treatment is to find efficient and equitable delivery alternatives and ways to finance a variety of mental health services in a changing mental health care system.

The economist researcher faces a number of challenges in attempting to meet the unmet need for treatment. These include:

- Defining the need for treatment
- Measuring need
- Identifying unmet need
- Establishing economic criteria for treatment
- Evaluating the economic effectiveness of treatment
- Estimating the cost of not treating treatable illnesses
- Reducing financial barriers to treatment

These challenges include methodological issues relating to definitions, measurement, and estimation techniques as well as conceptual issues involving the formulation of mental health policy and the establishment of priorities based on scientific knowledge.

Need and unmet need

Defining the need for treatment is the first requirement, which can be objectively addressed with epidemiological and utilization data on a population-wide basis. In developed countries, it is apparent that there is both under- and overutilization of mental health services. Underutilization is a relatively straightforward measure, which can be described as the mismatch between the epidemiological measures of a population with mental illness and the proportion of that population who receive appropriate treatment. This proportion is the basic measure of unmet need. Of course, it does not assume that all who receive treatment are treated appropriately, or even effectively.

Overutilization in the same population also occurs. In an economic sense, overutilization consists of the provision of services to people:

1. Not in need of treatment
2. Not in need of the type of treatment provided
3. Not in need of the intensity of treatment provided
4. With little chance of treatment being effective

The provision of such services inevitably reduces the availability of resources for those in need, in an area of health where there is significant unmet treatment needs, and also very few resources available for prevention. Unmet need may be the result of underprovision of mental health services, lack of financial access to services, lack of geographical access to services, or lack of knowledge of the existence of appropriate services.

Establishing economic criteria for treatment

From the economic point of view, the purpose of treating mental disorders is to reduce the economic burden of illness on the individual, the family, the community, and on society as a whole. The economic burden of a disorder is associated with morbidity, disability, and premature death. These have a negative impact on labor, a valuable economic resource, on economic capacity because of time spent away from work or a loss of effectiveness at work, and in other productive activities in the household and at school. Illness therefore creates an undeniable economic burden which is evident in the health sector, the welfare sector, and in prisons.

A number of methods have been developed by economists to measure the economic burden associated with the mortality and morbidity of illness. The most widely known of these methods are:

1. The human capital approach: developed by Mushkin (1962), Hodgkin &

Meiers (1982), and Rice (1966). This is the most widely used methodology to date.

2. The willingness to pay approach: developed by Schelling (1968) and Mishan (1971).

3. Quality-adjusted life years (QALYs): the application of this approach in the mental health field is widespread in schizophrenia treatment outcome research (Lehman, Thompson, Dixon & Scott, 1995).

4. Disability-adjusted life years (DALYs): developed by the World Bank, (Murray & Lopez, 1996).

Table 8.1 provides a comparison of these different approaches in measuring economic burden among seven dimensions. In general, according to the economic perspective, when treatment approaches with favorable cost-benefit, cost-effectiveness or cost-utility ratios are not utilized or are underutilized in mental health policy and practice, the economic burden imposed on the individual and on society is needlessly and unjustifiably high. This leads to another challenge in meeting the unmet need for treatment: how to evaluate the economic effectiveness of various treatment approaches and alternatives.

Evaluating the economic effectiveness of treatment

The economic literature has developed three basic methodologies which are used to evaluate the effectiveness of various treatment modalities. To date, Drummond, Stoddart & Torrance (1987) have provided one of the best descriptions of the three major methods of economic evaluation health care interventions. These are:

- Cost-benefit analysis: this evaluation compares those costs and benefits of a health care intervention that can be easily expressed in monetary terms. In most cost-benefit analyses the implicit 'do-nothing' alternative has some costs and benefits attached to it as well.
- Cost-effectiveness analysis: in this evaluation method, economic costs are related to a single, common effect of the intervention, the magnitude of which may differ among the alternative interventions.
- Cost-utility analysis: in this method the results of the economic evaluation of health care interventions are expressed in terms of the cost per QALY or DALY gained by undertaking one intervention instead of another.

Table 8.2 provides further information about these methods by comparing them in terms of three dimensions: measurement of costs, measurement of outcome, and effect of health care intervention.

Among policy makers and clinicians it is often believed that there are no well-designed economic evaluation studies in the mental health field which

Table 8.1. Comparison of alternative approaches in estimating the economic burden of mortality and morbidity

Approaches	Common denominator[a]	Assumptions[b]	Data requirements[c]	Weights used[d]	Equity/Efficiency[e]	Psycho-social[f]	Individual/Society[g]
Human capital	Monetary value	Productivity	Prevalence	Wages, employment	Efficiency	No	Population
Willingness to pay	Monetary value	Welfare/Well-being	Prevalence	Revealed preference/contingent preference	Efficiency	Yes	Individual
Quality-adjusted life years (QALYs)	Time (years)	Positive utility/quality of life	Prevalence/incidence	Delphi/expert assignment	Equity	Yes	Individual
Disability-adjusted life years (DALYs)	Time (years)	Negative utility/quality of life	Prevalence/incidence/duration/severity	Delphi/expert assignment	Equity	Yes	Individual/Population

[a] Indicates the unit of measurement.

[b] Assumptions will reflect different underlying philosophies and frameworks. The human capital approach is rooted in labor economics while the willingness to pay approach was developed within the framework of welfare economics. The QALYs and the DALYs were developed as global burden of disease measures based on various disciplines.

[c] Mostly epidemiological data requirements. Without epidemiological data the economic burden of an illness cannot be assessed.

[d] Weights used in measuring the burden of various disorders: researchers have been using different measures including lost wages due to illness, individual preferences for treating or not treating an illness and expert judgements on the basis of the Delphi method.

[e] This is an underlying economic value judgement about whether reducing the economic burden should focus primarily on efficiency or whether emphasis should be placed on equity issues for allocating scarce resources according to the burden of the illness.

[f] These may or may not be measured within a given approach.

[g] This describes the level of measurement/analysis, which can be the individual and/or the entire society.

Table 8.2. Basic types of economic evaluation of health care interventions

Type of analysis	Valuation of costs	Valuation of outcomes	Effects of interventions
Cost-benefit analysis	Monetary	Monetary	Single or multiple effects not necessarily the same for both alternatives, and same effects may be achieved to different degrees by the alternatives.
Cost-effectiveness analysis	Monetary	Natural medical units	Single effect of interest, same for both alternatives, but achieved to different degrees.
Cost-utility analysis	Monetary	QALYs, DALYs	Single or multiple effects, not necessarily the same for both alternatives, and same effects may be achieved to different degrees by the alternatives.

Source: Drummond, Stoddart & Torrance, 1987.

could aid decisions on resource allocation issues. A literature summary by Frank (1993) indicates that several well-designed studies have been conducted which have indicated the positive economic outcome of certain treatment approaches. They include:

Psychotropic medications
- Lithium (Reifman & Wyatt, 1980)
- Imipramine (Kamlet, 1992)
- Clozapine (Meltzer et al., 1993; Revicki, Luce, Weschler, Brown & Adler, 1990)
- Risperidone (Albright et al., 1996)

Therapies and treatment settings
- Partial hospitalization (Creed et al., 1990; Dickey et al., 1989)
- Psychotherapy (Kamlet, 1992; Miller & Magruder, in press)
- Vocational rehabilitation (Bond, 1992; Drake et al., 1994)
- Family management (Cardin, McGill & Falloon, 1985)

Treatment packages
- Program of assertive community treatment (Jerrell & Hu, 1989; Knapp et al., 1994)

The list has been selectively updated by studies on the cost-effectiveness of various new pharmacotherapies and other technological advancements for mental disorders, which post date Frank's paper. The major issue, according to Frank, is not the lack of economic evaluation studies but the lack of financial incentives to apply these new medical technologies in clinical practice. Evers, Van Wijk & Ament (1997), however, believe that there are still few good full economic evaluations of mental health care.

While Frank approaches the issue theoretically, the problem can be illustrated with a concrete example. During the 1980s, the total budget of the US public mental health system, which provides mental health care for the poor without private health insurance and the mentally disabled, did not increase after adjusting for inflation. The reaction of policy makers was that the available resources should be concentrated on the most severely ill. This was a priority decision. The decision, however, was one-sided: it did not take into consideration the new methodologies developed for treating the severely mentally ill, which were cost-effective. In certain cases they do not save economic resources but improve the clinical outcome of treatment, while in other cases positive economic savings can be demonstrated. Not introducing financial incentives to use economically effective treatment approaches led to a situation where the scarce public resources were spent inefficiently on one segment of the mentally ill population, while another segment of the population did not receive treatment. The introduction of cost-effective treatment approaches for the priority group could have led to savings in resources spent on this group, and to the use of resources for the treatment of those whose need was not met under the new policy.

A situation had developed where the allocation of scarce resources was neither efficient nor equitable, one of the worst possible scenarios in making resource allocation decisions. The economics of public finance usually assumes that there is a trade-off between equity and efficiency (Stiglitz, 1988); however, under certain circumstances suboptimal situations may develop without trade-offs. 'Fixing' these situations from a social and economic perspective is one of the most difficult tasks for health care expenditure policy.

Estimating the cost of not treating cost effectively treatable illnesses

If treatment approaches with favorable cost-benefit, cost-effectiveness and cost-utility ratios are underused, the economic burden imposed by the illness on the individual and on society is needlessly and unjustifiably high. This is illustrated by Rupp (1995), who focused on the economic consequences of not treating depression. This case study illustrates the major issues that need to be considered when conducting an analysis of the cost of not treating treatable illnesses; in other words, not meeting the unmet need for mental health treatment for certain segments of the population. The three major components of the methodology are summarized below.

1.   Estimating the incremental medical costs of treating previously untreated people
- the number and proportion of people with untreated disorders
- the diagnoses and severity of their disorders
- the treatment cost of high, moderate and low users
- reducing technical and fiscal inefficiencies in treatment
- the reduction in the use and cost of general medical services
- the cost of complications from untreated cases
- the proportion of treatment-resistant cases
- the help-seeking behavior of untreated people

2. Estimating the changes in costs related to mortality and morbidity
- reduction in suicide rate and associated life-time earning loss
- reduction in productivity loss due to: return to the labor force; reduction in dependence on public assistance; reduction in the disability period of the illness; reduction in absenteeism from the workplace; reduction in labor turnover rate; improved productivity level at the workplace, home and school; higher earning levels than for the nontreated population.
- increase in productivity loss due to negative side-effects of treatment

3. Estimating the cost-benefit ratio

- comparing the incremental costs of treatment with the monetary value of the reduction in lost productivity
- calculating the net loss due to untreated cases
- calculating the net economic return on a one-dollar investment in treating untreated people

It is clear from the items considered that in order for researchers to estimate the incremental mental health care costs of untreated cases, they must consider information on:

- epidemiological data (e.g., defining the number and severity of untreated cases)
- clinical data (e.g., proportion of treatment-resistant cases, reduction in the use and cost of general medical services (medical cost-offset), as well as complications from nontreatment)
- services research data (e.g., understanding help-seeking behavior and measuring the proportion of cases where patients will not seek help)
- economic data (estimating the technical and fiscal inefficiencies of treatment and the magnitude of their possible reduction, treatment-cost data and costing techniques). In the cited depression paper (Rupp, 1995), it was estimated that the incremental cost of treating untreated cases would be approximately US$4.2 billion (in 1985), an approximately 1% increase in total health care expenditure in the USA

Estimating the reduction of productivity loss related to morbidity and mortality is primarily the task of an economist, using economic values and measures for evaluation. Cost of illness studies can serve as a useful source for relevant data. The case study described by Rupp (1995) utilized the cost of depression studies conducted by Rice & Miller (1993), Stoudemire, Frank, Hedemark, Kamlet & Blazer (1986), and Greenberg, Stiglin, Finkelstein & Berndt (1993). According to Rupp's estimates, the total mortality- and morbidity-related productivity loss is $8.3 billion, while the net productivity loss if treatment is not provided is approximately $4 billion. Thus the net economic cost of not treating depression is approximately $4 billion lost to the US economy if treatable affective disorders remain untreated. Since the cost-benefit ratio is positive, every dollar spent on treating untreated affective disorder cases yields one dollar in the net economic return on employment earnings. The 'do-nothing' mental health policy in this situation results in economic losses.

The above calculations were based on aggregate or cost per capita average data. No individual data were available on epidemiological risk factors, clinical interventions, or the cost of treatment and reduced productivity. Collecting all of these data at the individual level is not impossible in large-scale epidemiological surveys. The ECA Study (Robins & Regier, 1991), the National Comorbidity Survey (Kessler et al., 1994), and the planned child mental health services research study (Hoagwood & Rupp, 1995), all took a significant step forward in collecting epidemiological, clinical and cost/ financing data within the framework of the same survey. Individual level data can also provide an opportunity for applying more sophisticated multivariate econometric analyses when conducting evaluation studies.

The findings of the cost-benefit study of nontreatment of treatable depression generate a special emphasis on the economics of secondary prevention. Not intervening with cost-effective treatment methods if they are available causes a greater financial loss to the economy than any saving in terms of incremental medical costs.

Financial barriers to treatment

From both individual and societal perspectives, financing and payment mechanisms have significant, sometimes overwhelming, effects on access to treatment. Methods of payment for medical practitioners, whether salaried, fee-for-service, capitation, or managed care, have impacts on the amount and types of services delivered to people with mental illness (Feldstein, 1993). Publicly provided services, while free at the point of delivery, are inevitably budget-capped, and implicitly rationed through waiting lists and waiting times for nonurgent treatment. At the same time, private health insurance schemes which are open-ended may result in some overutilization, unless clinical treatment guidelines are observed and treatment outcomes monitored. Particularly in the treatment of mental illness, the absence of a clear definition of the expected outcomes from episodes of care can result in extensive utilization of mental health services without concomitant effectiveness.

It has already been identified that untreated or undertreated mental illness results in a number of burdens to society, including publicly borne costs which may often be much greater than the initial costs of treatment. Underfunded public services can mean lack of access to appropriate care until the episode of illness becomes acute, and ultimately incurs much greater costs than early intervention. While mental health services continue to 'compete' with other acute health services for public funding, the need for good, rigorous economic evaluations of the effectiveness of mental health treatments cannot be overemphasized.

The type of funding, for example fee-for-service for medical practitioners, is an important determinant of the use of other health professionals in an episode of care, and can influence the cost-effectiveness of treatment. Inevitably, if a health professional is paid only for the direct care which he/she provides, there will be a financial disincentive to involve other, perhaps more appropriate professionals in the treatment. This is of course relevant for all health services, but the extent of unmet need in mental health emphasizes the importance of the efficient use of resources in the treatment of the mentally ill.

Cost comparisons and cost-effectiveness studies in relation to location of care have been undertaken, but more rigorous and complete ones are still required. Where funding is directly related to the type of treatment and location of care, the most cost-effective care environment may not be selected. Nonhospital care may be associated with different budgets and different responsibilities, thus financing mechanisms may inadvertently create structural barriers to the selection of the most appropriate and cost-effective care.

The impact of managed care on utilization and costs

Financing and delivery of mental health care are undergoing rapid change in the USA. Of particular importance are shifts in the health care system from an unmanaged fee-for-service basis to increased use of managed care. Managed care was almost entirely absent from the US mental health care system in the 1970s. Today the managed behavioral health care industry is estimated to cover approximately 170 million Americans for their mental health care. Managed care includes various organizational arrangements: Health Maintenance Organizations, Preferred Provider Organizations, and fee-for-service plans with managed behavioral health care contracts. It includes new financing mechanisms such as capitation and risk-sharing contracts with incentives to reduce the rate of increase or the absolute amount of mental health care and associated mental health care costs. Management techniques to reduce costs include imposing hospital preauthorization requirements, requiring concurrent utilization review, denying payment for research-related experimental care, instituting case management for high utilizers and substituting low-cost providers for high-cost providers.

To date, there have been several empirical studies conducted to estimate the impact of managed care on the utilization and cost of mental health services. These studies (e.g., Callahan, Shepard, Beinecke, Larson & Cavanaugh, 1995; Sturm, 1997; Stoner, Manning, Christianson, Gray & Marriott, 1997) all indicate that managed behavioral health care reduces the utilization and cost of inpatient services, and in general results in large cost savings. These radical changes in mental health service-use patterns and costs require that economists update the data used in econometric models of forecasting mental health care costs as well as those used in microsimulation models intended to estimate the cost of new programs or policies.

Currently in the USA, implementing mental health insurance parity in the private sector is the focus of mental health policy formulation. The term mental health insurance parity refers to insurance coverage for mental health services that is subject to the same benefits and restrictions as coverage for other health services. Lack of mental health insurance parity is not unique to private health insurance, this phenomenon exists in some national health insurance policies as well. Actuaries of private and public insurance policies have been concerned that mental health insurance parity may result in potentially high financial costs. As the National Advisory Mental Health Council (1997) report points out, these concerns are based on outmoded economic and actuarial models that do not consider the impact of managed care on reducing the utilization and costs of mental health services. The introduction of managed care in the USA raises the possibility of implementing mental health insurance parity and therefore reducing one of the major financial barriers to access to mental health care.

Summary

Two realities have provided a compelling economic perspective from which to write about how to meet the unmet need for treatment. First, the availability of new mental health interventions exceed our societal ability to pay for them. Second, decision-making rules are becoming more complex, guiding policy makers toward those interventions that are likely to yield the most benefit for the mentally ill population. Cost-benefit, cost-effectiveness, and cost-utility analyses are crucial to decisions about resource allocation in medical care. Whether policy makers choose explicit or implicit methods of reallocating financial resources among various subgroups of the mentally ill population, economic evaluation will provide critical information about the value of alternative investments in mental health service delivery.

References

Albright, P.S., Livingstone, S., Keegan, D.L., Ingham, M., Shrikhande, S. & Le Lorier, J. (1996). Reduction of healthcare resource utilisation and costs following the use of risperidone for patients with schizophrenia previously treated with standard antipsychotic therapy. *Clinical Drug Investigation*, 11, 289–99.

Bond, G.R. (1992). Vocational rehabilitation. In R.P. Liberman (ed.), *Handbook of Psychiatric Rehabilitation*, pp. 244–63. New York: Macmillan Press.

Callahan, J., Shepard, D., Beinecke, R., Larson, M.J. & Cavanaugh, D. (1995). Mental health/substance abuse treatment in managed care: the Massachusetts medicaid experience. *Health Affairs*, 14, 173–84.

Cardin, B., McGill, C.W. & Falloon, I.R.H. (1985). An economic analysis: costs, benefits and effectiveness. In I.R.H. Falloon (ed.), *Family Management of Schizo-phrenia – A Study of Clinical, Social, Family and Economic Benefits*, pp. 115–23. Baltimore, MD: Johns Hopkins University Press.

Creed, F., Balck, D., Anthony, P., Osborn, M., Thomas, P. & Tomenson, B. (1990). Randomized controlled trial of day patient versus inpatient psychiatric treatment. *British Medical Journal*, **300**, 1033–7.

Dickey, B., Binner, P.R., Leff, S., Uyeda, M.K., Schlesinger, M.J. & Gudeman, J.E. (1989). Containing mental health treatment costs through program design: a Massachusetts study. *American Journal of Public Health*, **79**, 863–7.

Drake, R.E., Becker, D.R., Biesanz, J.C., Torrey, W.C., McHugo, G.J. & Wyzik, P.F. (1994). Rehabilitative day treatment vs supported employment: I. Vocational outcomes. *Community Mental Health Journal*, **30**, 519–32.

Drummond, M.F., Stoddart, G.L. & Torrance, G.W. (1987). *Methods for the Economic Evaluation of Health Care Programmes*. New York: Oxford Medical Publications.

Evers, S.M., Van Wijk, A.S. & Ament, A.J. (1997). Economic evaluation of mental health interventions. A review. *Health Economics*, **6**, 161–77.

Feldstein, P.J. (1993). *Health Care Economics* (4th edition). New York: John Wiley.

Frank, R.G. (1993). Cost-benefit evaluations in mental health: implications for financing policy. In T.W. Hu & A. Rupp (eds.) *Research on the Economic of Mental Health*. Volume 14 in R.M. Scheffier & L.F. Rossiter (eds.) *Advances in Health Economics and Health Services Research*. JAI Press.

Greenberg, P.E., Stiglin, L.E., Finkelstein, S.N. & Berndt, E.R (1993). The economic burden of depression in 1990. *Journal of Clinical Psychiatry*, **54**, 405–18.

Hoagwood, K. & Rupp, A. (1995). Mental health service needs, use and costs for children and adolescents with mental disorders and their families: preliminary evidence. *Psychiatric Times*, March, 62–3.

Hodgkin, T.A. & Meiers, M. (1982). Cost of illness methodology: a guide to current practices. *Milbank Memorial Fund Quarterly*, **60**, 429–62.

Jerrell, J. & Hu, T.W. (1989). Cost-effectiveness of intensive clinical and case management compared with an existing system of care. *Inquiry*, **26**, 224–34.

Kamlet, M.S. (1992). Cost-utility analysis of maintenance treatment for recurrent depression: a theoretical framework and numerical illustration. In R.G. Frank & W.G. Manning (eds.), *Economics and Mental Health*, pp. 267–91. Baltimore, MD: Johns Hopkins University Press.

Kessler, R.C., McGonagle, K.A., Zhao, S., Nelson, C.B., Hughes, M., Eshleman, S., Wittchen, H-U. & Kendler, K.S. (1994). Lifetime and twelve month prevalence of DSM-III-R psychiatric disorders in the United States. *Archives of General Psychiatry*, **51**, 8–19.

Knapp, M., Beecham, J., Koutsogorgopoulou, V., Hallam, A., Fenyo, A., Marks, I.M., Connolly, J., Audini, B. & Muijen, M. (1994). Service use and costs of home-based vs hospital-based care for people with serious mental illness. *British Journal of Psychiatry*, **165**, 195–203.

Lehman, A.F., Thompson, J.W., Dixon, L.B. & Scott, J.E. (1995). Schizophrenia: treatment outcomes research, editor's introduction. *Schizophrenia Bulletin*, **21**, 561–6.

Meltzer, H.Y., Cola, P., Way, L., Thompson, P.A., Bastani, B., Davies, M.A. & Snitz, B.

(1993). Cost-effectiveness of clozapine in neuroleptic resistant schizophrenia. *American Journal of Psychiatry*, **150**, 1630–8.

Miller, N. & Magruder, K. (1999). *The Cost Effectiveness of Psychotherapy* (in press). London: John Wiley and Sons.

Mishan, E.J. (1971). Evaluation of life and limb: a theoretical approach. *Journal of Political Economy*, **79**, 687–705.

Murray, C.J.L. & Lopez, A.D. (eds.) (1996). *The Global Burden of Disease: a Comprehensive Assessment of Mortality and Disability from Diseases, Injuries, and Risk Factors in 1990 and Projected to 2020*. Cambridge, MA: Harvard University Press.

Mushkin, S.J. (1962). Health as an investment. *Journal of Political Economy*, **70**, 129–57.

National Advisory Mental Health Council (1997). *Parity Coverage of Mental Health Services in an Era of Managed Care*. Interim Report to Congress by NIH, April.

Reifman, A. & Wyatt, J. (1980). Lithium: brake in the rising cost of mental illness. *Archives of General Psychiatry*, **37**, 385–8.

Revicki, D., Luce, B.R., Weschler, J.M., Brown, R.E. & Adler, M.A. (1990). Cost-effectiveness of clozapine for treatment-resistant schizophrenic patients. *Hospital and Community Psychiatry*, **41**, 850–4.

Rice, D.P. (1966). Estimating the cost of illness. *Health Economics Series*, No. 6, DHEW Publication No. (PHS) 947-6. Rockville, MD: Department of Health, Education and Welfare.

Rice, D.P. & Miller, L.D. (1993). The economic burden of affective disorders. In T.W. Hu & A. Rupp (eds.) *Research on the Economics of Mental Health*. Volume 14 in R.M. Scheffier & L.F. Rossiter (eds.) *Advances in Health Economics and Health Services Research*. JAI Press.

Robins, L.N. & Regier, D.A. (eds.) (1991). *Psychiatric Disorders in America*. New York: The Free Press.

Rupp, A (1995). The economic consequences of not treating depression. *British Journal of Psychiatry*, **166** [Suppl. 27], 29–33.

Schelling, T.C. (1968). The life you save may be your own. In S.B. Chase (ed.), *Problems in Public Expenditure Analysis*, pp. 127–76. Washington, D.C.: The Brookings Institution.

Stiglitz, J.E. (1988). *Economics of the Public Sector* (2nd edition). New York: WW Norton and Company.

Stoner, T., Manning, W., Christianson, J., Gray, D.Z. & Marriott, S. (1997). Expenditures for mental health services in the Utah prepaid mental health plan. *Health Care Financing Review*, **18**, 73–94.

Stoudemire, A., Frank, R., Hedemark, N., Kamlet, M. & Blazer, D. (1986). The economic burden of depression. *General Hospital Psychiatry*, **8**, 387–94.

Sturm, R. (1997). How expensive is unlimited health care coverage under managed care? *Journal of the American Medical Association*, **278**, 18, 1533–7.

9

Unmet need for prevention

Beverley Raphael

Preventive as compared to treatment interventions should be considered in terms of the evidence of their effectiveness in achieving relevant outcomes. Barriers to a preventive approach are examined. Two main types of syndrome are thought to be suitable for preventive approaches. The first are the externalizing, aggressive, conduct, antisocial behavioral syndromes, while the second are the internalizing, withdrawing, depressive/anxiety syndromes. These syndromal patterns tend to continue throughout childhood, adolescence and into adult life, although there is overlap and comorbidity in many instances. Generic and specific risk and protective factors are examined as a background to preventive approaches.

Evidence shows that intervening with preventive measures in the prenatal, early infancy, preschool and school years reduces the severity of externalizing syndromes. Similarly, evidence shows that the severity of depressive/internalizing syndromes associated with postnatal depression and parental affective disorders can be reduced by preventive measures taken in school-based interventions, early intervention programs, and programs for children and adolescents encountering stressful life experiences. The evidence for the effectiveness of preventive as compared to treatment interventions is substantial and encompasses universal, selective and indicated interventions that have been tested in controlled trials. The potential gains from the systematic implementation of such interventions are substantial.

There is increasing recognition of the growing levels of morbidity associated with mental disorders and their major impact on public health, particularly when measured in terms of disability and the associated human and economic costs. A significant number of publications, research programs and health program initiatives demonstrate the scientific basis for prevention in the mental health field. Despite this, there is a reluctance to implement prevention programs, perhaps for the reasons suggested by Eisenberg (1995), i.e., they are often poorly understood and their benefits are seen as being uncertain or in the distant future. There has been little political commitment to these programs in the field of mental health, but awareness of the opportunities for prevention are growing. Mental health professionals who are trained in individual case-work may be reluctant to acknowledge the potential of prevention.

Just as the levels of morbidity may be investigated as representing levels of unmet need for treatment, the same process may reveal unmet needs for prevention. Preventive and treatment interventions operate at different stages of the vulnerability/prodrome/illness/recovery spectrum, and should be implemented according to the best available evidence as to what achieves the most favorable outcomes possible. In this context it is appropriate to consider the relative benefits of preventive as compared to treatment interventions, and the potential contribution of each.

Although there are a number of conditions or risk factors that could be considered when discussing the unmet need for preventive interventions, there are two major dimensions of morbidity that are particularly significant. These are conduct, antisocial, aggressive and violent behavioral syndromes or disorders, and internalizing, depressive, anxiety, withdrawal syndromes or disorders. These syndromes may coexist, or even change along the developmental trajectory.

Just as there is evidence that generic risk factors (see following paragraph) may increase susceptibility to a disease, there is also evidence that many factors interact in a 'causal chain', resulting in a person becoming unwell. In each instance further research is needed to clarify the nature of these risk factors and their relative contributions to morbidity, as well as the potential buffering provided by protective factors. The latter include having a warm, caring relationship with at least one parent; a positive, easy temperament; a good relationship with a peer or peers; experience of achievement and success during adolescence; a positive experience of school (Mrazek & Haggerty, 1994).

The generic risk factors that contribute to morbidity in childhood and adolescence include severe parental discord; coercive, cold and affectionless parental styles; parental mental illness or alcoholism (often maternal depression, paternal alcoholism or antisocial disorders), and adverse life events. A low birth weight and birth complications contribute generally to vulnerability, as does a shy, difficult or aggressive temperament. A low IQ may also contribute to general vulnerability. Mrazek & Haggerty (1994, p.182) emphasize the 'value in clarifying the role of those risk factors that appear to be common to many mental disorders, especially in view of the frequent comorbidity of these disorders'.

Community and social factors can also contribute generically; for instance, social disadvantage, poverty, poor housing, high level of community disorganization, and poor community institutions, especially schools. The converse of these can act as buffering or protective influences.

The relevance of genetic influences has also been highlighted in recent reviews (Rutter, 1997a,b). These findings emphasize how genetic factors contribute to a person's vulnerability to psychiatric disorders, and the interplay between nature and nurture. Rutter (1995) considers that genetic factors are important in all forms of psychopathology. It is also likely that genetic factors play a progressively greater role as children mature through adolescence to adulthood. Genetic research has shown the complexity of environmental influences, but also the opportunities for prevention if effective interventions can modify them.

Finally, preventive interventions can be focused on those symptoms or syndromes that start in childhood and persist into adulthood. Achenbach, Howell, McConaughty & Stranger (1995), using a study method based on syndromes (defined by parent, teacher and self ratings), showed the stability over time of five empirically based groups of symptoms: internalizing syndromes (withdrawn/anxious/depressed); externalizing syndromes (aggressive, oppositional, conduct, antisocial); attention problems; thought problems; and social problems. These persist through adolescence to adulthood, with adolescent anxious/depressed and aggressive behavior syndromes accounting for most of the variance in the corresponding adult syndromes. The studies also showed that patterns are influenced by gender, but that there may be considerable fluctuation and overlap. The two sets of syndromes are now considered in terms of a preventive approach.

Conduct, oppositional, antisocial, and aggressive syndromal patterns

It is difficult to find clear estimates of the burden and direct and indirect costs of these syndromes, but there is a great deal to suggest that they are substantial. For example, there are descriptions of the effects of oppositional and aggressive behavior on the child's development and family relationships; the cost of juvenile and adult justice systems dealing with conduct-disordered and antisocial youths; and the effects of violent and aggressive behaviors on the victims.

Risk and protective influences

Rutter (1997a) concluded that there are genetic influences, but that these may be associated more with pervasive and persistent antisocial behaviors and hyperactivity. These may include genetic susceptibility to environmental stressors and the two-way effects of adverse family environments on parent–child/child–parent interactions. Genetic findings may differ depending on whether the parent or child is reporting, with heritability being lower when based on child's reporting. Gender is also a risk factor, with even the earliest patterns of oppositional disorder being more likely to occur in boys than girls. Attention deficit hyperactivity disorder (ADHD) is also a risk factor in terms of comorbidity, with family functioning and interactions causing and maintaining problem behaviors. Cognitive and linguistic problems and having a low IQ may also be predictive, as may chronic ill health, especially if associated with impaired central nervous system and general functioning.

The early onset of aggressive and conduct symptoms is strongly predictive of conduct disorder, poorer outcomes, and chronic and serious antisocial behaviors (Mrazek & Haggerty, 1994). This finding links to the important influence of family adversity (relative risk = 3.1), specifically parental discord, inadequate parenting such as harsh, inconsistent and rejecting attitudes or abuse, and parental mental disorder (relative risk = 2.2), particularly maternal depression and/or antisocial personality disorder or alcoholism in the father. Community factors such as socioeconomic disadvantage, and living in a neighborhood with high levels of crime and social disintegration are likely to contribute further.

Evidence-based preventive interventions

Trials have shown that a number of approaches are effective, and may significantly lessen morbidity in childhood, and change the predicted pattern of morbidity and conduct disorder later in life. There are a number of illustrative projects targeting different developmental stages that represent both opportunity and unmet need.

Prenatal/Early Infancy project (Olds, Henderson, Tatelbaum & Chamberlain, 1988)

This combined approach to better prenatal and childbirth care, together with family support reduced the number of low-birth-weight deliveries and resulted in fewer instances of abuse. Similar projects include the studies of Gray, Cutler, Dean & Kempe (1979), and a number of others that examine the benefits of specific home visiting for parental support (e.g., Healthy Start, Hawaii). This is a generic intervention, but the reported results suggest that such interventions could enhance the protective factors. The Prenatal/Early Infancy program is a selective intervention in a randomized controlled trial targeting high-risk geographical areas and communities. The incidence of verified child abuse was reduced by 19% in the group visited by nurses, compared with a 4% reduction in the group who were not visited; the incidence of preterm delivery was also reduced by 75%. This type of program also links to those providing good support for pregnant women and mothers of young children, including projects such as the Infant Health and Development Project (1990) which showed better cognitive competence and fewer behavior problems in the intervention group.

Triple P: Positive Parenting for Preschoolers (Sanders, 1996)

This is an Australian program based on more than ten years of experimental clinical research that has established the effectiveness of intervention strategies in reducing oppositional behavior and conduct problems in a variety of populations: children from maritally discordant homes; children of depressed parents; children in step-families; developmentally disabled children and children in remote and rural areas. These studies have also been replicated in a number of contexts nationally (Sanders, 1996).

The intervention framework encompasses: training parents to implement behavior change and positive parenting strategies with their children in the home, with the effects being generalized to out-of-home situations; marital communication intervention for maritally discordant families to support parenting practices and reduce conflict; and enhanced behavioral interventions targeting maternal depression when this is a component (mood monitoring, cognitive restructuring, and coping skills techniques). Direct or enhanced intervention significantly reduced oppositional and aggressive behaviors and improved the parents' competence compared with control populations. Over 90% of the children in the intervention group improved so that their symptoms were no longer clinically significant. A self-directed intervention of the same type, supported by resources and telephone counseling, showed similar improvements. There is evidence for the long-term beneficial outcomes of such projects (e.g., Long, Forehand, Wierson & Morgan, 1994).

The other examples of interventions at the preschool level include the Perry Preschool Program, a selective intervention with trained teachers visiting home and school, which showed significantly fewer conduct, behavioral, and antisocial behaviors at all ages to 19, and a generally more positive outcome (Berrueta-Clement, Schweinhart, Barnett, Epstein & Weikart, 1984).

Second Step Violence Prevention Curriculum (Grossman et al., 1997)
This curriculum for elementary-grade children uses 30 specific lessons to teach social skills relating to anger management and impulse control. While significant changes were not observed on parent- or teacher-reported behavior scales, systematic observation showed decreases in physical aggression and increases in mental/prosocial behaviors in the children, which persisted for six months. It should also be noted that aggressive behavior increased in the control schools over the follow-up period. As these authors report, other studies support their findings (e.g., Dolan, Kellam, Brown & Werthamer-Larsson, 1993). In commenting on this report, Rosenberg, Powell & Hammond (1997) emphasize that this is part of a growing body of evidence showing that it is possible to reduce the level and cost of such violence. Another program of this kind is the intervention campaign against bullying and victim problems in children and adolescents developed in Norway by Olweus (1991). This is a universal preventive intervention using educational booklets, parent education booklets, a video, and self-report questionnaires for children in the program. This led to a 50% reduction in bully-victim

problems, decreased reports of antisocial behaviors, and increased satisfaction with school life. Similar programs have been replicated elsewhere.

Behaviorally Based Preventive Intervention (Bry, 1982)

This was a three-year preventive intervention using positive reinforcement for desirable school behaviors (report cards) for high-risk young people, with booster sessions following the initial intervention. The intervention appeared to prevent later delinquency as measured by both self-reports one year later and court reports five years later, i.e., 10% of the intervention group had court reports, as compared to 30% of the control group.

Other similar programs for the adolescent group include those targeting the prevention of substance abuse, programs dealing with school structures and organizations; school transition projects; and community-based programs directed at youth violence. Many of these latter require further study, but attest to the need for, and availability of, a range of interventions to target young people in different settings.

Conclusions about prevention of antisocial spectrum conditions

There are significant numbers of randomized controlled trials providing evidence for the effectiveness of prevention and the need for a prevention approach for this group of conditions. Offord & Bennett (1994) suggest that there is very little evidence for treatment effectiveness once the syndromes have stabilized and that prevention should be the approach of choice. There is much to support the need for a preventive approach commencing with perinatal care, but there is particular need for programs targeting preschool years to support more effective family functioning. A school-based, curriculum-oriented approach is likely to be effective with school-age children, and a more focused early intervention program with adolescents. Needless to say these would ideally be situated for improving the situation for the most socially disadvantaged – promoting social justice goals and altering the multiple risk factors that contribute in different sectors through multicomponent interventions.

Nevertheless, as with prevention of physical illness, there is likely to be considerable gain even when the interventions' effects are relatively small, simply because these problems are so prevalent. For instance, training community early-childhood nurses in 'Triple P' positive parenting frameworks has been shown to significantly reduce the symptoms of conduct disorder in a broader community sample. This shows the potential for substantial and positive prevention outcomes that are germane to this area of unmet need.

Depressive, internalizing, anxious, and withdrawing syndromal patterns

The burden and impact of depressive disorders in adult life is increasingly recognized. Indeed, measures such as disability-adjusted life years (DALYs) indicate that unipolar depression is currently one of the greatest causes of morbidity, and will have one of the greatest impacts on health worldwide by the year 2020. Even depressive symptoms at subsyndromal levels (for instance, two symptoms of depression) correlate with heightened health care utilization, poorer work and personal functioning and, for younger people, with vulnerabilities to hazardous levels of drug and alcohol use and a range of other pathologies. Up to 30% of adolescent females and 15% of adolescent males may suffer from clusters of symptoms of depression. Outcomes include not only morbidity, but also mortality due to suicide in a significant proportion of younger and older depressed persons.

Risk and protective influences

Rutter (1997*b*) reports that recent evidence supports earlier research and shows that a person is more susceptible to affective disorders if there is a history of them in their family. For disorders in childhood it is suggested that the genetic component is less significant, that there is potential comorbidity with antisocial behavior problems, as above, and that family discord is an environmental influence. The study of adults has shown that much of the genetic influence may be common to the trait of neuroticism and, as for conduct disorder, part of the susceptibility appears to involve vulnerability to environmental stressors. Gender is also an issue that requires further research, for a number of studies show that depressive symptoms and disorders are more prevalent in women, and that the increase in depressive symptomatology occurs in adolescence. The relationship between these symptoms and hormonal changes or subsequent patterns of depression in women requires further systematic clarification, but may provide opportunities for intervention. Social perceptions about gender roles may, of course, also be influential.

As noted above, being temperamental and vulnerable to environmental stressors may be personal traits that predispose to depression and anxiety syndromes, perhaps in the form of 'neuroticism'. Recent work indicates that having an optimistic explanatory style is likely to be protective against depression and anxiety syndromes, and that learned optimism may be protective. In contrast, negative explanatory styles, such as learned pessimism or helplessness, can increase the risk of depression (Seligman, 1993; Seligman, Reivich, Jaycox & Gillham, 1995).

Adverse environmental influences that increase a person's vulnerability to depression include: parental affective disorder, particularly maternal depression, or depression of both parents; disturbances in parenting (e.g., affectionless control); severe marital discord (which is likely to be interactive with depression in both directions); divorce; and other disruptions. The death of a parent in childhood, and childhood physical abuse or neglect, as well as sexual abuse, contribute to vulnerability in childhood or in later life. Other traumatic experiences, including separations or illness, can increase vulnerability in childhood and adult life. Experience of loss and failure – the break-up of a relationship, failure at school, and unemployment (particularly long-term unemployment) – are also associated with vulnerability to depression throughout the years of adolescence and adulthood. Depressive symptoms in old age may be linked to physical illness and dementia as well as a range of other factors.

Community factors tend to be generic, particularly poverty, but anomie, social isolation, and lack of paid employment are also important.

Protective factors throughout life include high intelligence, having an easy temperament, and having a good relationship with a supportive adult. In families with parental depression, resilience in adolescence is associated with having a good understanding of the parent's illness, good interpersonal relationships, and a strong sense of self (Beardslee & Podorefsky, 1988). Other work indicates that the negative influences associated with loss or abuse in childhood can be mitigated by experiences of academic or sporting achievement in adolescence, as well as a supportive relationship outside the home, and good interpersonal relationships.

Evidence-based interventions

A number of approaches offer important opportunities for prevention. These range from those focused on the management of parental depression and the mitigation of its potential effects on the child, to those aimed at enhancing optimism and positive explanatory styles in the child, to those promoting adaptation to stressful life experiences. There is also evidence that it may be possible to modify traits of vulnerability, such as neuroticism (Jorm, 1989).

Prenatal and postnatal depression and anxiety
Vulnerability to postnatal depression is increased if the woman has prenatal mood and anxiety problems, has a difficult labor, perceives or experiences her partner as not supportive, or if there is discord in their relationship. In some instances hormonal factors are important. What is clear is that this prevalent condition (one in ten women) can become chronic in many cases, and has profound negative effects on the infant's development, and responsiveness (Mrazek & Haggerty, 1994). Specific programs (including early and effective treatment) prevent the mother's depression from getting worse, and can

potentially benefit the relationship between the mother and her infant, and the infant's development. A brief psychosocial intervention of active listening, information, education, and support provided by midwives in the postnatal ward was effective in preventing postnatal depression (Boyce, in press). Interventions are also effective for maternal anxiety (Barnett, 1995). However, most of this simply represents good clinical care.

Specific treatment of maternal depression by appropriate and effective interventions is the key to preventing depression in the infant, and the earlier that effective prevention or treatment interventions are introduced, the less likely it is that prolonged withdrawal or developmental impairments will result.

Enhancing optimism and positive explanatory styles

Seligman's group (e.g., Gillham, Reivich, Jaycox & Seligman, 1995; Seligman et al., 1995) uses cognitive-behavioral formats and encourages self-competence through enhancing problem-solving abilities and positive explanatory styles. These interventions have been used for those with measurable symptoms of depression. Compared to nonintervention controls, the intervention group were less depressed and had fewer new episodes of depression in the follow-up period. These methods have been incorporated into general programs for a range of age groups, in terms of more broadly based interventions, and Seligman reports substantially and significantly lessened levels of onset and of depression in the follow-up period. The potential long-term benefits of this approach need to be followed up and the necessity of booster sessions investigated.

Shure and Spivac's Interpersonal Problem Solving Curriculum (1988) is another program of this type, with demonstrated benefits for high-risk children.

Dealing with stressful life experiences

A range of programs have been shown to be of benefit in these contexts.

The Children of Divorce Intervention Program was a selective intervention of ten one-hour weekly sessions for children aged 9–12. The intervention reduced anxiety, and improved indices of sociability and adaptation. The program focused on enhancing social competence (Pedro-Carroll & Cowen, 1985). These positive findings fit well with the work of Bloom, Hodges & Caldwell (1985), which showed positive effects over four years for a divorce intervention project. This project for children was replicated, with extensions for more disadvantaged groups, and once again showed beneficial effects (Alpert-Gillis, Pedro-Carroll & Cowen, 1989).

The Family Bereavement Program focused on the family environment with a three-session family grief workshop and 13 highly structured sessions with a family advisor who had personally suffered a similar bereavement

(Sandler et al., 1992). The intervention was shown to lessen depression and symptomatology of conduct disorder. Other preventive interventions have been reviewed by Black & Young (1995). Their findings endorse approaches that support the parents after the bereavement, prepare the child, ensure continuity of care through the period of loss, and encourage explaining to and talking with children. Black & Urbanowitz (1987) evaluated a brief family intervention of six counseling sessions and found beneficial outcomes at initial follow-up but no difference at two years, suggesting that, as with adults, the intervention may simply facilitate earlier resolution.

For children who have been traumatized, short-term cognitive-behavioral interventions may be indicated as suitable, and are effective in lessening the risk of posttraumatic stress disorder (PTSD) and anxiety disorders in some populations (Deblinger, McLeer & Henry, 1990). It is quite clear that regular treatment and management of sexually abused children do not lessen the risk of subsequent morbidity (Tebbutt, Swanston, Oates & O'Toole, 1997), and thus more specialized interventions are probably required. In this context, prevention of abuse in the first instance is important.

For children whose parents have affective disorder, a positive outcome is associated with treating the parents, and family interventions designed to help the child disengage from the parent's illness, to lessen family discord, and to increase parenting skills. Beardslee et al. (1993) conducted and reported on a specific trial that used a psycho-educational intervention. The outcomes of these studies, which link with demonstrated protective factors, have yet to be published.

Prevention and early intervention for depression and anxiety disorders

There are a number of important studies known as the Griffith Early Intervention Project (Dadds, Spence, Holland, Barrett & Laurens, 1997) which have shown that school-based programs building on cognitive-behavioral interventions can effectively intervene with children and adolescents who show early symptoms of anxiety and depression. These interventions benefit those with symptoms, and prevent the subsequent onset of symptoms. A range of other Australian projects are also underway, testing such models.

Clarke et al. (1992) have shown the effectiveness of cognitive-behavioral therapies as part of early intervention/prevention programs for depression in adolescence.

Conclusions about prevention of a related syndromes

It must be emphasized that generic interventions that modify parental discord and enhance parenting skills probably decrease vulnerability to depression, as do interventions that prevent abuse. There are also clear opportunities in the programs aimed at changing explanatory style and enhancing problem-solving and optimism, as these programs have demonstrated effectiveness in preventing depression.

Interventions aimed at children made vulnerable by stressful life experiences are also important opportunities for preventing depression. Curriculum-based programs, and more specific programs for early intervention and prevention of depression and related disorders can be used in school. Prevention, early detection and treatment of parental depression, with appropriate interventions for the child or children, contribute specifically and invaluably to prevent depression in infants, children, and young people. There is also ample evidence that depression is undertreated (e.g., Hirschfeld et al., 1997) and that national campaigns increase awareness and treatment levels. These national campaign initiatives should also encompass prevention, but should emphasize the psychological and social background, as well as other interventions.

Overview and conclusions

Two key syndrome areas evolve throughout childhood and are continuous with adult disorders. There is sound evidence of effective prevention which could contribute significantly to lessening morbidity, both in childhood and adolescence, as well as impacting on the cumulative developmental trajectory of vulnerability leading into adult life. Thus, the unmet need for prevention, as compared to treatment, interventions is established. Effective prevention should, in turn, lessen the burden of mental disorders in adults.

References

Achenbach, T.M., Howell, C.T., McConaughty, S.H. & Stranger, C. (1995). Six year predictors of problems in a national sample. III: Transitions to young adult syndromes. *Journal of the American Academy of Child and Adolescent Psychiatry*, 34, 658.

Alpert-Gillis, L.J., Pedro-Carroll, J.L. & Cowen, E.L. (1989). The children of divorce intervention program: development, implementation and evaluation of a program for young urban children. *Journal of Counselling and Clinical Psychology*, 57, 583–9.

Barnett, B. (1995). Preventive intervention: pregnancy and early parenting. In B. Raphael & G.D. Burrows (eds.), *Handbook of Studies on Preventive Psychiatry*. Amsterdam: Elsevier Science.

Beardslee, W.R. & Podorefsky, D. (1988). Resilient adolescents whose parents have serious affective and other psychiatric disorders: importance of self understanding and relationships. *American Journal of Psychiatry*, 145, 63–9.

Beardslee, W.R., Salt, P., Porterfield, K., Rothberg, P.C., van de Velde, P., Swatling, S., Hoke, L., Moilanen, D.L. & Wheelock, I. (1993). Comparison of preventive interventions for families with parental affective disorder. *Journal of the American Academy of Child and Adolescent Psychiatry*, **32**, 254–63.

Berrueta-Clement, J.R., Schweinhart, L.J., Barnett, W.S., Epstein, A.S. & Weikart, D.P. (1984). Changed lives: the effects of the Perry School Program on youth through age 19. (High/Scope Educational Research Foundation, Monograph 8.) Ypsilanti, MI: High/Scope Press.

Black, D. & Urbanowicz, M.A. (1987). Family intervention with bereaved children. *Journal of Child Psychology and Psychiatry*, **28**, 467–76.

Black, D. & Young, B. (1995). Bereaved children: risk and preventive intervention. In B. Raphael & G.D. Burrows (eds.), *Handbook of Studies on Preventive Psychiatry*. Amsterdam: Elsevier Science.

Bloom, B.L., Hodges, W.F. & Caldwell, R.A. (1985). A preventive intervention programme for the newly separated: final evaluations. *American Journal of Orthopsychiatry*, **55**, 9–26.

Boyce, P. (in press). Debriefing in obstetric settings. In B. Raphael & J. Wilson (eds.), *Stress Debriefing: Theory, Practice and Challenge*. Cambridge University Press.

Bry, B.H. (1982). Reducing the incidence of adolescent problems through preventive intervention: one-and five-year follow-up. *American Journal of Community Psychology*, **10**, 265–76.

Clarke, G., Hops, H., Lewinsohn, P.M., Andrews, J., Seeley, J.R. & Williams, J. (1992). Cognitive-behavioural group treatment of adolescent depression: prediction of outcome. *Behaviour Therapy*, **23**, 341–54.

Dadds, M., Spence, S., Holland, D.E., Barrett, P.M. & Laurens, K.R. (1997). Prevention and early intervention for anxiety disorders: a controlled trial. *Journal of Consulting and Clinical Psychology*, **65**, 627–35.

Deblinger, E., McLeer, S.V. & Henry, D. (1990). Cognitive behavioural treatment for sexually abused children suffering post traumatic stress: preliminary findings. *Journal of the American Academy of Child and Adolescent Psychiatry*, **29**, 747–52.

Dolan, L.J., Kellam, S.G., Brown, C.H. & Werthamer-Larsson, L. (1993). The short term impact of two classroom based prevention intervention on aggressive and shy behaviours and poor achievement. *Journal of Applied Developmental Psychology*, **14**, 317–45.

Eisenberg, L. (1995). Social policy and the reality of prevention. In B. Raphael & G.D. Burrows (eds.), *Handbook of Studies on Preventive Psychiatry*. Amsterdam: Elsevier Science.

Gillham, J.E., Reivich, K.J., Jaycox, L.H. & Seligman, M.E. (1995). Prevention of depressive symptoms in schoolchildren: two year follow up. *American Journal of Psychology*, **6**, 343–51.

Gray, J., Cutler, C., Dean, J. & Kempe, C.H. (1979). Prediction and prevention of child abuse and neglect. *Journal of Social Issues*, **35**, 127–39.

Grossman, D.C., Neckerman, H.J., Koepsell, T.D., Lui, P.-Y., Asher, K.N., Beland, K., Frey, K. & Rivara, F.P. (1997). Effectiveness of a violence prevention curriculum among children in elementary school: a randomised control trial. *Journal of the American Medical Association*, **277**, 1605–11.

Hirschfeld, R.M., Keller, M.B., Panico, S., Arons, B.S., Barlow, D., Davidoff, F., Endicott, J., Froom, J., Goldstein, M., Gorman, J.M., Marek, R.G., Maurer, T.A.,

Meyer, R., Phillips, K., Ross, J., Schwenk, T.L., Sharfstein, S.S., Thase, M.E. & Wyatt, R.J. (1997). The National Depressive and Manic Depressive Association Consensus Statement on the undertreatment of depression. *Journal of the American Medical Association*, **277**, 333–40.

Infant Health and Development Project (1990). Enhancing the outcomes of low birth weight premature infants: a multi-site randomised trial. *Journal of the American Medical Association*, **263**, 3035–42.

Jorm, A.F. (1989). Modifiability of trait anxiety and neuroticism: a meta-analysis of the literature. *Australian and New Zealand Journal of Psychiatry*, **23**, 21–9.

Long, P., Forehand, R., Wierson, M. & Morgan, A. (1994). Does parent training with young non compliant children have long term effects? *Behavioural Research and Therapy*, **32**, 101–7.

Mrazek, P.J. & Haggerty, R.J. (eds.) (1994). *Reducing Risks for Mental Disorders: Frontiers for Preventive Intervention Research*. Washington, D.C.: National Academy Press.

Offord, D.R. & Bennett, K.J. (1994). Conduct disorder: long term outcomes and intervention effectiveness. *Journal of the American Academy of Child and Adolescent Psychiatry*, **33**, 1069–78.

Olds, D., Henderson, C.R., Tatelbaum, R. & Chamberlain, R. (1988). Improving the life course development of socially disadvantaged mothers: a randomised trial of nurse home visitation. *American Journal of Public Health*, **78**, 1436–44.

Olweus, D. (1991). Bully/victim problems among schoolchildren: basic facts and effects of an intervention program. In D.J. Pepler & K.H. Rubin (eds.), *The Development and Treatment of Childhood Aggression*. Hillsdale: Lawrence Erlbaum Associates.

Pedro-Carroll, J.L. & Cowen, E.L. (1985). The children of divorce intervention program: an investigation of the efficiency of a school based prevention program. *Journal of Counselling and Clinical Psychology*, **53**, 603–11.

Rosenberg, M.L., Powell, K.E. & Hammond, R. (1997). Applying science to violence prevention. *Journal of the American Medical Association*, **277**, 1641–2.

Rutter, M. (1995). Relationships between mental disorders in childhood and adulthood. *Acta Psychiatrica Scandinavica*, **91**, 73–85.

Rutter, M. (1997a). Implications of genetic research for child psychiatry. *Canadian Journal of Psychiatry*, **42**, 569–76.

Rutter, M. (1997b). Child psychiatric disorder: measures, causal mechanisms and interventions. *Archives of General Psychiatry*, **54**, 785–9

Sanders, M. (ed.) (1996). *Healthy Families, Healthy Nation: Strategies for Promoting Family Mental Health in Australia*. Brisbane: Australian Academic Press.

Sandler, I.N., West, S.G., Baca, L., Pillow, D.R., Gersten, J.C., Rogosch, F., Virdin, L., Beals, J., Reynolds, K.D. & Kallgren, C. (1992). Linking empirically-based theory and evaluation: The Family Bereavement Program. *American Journal of Community Psychology*, **20**, 491–523.

Seligman, M. (1993). *Helplessness: On Depression, Development and Death*. San Francisco, CA: Freeman.

Seligman, M., Reivich, K., Jaycox, L. & Gillham, J. (1995). *The Optimistic Child*. Sydney: Random House.

Shure, M.B. & Spivak, G. (1988). Interpersonal cognitive problem solving. In R.H. Price, E.L. Cowen, R.P. Lorion, & J. Ramon-McKay (eds.), *Fourteen Ounces of Prevention: a Casebook for Practitioners.* Washington, D.C.: American Psychological Association.

Tebbutt, J., Swanston, H., Oates, R.K. & O'Toole, B.I. (1997). Five years after child sexual abuse: persisting dysfunction and problems of prediction. *Journal of the American Academy of Child and Adolescent Psychiatry,* **36**, 330–9.

10

Meeting unmet needs: can evidence-based approaches help?

Harold Alan Pincus and Deborah A. Zarin

In this chapter, we will discuss our attempt to develop evidence-based systems for defining, guiding, and monitoring aspects of psychiatric care in the USA; some of the limitations in these approaches (i.e., we should not get too overconfident about our capacities); and finally provide some recommendations about how to deal with some of these limitations – and particularly the role of a practice-based research network.

Basically, the problem put before contributors to this volume can be framed as four questions. Who gets treatment? What treatments are or should be provided? How are treatments provided – by whom, how much, and for how long? (and this ultimately translates into the economics). And, on what basis do we determine the above 'who', 'what', and 'how' – do we base it on tradition, on market values, or on evidence?

The *Diagnostic and Statistical Manual of Mental Disorders* (DSM-IV) introduction is clear in defining mental disorders as a grouping of symptoms plus either clinically significant distress or impairment in major role functioning [American Psychiatric Association (APA), 1994*a*]. The challenges are to determine which treatments are effective for whom, and to make sure that the people most in need get those treatments. It is important to define how we develop systems that encourage incentives for ensuring that the people in need of treatment receive the most appropriate medical care. In the USA there has been enormous growth in 'managed care' as a general approach for making these determinations. Our group has developed a model (Figure 10.1) of how managed care affects patient care, which can be applied to evaluating the processes of any health plan (Pincus, Zarin & West, 1996). The framework describes a model, in which an eligible population enters what has previously been called a 'black box', which encompasses different financial, organizational, contractual, and certain procedural elements. Examples of financial elements are financial incentives linked to capitation, or the fee-for-service scheme. Organizational and contractual elements include whether the primary health care is provided in the form of separate mental health components or in an integrated package. Finally, procedural elements limit the choices available to clinicians about who to treat and how (e.g., utilization management, clinical protocols, formulary management). These three el-

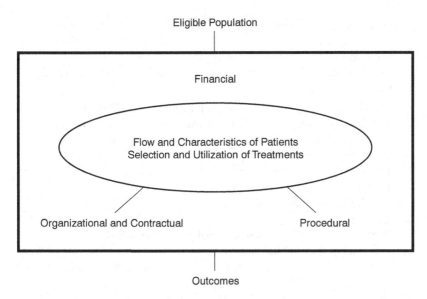

Figure 10.1 How: examining the 'black box' of health care plans.

ements – financial, organizational, and procedural – affect the flow and characteristics of patients through the system, and ultimately the selection and utilization of treatments for those patients. This process determines the outcome for both the individual and for the population under care. The question is, how do we determine the proper mix of these elements to meet the appropriate needs of a population and to achieve better outcomes for individuals?

Evidence-based medicine/evidence-based systems

We have been advocating a move toward evidence-based psychiatry, which is defined as 'decision-making based upon data regarding the likely impact of different treatments on specific outcomes for specific populations' (Sackett, Rosenberg, Gray, Haynes & Richardson, 1996). This is distinguished from tradition-based methods of using expert opinion or what has been termed the 'BOGSAT' method ('a bunch of guys sitting around a table'). An alternative is the market-based model. This model is reflected in the growth of managed health care in the USA. As an example of the market being more powerful than evidence, one of the largest managed care plans in the USA, Oxford Health Plans, recently announced that it was going to be covering alternative medicine treatments. The reason for doing this was not based upon evidence but the notion that this is likely to be attractive to a more healthy group of patients, therefore lowering their overall costs. At the other end of the spectrum, many health plans fail to cover treatments whose effectiveness has empirical support (e.g., certain types of psychiatric care; allergy medications).

We have embarked on an extensive process for developing evidence-based systems that involves:

1. Creating evidence-based diagnostic guidelines, as in DSM-IV.
2. Judging screening and assessment instruments for the application of those guidelines, i.e., the soon to be published *APA Handbook of Psychiatric Measures and Outcomes*.
3. Developing national practice guidelines, and then using them as a platform for developing local protocols.
4. Developing local protocols.
5. Ultimately proposing quality and outcome indicators to measure the degree of adherence to these national practice guidelines.
6. Influencing the establishment of systems that reinforce the use of these evidence-based approaches through reimbursement and other incentives.

Despite elements in psychiatry that have feared these approaches, this broad evidence-based strategy has the strong support of the APA.

The first step, which has resulted in considerable success, has been to try to develop more in the way of a science base. From 1984 to 1995, National Institutes of Health (NIH) funding for university departments of psychiatry rose from US$82 million to US$341 million, almost doubling the percentage of the NIH dollar received. In terms of research funding, psychiatry departments have moved from tenth to second position in medical schools (Author, 1995). Thus, the science base has expanded tremendously, though how much of that will be applicable to the development of some of these evidence-based procedures is an issue that is debatable and is discussed below.

We have also been developing a series of projects using evidence-based approaches that translate this expanded science base into clinical guidelines. We started implementing a formal evidence-based approach with the DSM-IV (and also by producing the Primary Care Version of the DSM-IV; APA, 1995a) and are in the process of developing the *Handbook of Psychiatric Measures and Outcomes*. The handbook includes systematic evidence reviews of over 270 different measures that could be applied in 38 different domains within psychiatry, both clinically and for research purposes. We have been developing practice guidelines, and now are beginning to embark on a process to develop evidence-based quality indicators.

Practice guidelines

APA practice guidelines are defined as strategies for the care of patients that

Table 10.1. American Psychiatric Association Practice Guidelines

Topic	Initial publication	Anticipated revision
Eating disorders	February 1993	1998
Major depressive disorder	April 1993	1998
Bipolar disorder	December 1994	1999
Substance-abuse disorder	November 1995	1999
Psychiatric evaluation	November 1995	2000
Nicotine dependence	September 1996	2000
Schizophrenia	April 1997	2001
Alzheimer's disease	May 1997	2001
Panic disorder	Spring 1998	
Delirium	Fall 1998	
Geriatric care	Fall 1998	
Mental retardation	1999	
HIV/AIDS	1999	
Obsessive-compulsive disorder	1999	
Posttraumatic stress disorder	1999	
Personality disorder	1999	

are developed by psychiatrists to assist psychiatrists in their clinical decision making (Zarin, Pincus & McIntyre, 1993). Practice guidelines adhere to the attributes developed by the U.S. Institute of Medicine (1992) (i.e., guidelines for guidelines) as described below. Table 10.1 lists the APA practice guidelines that have been developed or are in progress (APA, 1993a,b, 1994b, 1995b,c, 1996, 1997a,b).

Desired attributes of practice guidelines

1. Purpose – quality versus cost
2. Clear – written unambiguously
3. Credible – grounded in science
4. Valid – related to outcomes
5. Reliable – reproducible
6. Applicable – clinical and health systems management
7. Flexible – reflect clinical variations
8. Complete disclosure – development detailed
9. Disseminated – widely
10. Feedback – from clinical practitioners
11. Scheduled review – regular and frequent.

APA practice guidelines have the following components: (1) critical review and compilation of the literature on treatment; (2) a framework for clinical decision making; (3) treatment recommendation for a 'typical patient'; and (4) the implications for treatment of comorbidities and other complicating factors. They are developed and based on a standardized process. Topics are selected based on the prevalence of the disorder, the relevance to the field of psychiatry, and the likelihood that a practice guideline would improve practice in that particular area. Data extraction is done using an explicit and rigorous method. The specifications of the computerized literature searches are stated, the rules for reviewing specific articles are prescribed, and the extraction of data from articles is guided by the use of explicit extraction rules and evidence tables. The final version is published in the *American Journal of Psychiatry*, which subjects all practice guidelines to a peer review process. Practice guidelines undergo revision at three- to five-year intervals.

Typically, a guideline begins with a summary of recommendations, followed by sections on disease definition, epidemiology, and natural history; treatment principles and alternatives; the formulation of an individual treatment plan; clinical features influencing treatment; and research directions. 'Treatment principles' includes a discussion of psychiatric management and then a discussion of each specific treatment modality. Psychiatric management is defined as 'those activities that a psychiatrist would provide for every patient with this disorder regardless of the specific treatment modality which is chosen'. Psychiatric management typically consists of features that are, at times, called 'clinical management', 'medication management', 'supportive psychotherapy', and 'psychoeducation'. Both somatic and psychosocial treatment modalities are then reviewed. For each specific treatment modality the discussion follows the outline of: goals, efficacy, side-effects and toxicity, and issues in implementation. The section, 'formulation and implementation of a treatment plan', aims to provide a framework for individualized clinical decision making for a 'typical patient'. This section is frequently organized according to the phases of the illness. The section, 'clinical features influencing treatment' reviews those specific features that might affect the general treatment recommendations (e.g., the presence of a comorbid substance-use disorder).

Dissemination is accomplished through a variety of mechanisms: publication in the *American Journal of Psychiatry*, integration of practice guidelines into residency training programs; use of the guidelines for examinations (e.g., for residents and for recertification by the American Board of Psychiatry and Neurology); and by the development of 'companion' pieces for patients and physicians (e.g., patient guides and quick reference brochures, containing algorithms). In addition, if you have detailed treatment guidelines you will know how to manage your resources and pay your staff, and recent efforts have focused on the development of tools to assist systems of care in adapting APA guidelines for use with their providers.

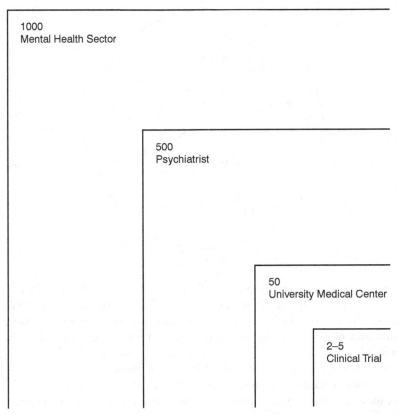

Figure 10.2 The ecology of mental health care. Figure adapted from Kerr-White et al., 1961.

Limitations in evidence-based approaches

In developing practice guidelines, we have found a number of limitations and problems: (1) the insufficiency of the evidence in many disorders – there are a lot of gaps; (2) the evidence is not relevant to both clinicians and staff; (3) limitations in the techniques for integrating evidence – how do we integrate evidence that may vary in terms of its findings and the quality of information it provides? (4) the difficulty of applying both social values and individual preferences when determining evidence-based guidelines; and (5) there is potential for misuse. For example, people often regard the lack of evidence of efficacy as being evidence of nonefficacy. We have to somehow guard against that misinterpretation, because there are many procedures throughout medicine for which there is simply no evidence, and nor is there ever likely to be, that they work.

The issue of generalization is depicted in Figure 10.2 as a modification of

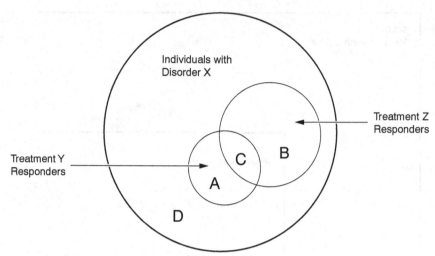

Figure 10.3 Clinical policy quandary number 1

Kerr-White's analysis of the ecology of medical care, essentially questioning the applicability of data from the very tiny fraction of individuals who participate in clinical trials to the average patient walking into the average clinician's office. Moreover, the information obtained from clinical trials cannot be applied to the average clinician's decision making. This is because, among other things, the clinical trials do not include a broad enough spectrum of conditions, patients, and treatment options. Furthermore there are the added issues of outcomes; for example, there is no one ideal outcome for all parties involved. Purchasers, providers, patients, families, and society may have different views. The development of clinical trials in each combination of patient and treatment factors would be enormously expensive and completely impractical. Thus, we are going to have to find acceptable ways of interpolating some of this information.

Evidence-based quandaries

Figure 10.3 depicts the results of clinical trials of two treatments. How does one decide between treatments A and B if making an evidence-based decision for an individual patient level or at a clinical policy level for national guidelines? How does one balance: (1) the proportion of responders to each possible treatment; (2) the degree of beneficial response; (3) the length of response; (4) the likelihood of adverse effects with each treatment; (5) other nonclinical costs; and (6) individual (or societal) preferences? An important issue from a guideline perspective is the question being asked. What is appropriate or necessary care, or is the aim to provide decision support for

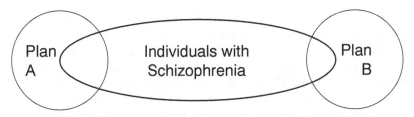

Figure 10.4 Risk adjustment. Total mental health costs, A > B. Mental health care costs for *n* individuals with schizophrenia, A < B. Average functional status for enrollees, A < B.

the clinician? (Kahan et al., 1994).

Another quandary relates to the issue of developing evidence-based approaches to compare the outcomes of different programs. For example, as depicted in Figure 10.4, two health care plans are competing against each other and Program A has 'the world's greatest treatment program for schizophrenia'. Assuring equal per capita resources, Program A is going to do poorly from a financial perspective and also in the measuring of outcomes. Program A will attract people with schizophrenia (and the more severe cases of schizophrenia), so that total mental health costs will be greater (although the total mental health costs for individuals with schizophrenia will be less), and the average mental health status of all enrollees will be less (although it will be higher for individuals with schizophrenia). It is essential that appropriate mechanisms for risk adjustment/case-mix severity be developed to permit more accurate comparisons.

Recommendations

Most importantly, we need more, and better, evidence. This will require overcoming major threats to clinical research. Currently in the USA, clinical research and academic centers are under a tremendous challenge, as managed care companies are channeling resources away from academic centers, and academics focus more on expanding clinical efficiency than academic pursuits (Tanne, 1997). It is also necessary to balance academic studies with those in industry (Zarin & Pincus, 1997). The pharmaceutical industry has invested immense resources in supporting research aimed at getting drugs to market. These industry studies do not necessarily aid clinicians in their individual clinical decision making. There is also a need for more relevant evidence, which is not only aimed at the kind of questions and decisions faced by practitioners, but which also draws subjects that are similar to patients in clinical practice. An important strategy is developing a practice-based research network as discussed below.

In developing evidence-based guidelines, there must be a 'truth-in-advertising' principle, with an open process and explicit documentation of that process, which honestly depicts the gaps in the evidence. We also need to improve how we integrate disparate research and clinical information within the evidence-based medicine doctrine. We need to involve patients and families, and also link clinicians and researchers more closely in this endeavor. Importantly, we ought to be sharing our efforts internationally. For example, the APA has been working together with the Royal College of Psychiatrists in Great Britain to aid in their development of practice guidelines, and we have begun discussions with the Royal Australia and New Zealand College of Psychiatrists on the development of practice guidelines and a practice research network. Ultimately, we have to improve the implementation of practice guidelines. There is ample evidence that it is necessary to actively implement, rather than simply publish, the practice guidelines if clinicians are to change their behavior (Asaph, Janoff, Wayson, Kilberg & Graham, 1991; Greco & Eisenberg, 1993; Mittman & Siu, 1992; Tunis et al., 1994). We have to continue to develop and test interventions, and see whether using these interventions changes clinicians' practices and ultimately improves outcomes. We need to design fair incentive systems, and apply new technologies, i.e., develop computer-based decision-support mechanisms.

The role of practice-based research

The APA has developed a practice research network (PRN) (Zarin, Pincus, West & McIntyre, 1997). The PRN is a group of clinical psychiatrists (currently 530, soon to be 1000) practising across the full range of clinical settings, who provide data about themselves, detailed information about the patients they see, the kind of treatments they provide, and patient outcomes. The PRN is able to generate a very large amount of clinically detailed data that goes well beyond that available in administrative data sets. For example, preliminary data indicate that a very extensive pattern of comorbidities (DSM-IV, Axis I, II and III) exists in psychiatric practice. This suggests that patients in routine clinical settings differ greatly from those taking part in clinical trials. Also, interestingly, the number of psychopharmacological agents prescribed per patient is much higher than would be expected from the published clinical trials. What is not known, but can be explored by the PRN, is whether this is inappropriate polypharmacy, or, given the kind of patients being seen in clinical practice, whether their symptoms are simply not responding to monotherapy, i.e., there are break-through symptoms that need to be treated with additional medications. The aim is to use these observational, naturalistic data (albeit imperfect since the patients and treatments are not randomized) to fill in some of the gaps as well as to try to better understand the systems and processes that occur in the context of health care plans.

References

American Psychiatric Association (1993a). Practice guideline for eating disorders. *American Journal of Psychiatry*, **150**, 212–28.

American Psychiatric Association (1993b). Practice guideline for major depressive disorders in adults. *American Journal of Psychiatry*, **150** [Suppl.], 1–26.

American Psychiatric Association (1994a). *Diagnostic and Statistical Manual of Mental Disorders* (4th edition). Washington, D.C.: American Psychiatric Association.

American Psychiatric Association (1994b). Practice guideline for the treatment of patients with bipolar disorder. *American Journal of Psychiatry*, **151** [Suppl.], 1–55.

American Psychiatric Association (1995a). *Diagnostic and Statistical Manual of Mental Disorders* (4th edition). Primary Care Version. Washington, D.C.: American Psychiatric Association.

American Psychiatric Association (1995b). Practice guideline for psychiatric evaluation of adults. *American Journal of Psychiatry*, **152** [Suppl.], 63–80.

American Psychiatric Association (1995c). Practice guideline for treatment of patients with substance use disorders, alcohol, cocaine, opioids. *American Journal of Psychiatry*, **152** [Suppl.], 1–59.

American Psychiatric Association (1996). Practice guideline for the treatment of patients with nicotine dependence. *American Journal of Psychiatry*, **153** [Suppl.], 1–31.

American Psychiatric Association (1997a). Practice guideline for the treatment of patients with schizophrenia. *American Journal of Psychiatry*, **154** [Suppl.], 1–63.

American Psychiatric Association (1997b). Practice guideline for the treatment of patients with Alzheimer's disease and other dementias of late life. *American Journal of Psychiatry*, **154** [Suppl.], 1–39.

Asaph, J.W., Janoff, K., Wayson, K., Kilberg, L. & Graham, M. (1991). Carotid endarterectomy in a community hospital: a change in physicians practice patterns. *American Journal of Surgery*, **161**, 616–18.

Author (1995). Datagram: NIH extramural support to institutions of higher education by department. *Psychiatric Research Report*, **10**, 19.

Greco, P.J. & Eisenberg, J.M. (1993). Changing physician practices. *New England Journal of Medicine*, **329**, 1271–3.

Institute of Medicine (1992). *Guidelines for Clinical Practice: From Development to Use*. Washington, D.C.: National Academy Press.

Kahan, J.P., Bernstein, S.J., Leape, L.L., Hilborne, L.H., Park, R.E., Parker, L., Kamberg, C.J. & Brook, R.H. (1994). Measuring the necessity of medical procedures. *Medical Care*, **32**, 357–65.

Kerr-White, (1961). *New England Journal of Medicine*, **265**, 885–92.

Mittman, B.S. & Siu, A. (1992). Changing provider behavior: applying research on outcomes and effectiveness in health care. In S. Shortell & U. Reinhardt (eds.),

Improving Health Policy and Management: Nine Critical Research Issues for the 1990s, pp. 195–226. Ann Arbor, MI: Health Administration Press.

Pincus, H.A., Zarin, D.A. & West, J. (1996). Peering into the 'black box': measuring outcomes of managed care. *Archives of General Psychiatry*, 53, 870–7.

Sackett, D.L., Rosenberg, W.M.C., Gray, J.A.M., Haynes, R.B. & Richardson, W.S. (1996). Evidence based medicine: what it is and what it isn't. *British Medical Journal*, 312, 71–2.

Tanne, J.H. (1997). US clinical research under threat. *British Medical Journal*, 315, 143.

Tunis, S.R., Hayward, R.S., Wilson, M.C., Rubin, H.R., Bass, E.B., Johnston, M. & Steinberg, E.P. (1994). Internist's attitude about clinical practice guidelines. *Annals of Internal Medicine*, 120, 956–63.

Zarin, D.A. & Pincus, H.A. (1997). From the Office of Research: risks in a public agenda. *Psychiatric Research Report*, 13, 2–8.

Zarin, D.A., Pincus, H.A. & McIntyre, J.S. (1993). Practice guidelines [editorial]. *American Journal of Psychiatry*, 150, 175–7.

Zarin, D.A., Pincus, H.A., West, J.C. & McIntyre, J.S. (1997). Practice-based research in psychiatry. *American Journal of Psychiatry*, 154, 1199–208.

11

Unmet need for management of mental disorders in primary care

T. Bedirhan Üstün

This chapter analyses the unmet need for management of mental disorders in primary care. It is written in light of the World Health Organization (WHO) Collaborative Study 'Psychological Problems in General Health Care', which was conducted in 14 countries. It focuses on the importance of primary care for mental health care; the definition of need; the current state of mental disorders in primary care; and implications for research and training. Three main parameters were utilized in the definition of need:

1. Clients. Mental health researchers have focused mainly on diagnosis to define need. However, primary care attenders and providers focus mainly on complaints that relate to daily functioning. While a diagnosis of the condition is necessary for the management of the patient, diagnosis alone does not provide the basis for understanding the patient's need. Both patients and primary care providers utilize the functioning/disability framework to make their encounter more meaningful.

2. Providers. For many providers, mental health problems are a nonissue: they are not considered a real problem, nor are they seen as remediable. Most primary care providers are not adequately trained or equipped with skills to manage mental health problems.

3. Services. Provision for need in primary care has often been seen as a result of the interaction between the client and the provider. However, the way the services are structured (e.g., appointment system, length of visit, numbers of patients, personal doctors) determines how a patient's needs can be expressed or modulated.

A new framework that uses models of the way the service functions is needed to understand the management of mental health problems in primary care.

What is primary care?

Primary care is 'first contact care' – in other words, it is where a 'need' is first objectified. Primary care, therefore, covers a wide range of health care needs – consumers can bring any health problems, physical, mental, emotional or social. Primary care is a heterogeneous set of services defined as having the following operational characteristics (Üstün, 1997):

- It is easily accessible and introduces the patients to the health care system.
- It provides integrated health care services (prevention, cure, promotion) that are comprehensive, simple, and continuous.
- It is serviced by primary care providers. These include doctors (basically general practitioners, family physicians and other physicians who give first contact care), nurses, counselors, social workers, and other health workers.
- It has a coordinator function as a gatekeeper or filter for referral of patients to other levels of health care and as a coordinator of long-term care.
- It provides a service in the context of family and community.
- It provides continued care and a more sustained relationship between the providers and consumers.

In summary, primary care is the basis of the health care system. It is the main vehicle for delivering care in response to the population's needs. Primary care is the arena where the needs and resources begin to match.

What makes primary care so special for mental health?

Primary care, given the above characteristics, is an essential environment in which to deliver mental health care. The WHO has long advocated the integration of mental health into primary care (Üstün & Gater, 1994). When one examines what really happens in primary care settings, one sees that it covers a whole range of health care needs that have psychosocial and behavioral components. In this sense, primary care should and often does consider mental health to be inseparable from physical health (Harding et al., 1983a, b; Murthy & Wig, 1983; Sartorius & Harding, 1983).

Primary care practice differs from specialty practice in a number of ways. First, patients seen in primary care frequently represent the less severe end of the disease spectrum. Usually they are at the early stages of illness, with less differentiated signs and symptoms. Second, primary care provides opportunities to promote health and prevent disease (Jenkins & Üstün, 1997). Consumers are generally seen regularly in primary care, whereas specialist services are usually prompted by a particular event. Primary care services can develop the long-term and integrative perspective that provides the basis for early detection, intervention, and long-term management.

This chapter will therefore focus on the burden of mental disorders in primary care and the unmet need. The facts from research will be summarized to identify unmet need in the primary care context.

What is a need? A need for what?

Need is difficult to define. It is usually described subjectively and is therefore in the eye of the beholder. An operational definition of need involves a number of complex parameters:

1. Need, on its own, is something that potentially could be satisfied. Physiological needs, e.g., need for food, can be defined in this way as 'basic needs'. One can identify daily requirements for water, food or shelter. When someone drinks, the need for water is satisfied. Similarly, need, in a health care context, refers to a change in the functional status and a possible remedy, e.g., when you cannot see clearly you may need eye-glasses. It is the actual dysfunction, not the mere diagnosis, which needs to be corrected.

2. Need is also 'managed' by providers. For example, the needs of a new-born are met by the mother who is the key provider of services and the mother becomes the 'need manager' of the infant by observing the levels of pleasure and pain. Likewise, providers of primary care services are powerful 'need managers' of their patients. What they provide as a solution, to some extent further defines the need (i.e., what constitutes a treatment may either be a life-saving solution, a cure, relief, stabilization, or assistance). Having a solution defines and reifies the problem, and puts the provider in a situation of defining the need, providing the solution, and managing the delivery schedule.

3. Need is also, to some extent, 'manufactured'. People's opinions as to what medical services they could possibly use are formed within the context of their view of the world. People are influenced by what they perceive as a need, and an ideological framework often defines that need. For example, in the 1990s, a three- to nine-fold increase in the recording of eating disorders occurred in British general practice (Turnbull, Ward, Treasure, Jick & Derby, 1996). This may be due to growing public recognition, rather than to a true increase in the number of people suffering from this group of disorders.

4. Consumers of services soon learn to 'demand'. A consumer may go on demanding whatever they are given. This may be seen as testing providers' resources and limits. It should be noted that while the object of need can be supplied completely, that of demand cannot be completely met. This is especially so when demand expresses itself as a 'desire' for some platonic ideal such as the 'complete state of well-being'. In short, while a need can be satisfied, a demand cannot always be met, and a desire can only sometimes be reached. We should make clear distinctions between need, demand, and desire.

Epidemiologists have naively equated need with diagnosis and then have rationally tried to base health care services on the prevalences of disorders in the population (Häfner, 1977; Kessler et al., 1994; Regier et al., 1993). Recent work has shown that diagnosis alone does not predict the need for care. Need is a function of both diagnosis and disability, that is, a product of functional limitations affecting the person in their interactions with society (World Health Organization, 1997).

To be relevant, estimation of need should be based on operational definitions:

1. There should be a problem with the person's level of functioning.
2. A problem should be objectively manifest, that is observable to the person or others.
3. There should be an effective and acceptable treatment or intervention.
4. Both the person in need and the provider should agree on the terms for the delivery of care.

Following such a definition, we can begin assessing the needs for adequate use and planning of resources, setting priorities on how needs will be met, and judging the costs and benefits. Needs can be defined either in terms of individuals or groups. *Individual-based needs assessment* leads to matching treatment provision to a consumer's need and ability to benefit (Thornicroft, Brewin & Wing, 1992). *Population-based needs assessment* leads to service planning and provision for populations and depends on that population's ability to benefit from the service. In this framework, when people have a mental disorder that alters their daily functioning, we are confronted with the following questions:

• What do primary care attenders need?
• How do primary care providers discover patients' or consumers' needs?
• Do consumers get what they need?
• Do consumers need what they get?

Unmet need for management of mental disorders in primary care

Current studies show that the global burden of mental disorders is considerable and should be a priority. The extent of disablement related to mental disorders throughout the world has been illustrated in a report prepared by the World Bank and the WHO (Murray & Lopez, 1996). This report calculated the global burden of disease by combining the years of life lost and the years lived with a disability to generate disability-adjusted life years (DALYs) lost, a metric which represents an attempt to quantify the burden of disease in terms of mortality and morbidity. According to this report, mental disorders are responsible for 10.5% of the global burden of disease (Murray & Lopez, 1997).

Since mental disorders are common, much of this global burden is treated in primary care. Worldwide, one in four primary care attenders has a diagnosable mental disorder such as a depressive, anxiety, or alcohol-use disorder. These common mental disorders are, on average, as disabling as physical disorders, and cause individuals, their families, and communities to suffer. There are acceptable and efficacious treatments for these common mental disorders, yet they are not sufficiently recognized and treated. Mental disorders in primary care constitute a major public health problem (Üstün & Sartorius, 1995).

How this burden is managed in primary care depends on many factors, such as the availability and accessibility of services, the availability of diagnostic tools and management interventions, models of service delivery including service structure and staffing, links to specialist care, the attitudinal environment of the service organization, and the general health status of the country.

Most patients with an identifiable mental disorder are seen in primary care

Epidemiological studies of the pathways followed by patients with mental disorders indicate that 60–96% of them who receive care visit a primary care setting first (Gater et al., 1991). If you take the whole spectrum of conditions, from minor anxiety or dysphoria to totally and permanently disabling conditions, the mental health needs requiring attention and care provision are extremely important in primary care (Goldberg & Huxley, 1992). One-quarter of patients seen in primary care have common mental disorders but chronic cases of severe mental disorders (e.g., schizophrenia, bipolar disorder) are now being referred for continuing care. Primary care has become the principal setting for the delivery of mental health care.

Caseness in primary care is not determined by diagnosis alone

Epidemiological surveys at the community level (e.g., Epidemiologic Catchment Area, UK and other national surveys) do not necessarily give a direct estimate of the needs for mental health services at the primary care level, because *diagnosis alone* in a community survey does not appear to predict mental health care needs. Data on the *functional status or disablement* of those with mental disorders are more useful in estimating health service utilization (Klerman, Olfson, Leon & Weissman, 1992; Knapp, Beecham, Fenyo & Hallam, 1995; Üstün, 1996). There are important research questions about what happens to cases in the community: what makes them decide to seek care and what determines the recognition of their condition? For example, if patients express their mental distress clearly or demand services, the recognition of caseness can be significantly improved.

Primary care providers are more likely to recognize and treat if their patient has a moderate or severe disability, that is when the mental disorder impairs social functioning, reduces efficiency, motivation and work productivity. This finding is consistent across centers, time, and individual diagnoses (Ormel et al., 1994; Von Korff, Üstün & Ormel, 1996).

The present system of primary mental health care is haphazard and inadequate

The WHO study (Üstün, 1994; Üstün & Sartorius, 1995) examined and compared the recognition of mental disorders by clinical and research methods, and found that the concordance rates varied between 5% and 60% across centers. Similarly, treatment rates for a given diagnosis varied between 2% and 45%. The monitoring and follow-up of the cases in primary care settings was inadequate and care between different agencies was often poorly coordinated.

At three months we found that 60% of those who had a mental disorder at intake remained ill, while at one year 46% remained ill. The patients who became well were those who were recognized by their primary care physician as ill, given appropriate treatment, and who complied with that treatment.

Predictors of outcome of common mental disorders in primary care
Predictors of good outcome include:

- A low level of disability
- A low level of severity of illness
- The physician correctly identifying the presenting symptoms
- Little comorbidity
- Good self-reported overall health
- Recommendation of counseling by physician
- The patient being well educated
- Being under 40 years old
- No current alcohol abuse

Efficacious treatments are available for common mental disorders

There are good drug treatments for depression, panic disorder, and obsess-ive-compulsive disorder, and good psychological treatments for depression, panic disorder and agoraphobia, obsessive compulsive disorder, generalized anxiety disorder, alcoholism, and chronic fatigue (Andrews, 1996). However, there is a huge gap between the expected efficacy and effectiveness of treatments in primary care.

Primary care providers are seldom provided with identification and management skills for common mental disorders

The primary care providers badly need the knowledge to provide the appropriate services for, and meet the needs of, the attenders. Many primary care providers have had little extra training in recognizing and treating patients with mental disorders since their initial clinical training. The continuing education that is available tends to be driven by the needs of the pharmaceutical industry or specialist mental health services, and is at variance with the practicalities of primary care. There is an urgent need to improve the knowledge and the skill base of primary care providers.

Innovative solutions are required to increase skills and knowledge. The WHO has developed a primary care education program to improve the recognition and management of common mental disorders in primary care (World Health Organization, 1996a). The WHO Collaborating Centre in Sydney has produced a practical workbook that is being published in Australian, UK, Canadian and Italian versions (Treatment Protocol Project, 1997). In summary, primary care providers need to be educated to recognize and treat people with mental disorders, be supported by ancillary staff to provide nondrug therapies, and be able to involve patients to increase their knowledge of, and compliance and collaboration with, self-management programs and groups.

Primary care services are not optimally organized to deliver mental health care

Primary care physicians are seldom given any structural incentives or appropriate reimbursement for providing mental health services. Short visits and the lack of continuous personal care for patients exhaust physicians and dissatisfy consumers. Several experimental approaches have demonstrated the successful use of auxiliary personnel (e.g., nurses, counselors) trained in mental health skills. Self-help programs for consumers could be equally effective for relatively mild cases, and computer programs could help by doing standard tasks such as screening, monitoring, or patient education.

General strategies of health care financing and organization

In this era when needs are growing and resources are limited a balance must be found between both the cost and affordability of services. Hence managing care has become inevitable. Previously, the doctor made a plan and the patient agreed to it and either the patient or the insurer paid the bill. This open-ended approach often led to increased premiums and spiraling health care costs. No country is able to afford this arrangement and rationing is inevitable (Andrews, 1997; Bobadilla, Cowley, Musgrove & Saxenian, 1994). What has emerged is a replacement of the clinician as the ultimate decision maker with the most stringent criteria for medical necessity that defines need. The control is shifted upwards, from the provider-client to the third party insurance companies, to fourth party 'utilization review firms', and fifth party 'payers of bills'. Mega-systems are emerging to finance, provide, and manage health care services, systems that are quite remote from considerations of the patient's need and the clinician's ability to meet that need.

Instead of emphasis on cost-effectiveness the emphasis may be placed on cutting costs and providing a less intensive style of care for a sick population. On the good side, this system may bring rational planning and parity of mental and physical disorders. Nevertheless many of the developments have not resulted in a rational treatment policy based on routine outcome assessment. How should we organize society's resources to get the most health gain, most equitable deployment of resources, and to serve those who are in greatest need? Certainly primary care and mental health care delivery will be at the core of this development (Rice, Kelman & Miller, 1992) for primary care is the place where the 'rubber hits the road'.

The needs assessment strategy is changing

Needs assessment was once to be understood in the context of hospital-based care, with a single portion of the health care sector being the focus for needs assessment. The parameters of this model were things such as availability of services, expressed in terms of the number of psychiatric beds, distribution of psychiatrists, staffing requirements, and funding allotments from national and local agencies. It examined the magnitude of the illness in the community and estimated the proportion seeking health care from primary care or emergency services. Some exemplary work was done in the early detection of new cases, continued care of stable older cases, prevention of illness in at-risk populations, and health promotion among the overall population. This systematic needs-assessment approach was mainly focused on whether severely ill, usually psychotic, patients could be placed in the community (Phelan et al., 1995). What were these patients not able to do? What could be done in terms of service provision to make them able to participate in the community and remain out of asylums? The answers were mainly to provide a protected environment, possibly family care, effective treatment, rehabilitation programs, and to make services available for support and crisis intervention (Bebbinton, Brewin, Marsden & Lesage, 1996; el-Guebaly, Kingstone, Rae-Grant & Fyfe, 1993; Ferguson, Cooper, Brothwell, Markantonakis & Tyrer, 1992). Primary care services were not considered providers of these types of service, since primary care physicians were not properly trained and were already overburdened by patients with other types of mental disorders.

While this approach was useful, it is important to explore needs more comprehensively. In a framework of competing demands, we need a single currency to evaluate and compare needs, a currency in which objective indicators are presented in an integrated fashion. In other words, should we base the need-resource equation on specific mental health care needs, or see it in the context of the whole global burden of disease argument?

Introduction of the DALY concept

Estimation of needs for health services, their cost and effectiveness require indicators that go beyond measures of death rates or diagnosis, and include the functioning of individuals. The Global Burden of Disease (GBD) project was carried out by the World Bank in collaboration with the World Health Organization (World Bank, 1993; World Health Organization, 1996b) and was designed to address three main goals:

- To provide information on *nonfatal health outcomes* to inform international health policy which until then had focused on mortality.
- To develop *unbiased epidemiological assessments* of the frequency of major disorders.
- To *quantify the burden of disease* with a measure that could also be used *for cost-effectiveness analysis.*

The GBD project aimed to produce internally consistent estimates of mortality and the disabling sequelae of the 107 major diseases, divided into three large groups: communicable, maternal and perinatal diseases; noncommunicable diseases; and injuries. The study also estimated the fraction of mortality and disability attributable to ten major risk factors. It developed various projections of mortality and disability for 2020 by cause, age, sex, and region. The results of the GBD project were presented using a common metric of disability-adjusted life years (DALYs). DALYs are time-based health-outcome measures, the inverse of quality-adjusted life years, that include weights for time spent in less-than-perfect health. The results were based on *years of life lost* because of premature death (YLLs) and *years of life lived with disability* (YLDs). In summary, one DALY is one lost year of healthy life (Murray, 1994): DALY = YLL + YLD (burden = mortality + disability).

As this approach shows, DALYs reflect the total burden by taking into account mortality and disability, which is argued to be a sound approach for setting priorities in health resource allocation (Murray & Lopez, 1996). The GBD project provides a framework for estimating the portion of the burden that could be averted by increasing the coverage and effectiveness of services, and the use of cost-effective interventions (Jamison, Saxenian & Bergevin, 1995; World Health Organization, 1996b).

Conclusions

The burden of mental disorders in primary care constitutes a public health priority (Jenkins, 1997). Most cases of common mental disorders in primary care settings are not adequately recognized and treated (Üstün, 1993). Common mental disorders are often persistent, long-term or relapsing conditions. The public health burden of mental disorders calls for an immediate implementation of available tools. The implementation should go hand-in-hand with constant monitoring and evaluation as to whether training and implementation programs are effective. The following suggestions can be made regarding possible developments to deal with the unmet need for mental disorders in primary care.

1. Primary care should be seen as an important setting in which to deliver mental health care. Primary care should be seen as the first and foremost layer of the health care system and, as such, the structure should be organized to deliver mental health care. There should be incentives to provide mental health services and to promote mental health. The system should be evaluated and updated regularly.

2. Primary care should be seen as requiring *teamwork*. No single primary care provider in solo practice can possibly handle all the services necessary to meet the mental health care needs of a community. In the primary care team, physicians, physician assistants, nurses, and community health workers should combine their skills and efforts to appropriately provide services. They should be trained as a workforce that delivers these services in response to the health care needs of the community. Their *training* should be focused on the *skills and competencies* that match these needs.

3. Creation of a *Management Strategy* for common mental disorders in primary care is essential. These disorders require long-term care and carefully planned management strategies. We need to link detection and classification tools with management tools. This linkage has proved to be useful in the example of ICD-10 PC (Üstün, Goldberg, Cooper, Simon & Sartorius, 1995; World Health Organization, 1996a). In addition, local adaptations of management guidelines are necessary to develop best practice (Treatment Protocol Project, 1997). Management strategies should include the use of psychosocial interventions and cognitive-behavioral techniques.

4. The training and services provided should be based on state-of-the-art reviews of available knowledge, tailored for the primary care level. Wherever possible this information should be *evidence-based* with proof of effectiveness in primary care settings. Whenever such data are not available, there should be *consensus-based guidelines* for standard procedures that involve primary care providers, mental health experts, and staff from related agencies.

5. These diagnostic and management guidelines, and the training programs should be continuously evaluated for their accuracy, applicability, efficacy, and effectiveness. These guidelines should be periodically revised in light of the experience gained in their use, and innovations in practice.

6. Programs directed at increasing public awareness and reducing stigma

are important at a local level. The composition of a *primary care team* (e.g., physicians, nurses, other social work personnel, information officers) and its impact on service delivery and outcomes of treatment should be studied for alternative models.

7. These strategies should be incorporated in overall primary care programs which include components such as *screening of high-risk groups* (e.g., screening for depression in multiparous pregnant women) and *prevention of a relapse* in recurrent disorders.

8. Evaluation of the effectiveness of treatments should be identified and primary care teams should be encouraged to explore the best ways of achieving their targets. These outcome criteria may include reducing symptoms, disability, the duration of the illness, as well as direct and indirect costs, and increasing the quality of life, and patient satisfaction. The measurement of outcome should be routine.

More information is needed on:

- The *decision to seek care* by those people who are identified as cases in community surveys (Jacomb et al., 1997). We need to know their pathways to primary care and alternative carers, and the barriers to seeking care.
- The mental health needs of *children and adolescents* (Burns et al., 1995).
- The *routine use of screening* for mental disorders in primary care. While there is a need for *rapid identification* of patients with mental health problems, the effectiveness and efficiency of this process needs to be demonstrated.
- The structure and organization of primary care, i.e., *descriptive parameters*. Since primary care is heterogeneous, one needs a system to identify whether this is a personal care appointment system or a clinical care walk-in system; one needs to record the *time* allocated for each encounter, the *volume and flow* of patients, and the *linkage with specialty settings*.

In addition to the above, systems for auditing primary care services for *quality assurance* purposes have to be developed and implemented (Marks, 1992; Tien, 1992). The direct and indirect costs and gains of primary care mental health services (per intervention, per disorder) should be measured routinely in research on interventions. These are important for informing planning and priority setting. The impact of *reimbursement schemes* on the *process of primary mental health care* should also be systematically reviewed in an attempt to identify better methods of service delivery.

In conclusion, mental disorders constitute a public health problem as reflected by their significant contribution to the global burden of disease. Primary care is the principal tool with which to deal with this burden. Mental health must be an integral component of primary care. We have the knowledge base and the evidence base to avert some of this burden through primary care. We need to extend the coverage and effectiveness of interventions for mental disorders in primary care. The response to this public health problem should go beyond the traditional 'lip-service' of sporadic studies and should be conceived as a global strategy. There is considerable experience and knowledge of the mental health components in primary care gained from a worldwide network of centers (Üstün and Jenkins, 1997). Once this knowledge and experience is integrated into practice, we will have more comprehensive services and more meaningful and satisfactory outcomes.

References

Andrews, G. (1996). Talk that works: the rise of cognitive behavioural therapy. *British Medical Journal*, **313**, 1501–2.

Andrews, G. (1997). Managing scarcity: a worked example using burden and efficacy. *Australian Psychiatry*, **5**, 225–7.

Bebbington, P., Brewin, C.R., Marsden, L. & Lesage, A. (1996). Measuring the need for psychiatric treatment in the general population: the community version of the MRC needs for care assessment. *Psychological Medicine*, **26**, 229–36.

Bobadilla, J.-L., Cowley, P., Musgrove, P. & Saxenian, H. (1994). Design, content and financing of an essential national package of health services. In C.J.L. Murray & A.D. Lopez (eds.), *Global Comparative Assessments in the Health Sector: Disease Burden, Expenditures and Intervention Packages*. Geneva: World Health Organization.

Burns, B.J., Costello, E.J., Angold, A., Tweed, D., Stangl, D., Farmer, E.M. & Erkanli, A. (1995). Children's mental health service use across service sectors. *Health Affairs*, **14**, 147–59.

el-Guebaly, N., Kingstone, E., Rae-Grant, Q. & Fyfe, I. (1993). The geographical distribution of psychiatrists in Canada: unmet needs and remedial strategies. *Canadian Journal Psychiatry*, **38**, 212–16.

Ferguson, B., Cooper, S., Brothwell, J., Markantonakis, A. & Tyrer, P. (1992). The clinical evaluation of a new community psychiatric service based on general practice psychiatric clinics. *British Journal of Psychiatry*, **160**, 493–7.

Gater, R., de Almeida e Sousa, B., Barrientos, G., Caraveo, J., Chandrashekar, C.R., Dhadphale, M., Goldberg, D., al Kathiri, A.H., Mubbashar, M., Silhan, K. et al. (1991). The pathways to psychiatric care: a cross cultural study. *Psychological Medicine*, **21**, 761–74.

Goldberg, D.P. & Huxley, P. (1992). *Common Mental Disorders: A Biosocial Model*. London: Routledge & Kegan Paul.

Häfner, H. (1977). *Epidemiologically Based Needs Assessment*. Berlin: Springer-Verlag.

Harding, T.W., Climent, C.E., Diop, M., Giel, R., Ibrahim, H.H.A., Murthy, R.S., Suleiman, M.A. & Wig, N.N. (1983a). The WHO collaborative study on strategies for extending mental health care. II: The development of new research methods. *American Journal of Psychiatry*, **140**, 1474–80.

Harding, T.W., d'Arrigo Busnello, E., Climent, C.E., Diop, M., El-Hakim, A., Giel, R., Ibrahim, H.H.A., Ladrigo-Ignacio, L. & Wig, N.N. (1983b). The WHO collaborative study on strategies for extending mental health care. III: Evaluative design and illustrative results. *American Journal of Psychiatry*, 140, 1481–5.

Jacomb, P.A., Jorm, A.F., Korten, A.E., Rodgers, B., Henderson, S. & Christensen, H. (1997). GP attendance by elderly Australians: evidence for unmet need in elderly men. *Medical Journal of Australia*, 166, 123–6.

Jamison, D.T., Saxenian, H. & Bergevin, Y. (1995). Investing in health wisely. The role of needs-based technology assessment. *International Journal of Technology Assessment in Health Care*, 11, 673–84.

Jenkins, R. (1997). Reducing the burden of mental illness. *Lancet*, 349, 1340.

Jenkins, R. & Üstün, T.B. (eds.) (1997). *Preventing Mental Illness: Mental Health Promotion in Primary Care*. Chichester: John Wiley & Sons.

Kessler, R.C., McGonagle, K.A., Zhao, S., Nelson, C.B., Hughes, M., Eshleman, S., Wittchen, H-U. & Kendler, K.S. (1994). Lifetime and twelve month prevalence of DSM-III-R psychiatric disorders in the United States. *Archives of General Psychiatry*, 51, 8–19.

Klerman, G.L., Olfson, M., Leon, A.C. & Weissman, M.M. (1992). Measuring the need for mental health care. *Health Affairs*, 11, 23–33.

Knapp, M., Beecham, J., Fenyo, A. & Hallam, A. (1995). Community mental health care for former hospital in-patients. Predicting costs from needs and diagnoses. *British Journal of Psychiatry, Supplement*, 27, 10–18.

Lesage, A.D., Fournier, L., Cyr, M., Toupin, J., Fabian, J., Gaudette, G., Vanier, C., Bebbington, P.E. & Brewin, C.R. (1996). The reliability of the community version of the MRC needs for care assessment. *Psychological Medicine*, 26, 237–43.

Marks, I. (1992). Innovations in mental health care delivery. *British Journal of Psychiatry*, 160, 589–97.

Murray, C.J.L. (1994). Quantifying the burden of disease: the technical basis for disability-adjusted life years. *Bulletin of the World Health Organization*, 72, 429–45.

Murray, C.J.L. & Lopez, A.D. (1996). Evidence-based health policy – lessons from the Global Burden of Disease Study. *Science*, 274, 740–3.

Murray, C.J.L. & Lopez, A.D. (1997). Global mortality, disability, and the contribution of risk factors: Global Burden of Disease Study. *Lancet*, 349, 1436–42.

Murthy, R.S. & Wig, N.N. (1983). The WHO collaborative study on strategies for extending mental health care. IV: A training approach to enhancing the availability of mental health manpower in a developing country. *American Journal of Psychiatry*, 140, 1486–90.

Ormel, J., Von Korff, M., Üstün, T.B., Pini, S., Korten, A. & Oldehinkel, T. (1994). Common mental disorders and disability across cultures. Results from the WHO collaborative study on psychological problems in general health care. *Journal of the American Medical Association*, 272, 1741–8.

Phelan, M., Slade, M., Thornicroft, G., Dunn, G., Holloway, F., Wykes, T., Strathdee, G., Loftus, L., McCrone, P. & Hayward, P. (1995). The Camberwell Assessment of Need: the validity and reliability of an instrument to assess the needs of people with severe mental illness. *British Journal of Psychiatry*, 167, 589–95.

Regier, D.A., Narrow, W.E., Rae, D.S., Manderscheid, R.W., Locke, B.Z. & Goodwin, F.K. (1993). The DeFacto US Mental and Addictive Disorders System. *Archives of General Psychiatry*, 50, 85–94.

Rice, D.P., Kelman, S. & Miller, L.S. (1992). The economic burden of mental illness. *Hospital and Community Psychiatry*, **43**, 1227–32.

Sartorius, N. & Harding, T.W. (1983). The WHO collaborative study on strategies for extending mental health care. I: The genesis of the study. *American Journal of Psychiatry*, **140**, 1470–3.

Thornicroft, G., Brewin, C.R. & Wing, J. (1992). *Measuring Mental Health Needs.* London: Gaskell.

Tien, L. (1992). Determinants of equality and equity for special populations served by public mental health systems. *Hospital and Community Psychiatry*, **43**, 1104–8.

Treatment Protocol Project (1997). *The Management of Mental Disorders* (2nd edition). Sydney: World Health Organization Collaborating Centre for Mental Health and Substance Abuse.

Turnbull, S., Ward, A., Treasure, J., Jick, H. & Derby, L. (1996). The demand for eating disorder care. An epidemiological study using the general practice research database. *British Journal of Psychiatry*, **169**, 705–12.

Üstün, T.B. (1993). Public health aspects of anxiety and depressive disorders. *International Clinical Psychopharmacology*, **8**, 15–20.

Üstün, T.B. (1994). WHO Collaborative Study: an epidemiological survey of psychological problems in general health care in 15 centers worldwide. *International Review of Psychiatry*, **6**, 357–63.

Üstün, T.B. (1996). A new paradigm – assessment of functioning and the WHO's ICIDH (editorial). *South African Medical Journal*, **86** [Suppl. 12], 1575.

Üstün, T.B. (1997). The primary care setting relevance, advantages, challenges. In R. Jenkins & T.B. Üstün (eds.), *Preventing Mental Illness: Mental Health Promotion in Primary Care.* Chichester: John Wiley & Sons.

Üstün, T.B. & Gater, R. (1994). Integrating mental health into primary care. *Current Opinion in Psychiatry*, **7**, 173–80.

Üstün, T.B. & Jenkins, R. (1997). Epilogue: the way forward – proposals for action. In R. Jenkins & T.B. Üstün (eds.), *Preventing Mental Illness: Mental Health Promotion in Primary Care.* Chichester: John Wiley & Sons.

Üstün, T.B. & Sartorius, N. (1995). *Mental Illness in General Health Care: An International Study.* Chichester: Wiley & Sons (for the World Health Organization).

Üstün, T.B., Goldberg, D., Cooper, J., Simon, G.E. & Sartorius, N. (1995). New classification for mental disorders with management guidelines for use in primary care: ICD-10 PHC chapter five. *British Journal of General Practice*, April, 211–15.

Von Korff, M., Üstün, T.B. & Ormel, J. (1996). Self-report disability in an international primary care study of psychological illness. *Journal of Clinical Epidemiology*, **49**, 297–303.

World Bank (1993). *World Development Report, 1993: Investing in Health.* Oxford: Oxford University Press.

World Health Organization (1996a). *Diagnostic and Management Guidelines for Mental Disorders in Primary Care. ICD-10 Chapter V Primary Care Version.* Göttingen: Hogrefe & Huber Publishers (for the World Health Organization).

World Health Organization (1996b). *Investing in Health Research and Development: Report of the Ad Hoc Committee on Health Research Relating to Future Intervention*

Options. Geneva: World Health Organization.

World Health Organization (1997). *International Classification of Impairments, Activities and Participation. A Manual of Dimensions of Disablement and Functioning. Beta-1 draft for field trials*, pp. 1–272. Geneva: World Health Organization.

12

Is complementary medicine filling needs that could be met by orthodox medicine?

John E. Cooper

Summary

Some aspects of complementary (or alternative) medicine are examined in the social and cultural settings of countries that also have an elaborate and widely available medical service based upon modern scientific medicine (called 'orthodox' medicine). It is often thought that complementary treatments can have a good effect, although brief, on almost anybody who uses them. It is also likely that persons with certain psychiatric disorders get a more lasting benefit from some types of complementary treatments, although not always for the reasons assumed by either the user or the therapist. As yet, no studies have been done to test these suggestions, but the case seems strong enough to justify the effort and expense of collaborative investigations. There is also a good case for regularly including some systematic information about complementary treatments in the curriculum of orthodox medical schools, rather than to continue the current practice of ignoring the subject.

Introduction

The results of recent surveys in Europe, the USA, and Australia show that complementary treatments must be providing something that is regarded as important by large sections of the adult population of those countries (Eisenberg et al., 1993; Fisher & Ward, 1994; MacLennan, Wilson & Tatlor, 1996; 'Which?', 1995). The findings are so striking and consistent that the orthodox medical profession would be well advised to try to assess how much the large and increasing industry of complementary medicine is meeting needs that could or should be met by orthodox medical services. For instance:

1. All the surveys agree that about one-half of the adult population uses complementary treatments at some time in their life, and that as many as one-third uses them repeatedly or even regularly. About half of these users are dissatisfied with the orthodox treatment they have received, often for

long-standing conditions. Many are comparatively young, and all need to pay for the treatment.

2. Estimates from the same surveys suggest that the total amount spent on complementary treatments is of the same order of magnitude as the amount spent on orthodox medical treatments. The most recent survey, in Australia, estimated that more was spent on complementary treatments than on orthodox ones (MacLennan et al., 1996).

3. More than half of all medical students would like to learn something about complementary treatments during their orthodox training (Furnham, 1993), and in the UK about half of the general public would like complementary treatments to be available on the National Health Service.

4. Increasing demands are being made for the inclusion of some teaching on complementary treatments in the curriculum in orthodox medical schools (Goodman, 1997; Rampes, Sharples, Maragh & Fisher, 1997).

Some selected aspects of complementary treatments will be discussed here, but no attempt will be made to comprehensively describe or classify the large number of different treatments that come under the general term. A list provided later in the chapter contains most of the better known types, and is sufficient for the present purposes. A useful account of these and others can be found in a recent publication by the Consumers Association of the UK ('Which?', 1996), and in the latest publication by the British Medical Association on this subject (British Medical Association, 1993) and journals devoted to complementary medicine, such as *Acupuncture in Medicine, Alternative Therapies in Health and Medicine, American Journal of Chinese Medicine, British Homeopathic Journal, Complementary Therapies in Medicine, Complementary Medical Research, European Journal of Oriental Medicine, European Journal of Herbal Medicine, Journal of the American Osteopathic Association, Journal of Alternative and Complementary Medicine, Journal of Manipulative and Physiological Therapeutics,* and *The Homeopath*.

The term 'complementary' is used here in preference to 'alternative', since alternative implies that it might be reasonable to use such treatments instead of orthodox treatments, rather than after an orthodox treatment has been tried. Since there is no robust evidence that the majority of complementary treatments have any effect upon physical disorders, there are clear dangers of delayed identification of potentially dangerous disorders if orthodox services are not used first.

This chapter is in three parts: first, a brief discussion of what comes under the general term of complementary medicine, with a small number of examples; second, a general discussion of why people believe things to be true; and, third, suggestions about why complementary treatments may have good effects for some people.

Varieties of complementary treatments

There is a major problem in that it is currently conventional to include a wide variety of procedures in the term complementary treatments. Their most obvious shared feature is that they are types of treatment or healing that are not part of the medical curriculum in orthodox medical schools, but much would be gained if a more informative and rational classification or grouping could be agreed. Some complementary treatments have organizations that look after standards of training, and some, such as osteopathy and chiropractic, are offshoots of some parts of orthodox medicine. Many others are completely different to, and separate from, any aspects of orthodox medicine, and are based upon ideas about vibrations or life forces for which there is no scientific evidence.

Currently available complementary therapies

Group 1. Complete traditional systems available before 1790:

1. Traditional Chinese medicine (acupuncture, moxibustion, herbal remedies, shiatsu, tai-chi-chuan).
2. Ayurvedic medicine (India).
3. Western herbal medicine.

Group 2. Systems developed after 1790:

1. Emphasis on the technique (useful for anything): hypnosis and relaxation, laying on of hands (spirit healing), naturopathy, crystal therapy, iridology (iris of eye), metamorphic technique, reflexology (soles of feet).
2. Emphasis on specific remedies for particular ailments: homeopathy, bach flower remedies, aromatherapy, color therapy.
3. Effect limited to one system or one part of body: osteopathy, chiropractic, colonic lavage, Alexander technique (posture), rolfing (a form of painful massage intended to relieve tensions by relaxing and repositioning muscles).
4. Distant healing (most of these act by facilitating or rebalancing a 'life-force' or vibrations): radiesthesia; radionics.

The date of 1790 has no great significance, but is chosen for convenience partly because homeopathy was developed around that time. In addition, what we now call the scientific method of investigation began about then. The members of Group 1 are several thousand years old, but are still widely used. In their countries of origin, traditional Chinese medicine and Ayurvedic medicine (from the Indian subcontinent) are still taught as formal systems of healing in special colleges that award degrees recognized by their respective governments.

Group 2 is subdivided by: (1) emphasis on the technique, which is useful for almost anything; (2) emphasis on specific remedies for particular ailments; (3) emphasis on one system or part of the body; and (4) the unique fact that the physical presence of the person being healed is not required. They are grouped merely for convenience, and there is considerable overlap. Many of these treatments are believed to act by means of rebalancing a 'life-force', or through vibrations and fundamental powers that pervade and affect everything.

This list does not include a large number of spurious treatments for cancer; these appear from time to time, and disappear equally quickly. They are usually promulgated by one individual for obvious profit, and are quite separate from established complementary systems and practitioners. There is also no mention in this chapter of religious healing carried out within an accepted religious framework. No comments are made, or implied, about what might or might not happen in the setting of sincere religious faith of any denomination.

Only brief comments will be made on a few selected complementary treatments, chosen to illustrate why so many orthodox doctors find it difficult to take this whole subject seriously, particularly if they are interested in medical research.

Acupuncture has always been an important part of traditional Chinese medicine, along with moxibustion, the feeling of the pulse at the wrist, and Chinese herbal remedies. These are all linked together by the principles of life-energy, *qi*, which has two component forces, *yin* and *yan*. These are opposites, and exist in all of nature. *Yin* is associated with darkness, rest, earth, inwardness, downwardness, femaleness, and water; whereas *Yan* is associated with light, activity, energy, expansion, upwards, maleness, and fire. The human body is supposed to contain a large number of invisible channels or meridians, along which these two components of the life-energy *qi* must flow for normal life and functioning. When the *yin* and *yan* are in balance, all is well. When *qi* becomes blocked, deficient or stagnant because of imbalance of the flow of *yin* and *yan*, illness results.

It is believed that by placing fine needles in special points along the meridians, the *qi* can be stimulated to get the flow and balance back to normal. In *moxibustion*, the same points are stimulated by burning a very small piece of dry vegetable fluff on them for a few seconds. The same points can also be stimulated by pressure, massage, or electricity. The meridians have names and many points; over 200 points have to be learned if the traditional approach is taken seriously. The meridians are invisible, and do not correspond with any known anatomical structures.

Ayurvedic medicine, originating in India and Sri Lanka, is, like traditional

Chinese medicine, a comprehensive system of ideas based upon a concept of a life force (*ojas*) which needs to be in balance for good health to be achieved and maintained. The five basic elements of fire, water, earth, air, and ether are combined in the human body in various and individually different proportions to produce three 'humors' which influence the health and temperament of each person. The balance of these for each person can be corrected by such things as certain foods, drinks, sexual gratification, light, fresh air, and spiritual activities. A process of 'detoxification' by warmth, massage with special oils, special diets, various herbal remedies, yoga exercises, and meditation are also commonly used. Ayurvedic medicine is possibly even older than the Chinese system.

Homeopathy (originally and often still spelt homoeopathy) is based on the principle 'let like be treated by like', an ancient folk belief that can be traced back to the Delphic Oracle and Hippocrates. Administration of a substance that produces effects similar to the symptoms of a disease is supposed to help a person with that disease to fight against it. This idea is certainly ancient, but it has no logical or scientific justification. The reasonable precaution is taken of diluting the supposedly active substances used as medicines before giving them to the patient, but herein lies another difficulty for the orthodox doctor. A commonly used technique is to dilute the active principle 1 in 99, thirty times in sequence, shaking the solution vigorously between each process of dilution. This gives a final dilution of 10^{-60}, which means that it is unlikely for even one molecule of the original active agent to be present in a dose given to a patient. This is not a problem for the homeopathic therapist, because the dilution is compensated for by a parallel belief that the solution has become 'potentiated' by the shaking after each dilution, and that the curative power is somehow carried through to the next stage.

Iridology and *reflexology* have a major principle in common, in that both depend upon the idea that the whole body is represented in miniature on one small part of itself; for iridology, this is the iris of the eyes; and for reflexology, it is the soles of the feet. For reflexology, massage of the specific areas that represent the various organs of the body is supposed to produce a restorative effect.

Common features of complementary treatments

The treatments on this list are so varied and different that it is natural to ask whether they have anything in common that can be usefully identified, apart from the point, already noted, that none are taught in orthodox medical schools. One basic feature stands out: that the concepts of life-force, vibrations, energies, balances and such-like, upon which these complementary treatments are based, are fixed and unchanging for all time. These ideas are not expected to be developed or to change as new discoveries are made about the nature of ourselves and the world around us. This contrasts fundamentally with orthodox anatomy, physiology, and biochemistry, which are continually changing as new discoveries are made; discoveries that result in new treatments being devised and tested, and in old treatments being discarded.

To some users of complementary medicine, this quality of a supposed timeless, eternal truthfulness is an attractive feature rather than a disadvantage. Other differences with orthodox medicine (see below) are to do with the self-selection of users of complementary medicine. Orthodox medical services have to deal with all comers from total populations, and are the basis of successful public health campaigns, ranging from the importance of clean water to mass immunization and vaccination of children. These are not features of complementary medicine. For interested readers, Ernst (1995) discusses some common misconceptions about complementary treatments.

Some differences between orthodox and complementary systems and treatments

Orthodox medicine
1. Orthodox medicine is based on current scientific concepts of anatomy, physiology, biochemistry, etc.
2. The basis of orthodox medicine and its treatments are expected to evolve and change.
3. Orthodox medicine serves whole populations.
4. Orthodox medicine is the basis of successful preventative and prophylactic health campaigns.

Complementary medicine
1. Complementary medicine is based on beliefs for which there is no scientific evidence.
2. The beliefs and the treatments do not change.
3. Users are self-selected.
4. No use of prevention or prophylaxis.

The popularity of complementary medicine

The size and costs of the complementary medicine industry have already been noted, and it is important to try to understand why the present degree of popularity has been reached. Some positive reasons for this arise from the nature of the consultation. This will be examined in detail later, but there are also several more general reasons worth noting.

Whatever the type of complementary medicine being used, it is common to find that the consultation lasts for 45–60 minutes, and that a very personal approach is used. Often the individual's uniqueness is emphasized, as is the need to tailor the details of the treatment to the patient's particular personality and background. In other words, from the customer's viewpoint, the face value and acceptability of the whole procedure are likely to be high, even though the eventual effectiveness may be low. This contrasts with many consultations with orthodox doctors, where these qualities may be reversed; an effective remedy may be rapidly prescribed for an identified physical or psychiatric disorder, but the patient may not be given much information about either the nature of the illness or the reasons why the treatment will be effective (Ernst, Resch & Hill, 1997).

Another reason for the popularity of complementary therapies is that famous and respected people have often stated publicly that they use and recommend them. Homeopathy, for instance, has been associated with various members of the British Royal Family since the 1830s (manifest in the continued and prosperous presence of the Royal Homeopathic Hospital in London). Other declared enthusiasts over the years include John D. Rockefeller Snr., Mahatma Ghandi, Yehudi Menuhin, and Tina Turner.

The views of orthodox doctors and their organizations about complementary medicine

Some orthodox doctors reject this subject completely, and say openly and forcefully that any investigation of complementary treatments is a waste of time because of the ridiculous theories upon which they are based (Baum, 1989; Skrabenek, 1986). At the other extreme are those doctors who, after qualifying in the usual way in orthodox medicine, then study and take some sort of diploma or certificate in an alternative system, such as homeopathy, acupuncture, chiropractic or osteopathy; they then add these to the range of treatments that they offer to their patients, or they may become specialists in the subject.

Most orthodox medical practitioners are probably somewhere in the middle, accepting that perhaps some of the treatments are occasionally useful for some people, although not having much faith in the mysterious mechanisms that are claimed to be responsible. The attitude of medical organizations such as the British Medical Association (BMA) has changed a great deal in the last ten years or so. A BMA publication in 1986 was rather disapproving, but in 1993 the BMA published 'Complementary Medicine: a Guide to Good Practice' which accepts that cautious collaboration between general practitioners and selected complementary practitioners may be appropriate if the patient so requests. It recommends that the orthodox general practitioner keeps clinical responsibility for the patient and is kept informed of progress (British Medical Association, 1993).

The World Health Organization (WHO) is responsible for providing all countries with advice about health services, and since what we are calling complementary treatment is all that is easily available to many of the world's population, its policies are naturally sympathetic. Since WHO must also be committed to scientific advances in health care (seen, for instance, in the remarkably successful smallpox vaccination campaign and in efforts to improve infant and child health), some uneasy compromises have to be achieved if traditional and orthodox medical care have to be integrated. A series of publications has been produced over the last 15 years or so by a small Traditional Medicine Unit at WHO Geneva, and some of their titles, indicating the contents of this program, are given below:

- 1991 A proposed standard international acupuncture nomenclature.
- 1991 Guidelines for the assessment of herbal medicines.
- 1995 Guidelines for clinical research on acupuncture.
- 1995 Guidelines for safe acupuncture treatment.
- 1996 Guidelines for training traditional health practitioners in primary health care.

This present chapter is based on the view that intolerant rejection is an error, and shows a misunderstanding of the nature of scientific knowledge and the purposes of scientific enquiry. The history of scientific investigation contains many instances of the arrogant dismissal by prominent scientists of unexpected new discoveries (and the abuse of those who made them) on the grounds that the new and surprising findings could not possibly be true since they did not fit in with the currently accepted orthodoxy of the day. There is an important difference between scepticism (healthy and useful), and dogmatism (arrogant and blinkered). Healthy scepticism should also be tempered by a degree of tolerance, and by an acceptance that it is often wise to say, 'I don't know, and surprising things occasionally turn out to be true'.

The beliefs of complementary practitioners about how their remedies work

Some common themes emerge: first, almost always treatment of the whole person is emphasized (that is, no separation of mind from body, together with adjustment of balance or harmony with the environment). Nowadays, almost all orthodox doctors also claim to treat the whole person, but there is an important difference here – most orthodox treatments or operations are directed at a specific function or part of the person, and it is the doctor who claims to bear the whole person (or family) in mind when deciding on the various parts of the overall management and treatment program. Even when this is genuinely the case, it may not be evident to the patient, particularly when the orthodox doctor tries to explain how the specific treatment or operation works. The concept of the patient, family, and environment as a complex interactive system may well be guiding the treatment decisions of an orthodox doctor, but this is easily obscured from the patient's viewpoint by the attention given to technical details (often necessary to ensure that the treatment is correctly administered). In contrast, for most of the complementary therapies it is the treatment itself that is supposed to act on the whole person and the balance between person and environment. This point is usually declared early, and often emphasized repeatedly by the therapist – indeed, it is often one of the main reasons why complementary treatment is being sought by the patient.

Second, authors of books and papers on complementary treatments usually make it abundantly clear that they believe without a shadow of doubt in the truth of their theories and the effectiveness of their treatments. They are entitled to believe whatever they like, but it is necessary to be clear about the basis of these beliefs. A frequent problem is that such books and articles almost always claim that there is abundant *scientific* evidence for these treatments, and that therefore other people should agree to their having the same status as orthodox treatments. This assertion is strongly refuted by orthodox medical scientists and educators. In this disagreement about what is 'scientific' evidence, we find one of the key issues that must be faced when trying to understand the nature and popularity of complementary medicines. A brief diversion into a discussion of what people regard as evidence, or, in other words, the reasons why people believe things to be true, is justified here.

Reasons why people believe things to be true

A. Inner certainty (a personal belief that is usually neither caused nor changed by experience of specific events, and that is not changed by any sort of evidence).
B. Statements by an accepted authority.
C. The personal experience of one person (sincere personal testimony) – *subjective evidence.*
D. The agreed opinion of several people, based on their own experience and/or general knowledge (everybody knows; stands to reason; commonsense) – *objective evidence.*
E. A set of observations that are consistent with a stated aim or hypothesis, made by one or more persons (usually professionals) using agreed methods/techniques – *systematic evidence.*
F. Repeated observations by several professional workers involving controlled comparisons that are subject to statistical analysis – *scientific evidence.*

Above is a list of reasons why people accept as true what other people tell them. It is, of course, a rather crude summary of many difficult and complicated issues. The categories A to F can all be subdivided in various ways, but this is not necessary for the purposes of this present discussion. Most decisions in everyday life, when dealing with other ordinary individuals with whom there is no quarrel, are determined by variable mixtures of A, B, C, and D. This is reasonable and practical, since most people can be trusted and believed.

These categories are adequate for most daily decisions, but something more elaborate is needed for the study and understanding of the disciplines often called 'the humanities', such as history, economics, social psychology, and social anthropology. Category E (called 'systematic' for convenience) comes into play here; it is also the basis of evidence for much of clinical psychopathology and many types of psychotherapy (including psychoanalysis). However, the position is quite different when we come to learning about how to understand, control, and use the physical world around us with modern technology (for example, motor cars, airplanes, electricity, television, and computers), and how to understand the strange and delicate processes hidden inside our minds and bodies which determine whether we are healthy and happy, or miserable.

The development of modern technology depends on the use of category F, that is the accumulation and use of scientific (or controlled) evidence. This is very different from the usually acceptable categories A to D, and also different from the more elaborately constructed 'systematic' category E. Historically, while the body of knowledge about the world and ourselves remained at or above the level of E, progress in understanding it was very slow, and technology quite limited. When category F became widely recognized and applied to establish the beginnings of physics and chemistry about 200 years ago, powerful technology was also able to develop, and our daily lives (and later our medical treatments) were progressively transformed. The word progressive is the key to a great deal of the difference between the slow changes of the prescientific eras, and what we are now faced with in the modern era of information explosions and technical developments.

The difference between E and F is of special importance for the present discussion. A key aspect of category F is that the observations can be repeated by other people. Anything that fails to be confirmed by people other than those who made the original observation is not included in this category. In addition, other possible explanations for whatever effect is being studied are eliminated as far as possible by designing the experiment with this in mind; this is what is meant by the perhaps rather optimistic term 'controlled'. In assessing medical treatments, it is particularly important to try to eliminate observer bias (honest and nonpurposeful), and also the natural tendency for symptoms to change that is always present to some degree. There are several other and unavoidable sources of variation in measurements of change in controlled experiment, but, since they are usually small and may go either way, for simplicity they can be left out of the present discussion. They are well summarized in Resch & Ernst (1996).

There are, of course, many decisions made during orthodox medical practice and general patient management that cannot and should not fulfil the conditions of F. This, however, is another subject and not what is being discussed here. As noted above, a major problem arises because claims are often made that 'scientific evidence' exists to demonstrate the effectiveness of many complementary treatments. However, in the terms we are using here, one or more of categories A, B, C or D usually apply. Occasionally the systematic category E applies (for instance, for homeopathy), but evidence in the scientific category F is found very rarely. When category F does occur, however, it must be taken seriously. Such instances will be discussed first for physical illnesses.

The scientific evidence (category F) for the effectiveness of complementary treatments on the physical illnesses to which they are applied

Published papers containing such evidence fall into two main groups – a large number in the journals devoted to complementary treatments (some of which are listed above to illustrate the amount of literature available), and a much smaller number published in orthodox general medical journals of international status, such as *The Lancet*, and the journals of the British, American, and Australian and New Zealand Medical Associations. The *Journal of the Royal Society of Medicine* of the UK has also recently published an extensive series of comments on this whole subject in its correspondence section (see Goodman, 1997).

Papers in the specialist complementary journals show a great deal of enthusiasm, and usually contain two uncritical assumptions: first, that complementary treatments actually do what they are supposed to do; and second, that there is no need to examine the truth of the various underlying theories. Most of the papers are written (and accepted by these journals) in this spirit. Except for acupuncture and homeopathy, rigorous attempts to 'control' studies are rare, and anecdotal accounts of single cases are common.

The orthodox international medical journals contain only a few papers on complementary treatments, but the number is increasing. Since 1966 the number of papers appearing on complementary treatments is said to have increased sixfold (Ernst, 1996). The still comparatively small number is no doubt connected with the pressure on publication space, and the stringent requirements of peer review. Some of the papers are surveys on how many people use complementary treatments and why, as already noted. The complementary treatments reported upon most frequently are acupuncture, homeopathy, and the similar osteopathy and chiropractic. This is not the place to attempt a comprehensive review of evidence, but, in summary, it seems clear that:

1. For homeopathy, there are some investigations that meet high standards, and whose results show a beneficial effect for some patients with asthma, some forms of arthritis, and various allergies (Reilly et al., 1994).

2. Acupuncture may affect various types of pain, and may be effective in lessening nausea and vomiting (Deluze, Bosia, Zirbs, Chantraine & Visher, 1992; Patel, Gutzwiller, Paccaud & Marrazi, 1989; Vickers, 1996).

3. Chiropractic and osteopathic manipulations (mainly of the spine and neck) appear to be more effective than conventional treatments for many patients troubled by backache and various other musculoskeletal aches and pains (Meade, Dyer, Browne & Frank,1995; Shekelle, Adams, Chassin, Hurwitz & Brook, 1992).

Having said this, it is necessary to note that a number of well-conducted investigations of the same treatments also found no benefit for the patients. The most that can be said is that the number of positive reports is large enough to justify further studies. The purpose of these should be to try to discover under what conditions and for which patients the treatment investigated can be made consistently helpful; as already noted, this is a separate issue from whether there is any support for the principles supposed to underlie a complementary treatment. It could be that the more rigorous the controls and the better the methods of assessment, the less likely it is that a beneficial effect will be found. At the very least, more will have been learned about the problems of how to conduct clinical trials.

How may complementary treatments be effective for people with psychiatric disorders?

There is one beneficial effect common to many complementary treatments that needs to be mentioned first, since there is not likely to be disagreement about it, namely the generally good effect of a session of deep relaxation. This is part of many complementary treatments, and in some it is accompanied by massage and pleasant aromas. Relaxation is also part of several forms of orthodox therapy for a variety of disorders. The point at issue is whether complementary treatments can produce additional benefits.

The discussion here will not be referring to people with psychiatric disorders such as schizophrenia and depressive psychoses, but to the much larger number with various forms of less severe depression, dysthymia, and anxiety states. Also included are those with somatic symptoms who may well not qualify for a diagnosis, but who nevertheless may feel far from well. These points are discussed in more detail later.

The first issue in the line of reasoning to be developed here rests on a detailed examination of some of the components of the consultation process. The specific content of intended treatments, whether orthodox or complementary, is not important at this stage. The example is of a person with an identifiable and treatable physical illness who consults an orthodox doctor. In a consultation, the patient is likely to present:

1. Physical symptoms caused directly by the physical illness.
2. Psychological symptoms and/or emotional feelings that are a reaction to the physical symptoms of the disease.
3. Illness behavior appropriate to the social and cultural setting.

If the doctor identifies the disease and acts appropriately, then all of these three components are likely to change for the better, but in different ways and at different speeds. Even if effective treatment for the physical disease is started at once, it is unlikely that there will be much immediate change in the physical symptoms caused directly by the physical illness. Therefore, most of the good direct effects of treatment will probably be delayed for at least a few days, although these will be the most important components of the overall improvement in the long run.

There can, however, be an immediate improvement in the emotional symptoms and illness behavior, due to:

1. Lessening of the fear induced by not knowing what is wrong.
2. Knowing that something is being done that should soon produce improvement.
3. The feeling of having been accepted as a patient by the doctor (and therefore also by family and friends) and cooperating in the treatment regimen (as good patients should).

These three types of improvement, that are not due to the direct physical treatment, will be lumped together and called 'the consultation effect'. This effect is an important experience for the patient, often underestimated by modern doctors working under pressure in busy health services (but rarely neglected by specialists working in private practice). It is likely to be enhanced by impressive surroundings, a distinguished therapist with a personal approach, a significant amount of time being spent on the consultation and on discussion of any investigative procedures, and anything else that increases the patient's hopes and expectations.

In other words, there is likely to be an immediate improvement in the emotional and behavioral components due to the consultation effect, but this is less fundamental, and in the long run less important, than the improvement in the physical symptoms. An advantage of this type of analysis of a consultation is that terms such as 'placebo' and 'nonspecific treatment effect' are avoided. If the same reasoning is applied to a consultation in which the orthodox doctor gets the treatment wrong, it is quite possible to see how the consultation effect could produce some immediate improvement in the emotional and behavioral components, but this would probably fade away as the physically caused symptoms persist and the patient's fears then return.

If the same model is applied to a consultation between the same patient with a physical illness and a complementary practitioner who offers an ineffective treatment (that is, wrong in the same sense as the model just discussed), it is very likely that, in just the same way, the patient will experience a temporary improvement due to the consultation effect. In other words, the patient will probably be satisfied in the short term with the overall experience of the complementary consultation.

Applying this reasoning to a patient with a psychological disorder seeking a consultation with either an orthodox doctor or a complementary practitioner requires an amplified model of a consultation because of two additional points. First, many psychiatric disorders are characterized by both physical and psychological symptoms. The physical symptoms, such as tiredness, aches and pains, loss of appetite and loss of weight, are not caused by any detectable physical abnormalities, and are part of the basically psychological illness. They can be just as troublesome to the patient as more obviously psychological symptoms such as depression and anxiety, and to both the patient and the family they appear to be convincingly physical in nature. These psychologically caused physical-seeming symptoms are known as 'somatoform' or 'somatic' in current psychiatric practice, and somatic will be used here.

There is therefore a possibility that a patient with a psychological disorder will present at a consultation with three types of symptoms, all of psychological origin:

1. Symptoms such as anxiety and depression.
2. Somatic symptoms, as just described.
3. Psychological symptoms and/or emotional feelings that are a reaction to the idea of being ill now, and possibly staying ill or getting worse in the future (as for the physical symptoms in the first model discussed).

In addition, there are two types of treatment that can be effective for psychological disorders. First, medication, which acts directly on the central nervous system, and, second, psychological treatments such as psychotherapy and behavioral therapies which change thoughts, feelings and behavior in other (but largely unknown) ways. An important difference between these two is that the psychological treatments can be effective only if the patient accepts and understands to some degree what is involved, whereas for medication to be successful the patient merely has to take it.

Depending on the nature of the psychological disorder, all of these components may be improved by appropriate medication, and all may be improved by appropriate psychological treatment – but, as already noted, this latter can be effective only if it is acceptable to the patient (see also Chapter 13).

It is very likely that many contemporary orthodox psychiatrists underestimate the degree to which the patient, rather than the psychiatrist, decides what can be regarded as an appropriate psychological treatment. Something that the patient does not want or understand cannot be effective psychologically, whatever the doctor may believe or intend.

A commonly observed extension of this point is that some of the transactions and interactions of the consultation, that are not part of the treatment in the doctor's view, may have a considerable beneficial impact on the patient. This is because they fit in with the patient's expectations and concepts of what might be treatment, and how their illness might be put right. Examples of these inadvertent treatment effects are the spending of time and effort on obtaining details of the patient's family history and personal development, impressive investigatory procedures such as radiographs, the simple act of referral to a hospital specialist, and the formal naming of the disorder (giving an official diagnosis).

To put this important point in another way, when we are dealing with psychological treatments for psychological disorders, only things that have some meaning and appeal to the patient are likely to have an impact, and so are able to produce the desired change. If we apply this line of reasoning to a patient with a psychological illness whose outward signs include some somatic symptoms, treatment from a complementary practitioner that is directed at these somatic symptoms may well be effective, as long as the whole experience is what the patient regards as appropriate. The point that, in terms of an orthodox view of the illness, both the patient and the complementary practitioner are mistaken in regarding the illness as basically physical does not necessarily detract from some aspects of the healing power of the consultation; what matters is that a psychological illness is being treated by a self-chosen and therefore acceptable and appealing psychological experience. This extra healing effect is likely to be more powerful and long-lasting than the consultation effect (present even when the treatment for a disorder is wrong) that has already been discussed.

Whether this extra improvement would be sustained or even become progressive and constitute a cure would depend upon at least two other influences. One of these is the original cause (or causes) of the psychological illness; if this is still present, then only short-lived improvement is likely. The other influence may come from changed circumstances in those cases where the original cause or causes have already diminished or disappeared for reasons not connected with the consultation, but the patient is stuck for some reason in the sick role. For instance, a patient who was incapacitated for a long time, but whose disorder has naturally improved or resolved, may not be able to get out of the sick role without being ridiculed or losing face until an acceptable healing procedure has been experienced and recognized as such by friends and family. Under these circumstances, a complementary consultation could be exactly what is needed for recovery. This example applies particularly to people for whom social stresses or poor physical health contributed to their illness, but whose social support network or physical health has changed for the better with the passage of time.

Psychiatric disorders associated with somatic symptoms

Evidence has been available for many years about the high frequency of such disorders in people seen in primary care, and a recently published collaborative study organized by the WHO confirms the previous findings (Üstün & Sartorius, 1995). This study involved centers in 14 different countries, and was based upon series of consecutive attenders at general health facilities. The summed frequency of the disorders of interest to this present discussion across the centers was 21.4% (depression 10.4%, neurasthenia 5.4%, somatoform disorder 2.7%, dysthymia 2.1%, hypochondriasis 0.8%).

These figures apply to clinic attenders, so there are probably many more similar people in the community with similar disorders and symptoms who do not come forward seeking orthodox medical help.

Below is a list of psychiatric disorders that are particularly closely associated with somatic symptoms. Some of these are quite common, and are often found in people not in contact with the orthodox medical or psychiatric services. It is therefore quite likely that there are many individuals in the community of this type who might benefit from complementary treatment. Some of these are comparatively rare, such as dissociative disorders (previously known as conversion hysteria), but all are well known in psychiatric and medical practice. Individuals with mild or subdiagnostic forms of neurasthenia, hypochondriasis and somatization disorder must be even more frequent in the community than those with a sufficient number of symptoms to allow a diagnosis to be made, already noted in the WHO study. Item 7 is one of the most common disorders seen in patients in primary care worldwide.

Item 5 on the list, 'Elaboration of physically caused symptoms for psychological reasons' is a new category in ICD-10, chapter V (F68.0). Its most common form is well recognized by psychiatrists who work in liaison services in medical and surgical wards, since the category applies to patients who have a confirmed physical disorder, disease or disability. To quote from the ICD-10 glossary – 'dissatisfaction with the results of treatment or investigations, or disappointment with the amount of personal attention received in wards or clinics, may be a motivating factor'. Item 6 covers some aspects of prolongation of the sick role already mentioned.

Conditions that may respond to a psychological stimulus

The physical behavior of a person with any of the following psychological disorders:

1. Dissociative disorders (conversion).
2. Neurasthenia.
3. Hypochondriasis.
4. Somatoform disorders.
5. Elaboration of physically caused symptoms for psychological reasons.
6. Learned motor behavior prolonged for psychological reasons.
7. Episodes of mild and moderate anxiety and/or depression with somatic symptoms.

Conclusions

There seems to be a good case for concluding that one important reason why complementary treatments are so popular is that the consultation effect as described here provides an acceptable 'treatment experience' for many people who have not been satisfied by the orthodox medical services. The benefit they obtain from a complementary consultation may not often be fundamental or long-lasting, but it can be immediately obvious and therefore gratifying, even for patients with physical disorders not affected by the treatment itself. For some patients with psychiatric disorders presenting with somatic symptoms, it is possible that there could be extra benefits that are more powerful and long-lasting than the short-term consultation effect.

Complementary treatment is usually obtained in a setting which has several attractions for the patient – it is self-chosen, and probably involves a more personal and sympathetic approach and a longer consultation by the complementary therapist than was experienced in previous orthodox medical contacts. All of these attributes can, and should, be a part of orthodox consultations, but it is easy to see how they can sometimes be obscured by the pressure of numbers often experienced by doctors and other medical professionals who work in the orthodox services. Orthodox medical practitioners must give a necessary priority to the early detection of dangerous medical diseases and must also deal with acutely dangerous situations. Those who work in the setting of comprehensive national or regional medical services must also deal with all comers, including the poor, the chronically disabled and the badly organized. These conditions are very different from the settings in which complementary therapists practice.

Implications for medical education and research

These conclusions suggest that it is appropriate to treat with respect those who seek complementary therapies, and also to respect those who offer the therapies in good faith and with due professional behavior. The systematic and critical evaluation of complementary therapies, therapists and their customers seems to be justified, first as issues of medical and scientific importance, and second because of the increasing size and costs of the whole complementary treatment industry. The standards applied to these investigations should be just the same as those used in the tests of conventional therapies.

To investigate these therapies for reasons that are at odds with the beliefs of the therapists (and probably most of their patients) sets some unusual problems for the investigators. There are also problems of limited research resources, conflicting priorities, and risk to professional reputations. Nevertheless, there are now some signs that investigators with a serious interest and a rigorous approach are beginning to emerge. For instance, in the UK there is now a Department of Complementary Medicine in the Postgraduate Medical School at Exeter that has recently produced a very useful set of commentaries and reviews (Ernst, 1996), and it is to be hoped that this group and others will be able to find both resources and collaborators in the near future.

Quite different types of investigations are needed to test the main issues that have been discussed here. The suggestion that substantial proportions of those obtaining benefit from complementary treatments will be found to be suffering from somatic symptoms that are part of a psychiatric disorder requires detailed study of those receiving treatment, but not much else. No interference with or assessment of the treatment received would be involved, and the complementary therapists would only have to give their consent to the study being undertaken. Access to their own records of treatment given and improvement recorded would be an advantage, but not essential.

Study of the effectiveness of complementary treatments by rigorous double-blind controlled clinical trials is an altogether more difficult problem, but a sufficient number have already been done to show that further studies are possible. Many authors in this field have already emphasized that the first requirement for studies of all types is a willingness for close and constructive collaboration between orthodox clinical scientists and complementary practitioners.

Implications for medical services

Recently, many managers and accountants have been appointed in the UK's NHS, and have been given unprecedented powers over finances and the design of the health service. Now the same is happening in other countries. The comparative cheapness of many complementary remedies (and the not always justified claims of their being free from dangerous side-effects) makes them attractive to those responsible for limited budgets, particularly if the budget holders have little or no knowledge of the differences between orthodox and complementary treatments. Budget holders who do not have the necessary knowledge are starting to comment on the desirability of making some complementary treatments available within the NHS in the UK for those who want it, and complementary practitioners will not be slow to see great opportunities for themselves. Furthermore, in the UK, one recent survey showed that the majority of the general public who responded to the survey questions were in favor of complementary treatments being available on the NHS ('Which?', 1995). One implication of this is that, on a limited budget with decisions being made by nonmedically qualified managers (or a committee with minimal input from the medically qualified), decisions on cost alone could result in some complementary treatments displacing some orthodox treatments. Educating all those in charge of the health services would appear to be the best counter to this possibility.

The future policy of medical educators about complementary treatments with respect to undergraduate and postgraduate teaching

In the UK, a survey in 1996 showed that of 24 medical schools, three offered small amounts of teaching on complementary medicine, four were considering it, and the other 17 had none. However, the same survey showed that more than half the medical students would like to be told something about the topic, particularly on hypnosis and acupuncture (Rampes et al., 1997).

Rather more seems to be happening in the USA than in the UK and Europe. Reports show that about one-third of medical schools in the USA have something about complementary treatments in their curriculum, although probably not much more than recommended reading.

More needs to be done, and the first step would be for some information and discussion on complementary medicine to be widely accepted as a legitimate part of the curriculum in orthodox medical schools. The objective should be to encourage the students to apply their own critical faculties to the problem, in the hope of helping them to decide what to say to future patients when asked for advice about complementary treatments. Debates will be needed to achieve even the small amount of time required. Anybody who is responsible for overseeing the teaching timetables of a medical school is well aware of the constant pressure from enthusiasts of many disciplines for more and more teaching time in curricula, even though they are already acknowledged to be overcrowded with scientifically based topics. However, even medical curricula have to move with the times, and the case for complementary medicine is now strong.

It is important that any such teaching should not be done by overenthusiastic and committed complementary practitioners, who are likely to want to talk about vibrations, life-forces and similar concepts. There is a need to find orthodox medical scientists and doctors who are willing to collaborate with doubly qualified complementary practitioners, and all must have a constructive but critical approach. There are a few such individuals around, but nevertheless it is likely that most medical schools already contain the small number of academic staff sufficiently interested to cope with the small but regular teaching input needed.

References

Baum, M. (1989). Rationalism versus irrationalism in the care of the sick: science versus the absurd (Editorial). *Medical Journal of Australia*, **151**, 607–8.

British Medical Association (1993). *Complementary Medicine: New Approaches to Good Practice*. Oxford: Oxford University Press.

Deluze, C., Bosia, L., Zirbs, A., Chantraine, A. & Vischer, T.L. (1992). Electroacupuncture in fibromyalgia: results of a controlled trial. *British Medical Journal*, **305**, 1249–52.

Eisenberg, D.M., Kessler, R.C., Foster, C., Norlock. F.E., Collins, D.R. & Delbano, T.L. (1993). Unconventional medicine in the United States: prevalence, costs and pattern of use. *New England Journal of Medicine*, **328**, 246–52.

Ernst, E. (1995). Complementary medicine: common misconceptions. *Journal of the Royal Society of Medicine*, **88**, 244–7.

Ernst, E. (ed.) (1996). *Complementary Medicine: an Objective Appraisal*. Oxford: Butterworth-Heinemann.

Ernst, E., Resch, K.L. & Hill, S. (1997). Do complementary practitioners have a better bedside manner than physicians? *Journal of the Royal Society of Medicine*, **90**, 118–19.

Fisher, P. & Ward, A. (1994). Complementary medicine in Europe. *British Medical Journal*, **309**, 107–11.

Furnham, A. (1993). Attitudes to alternative medicine: a study of the perceptions of those studying orthodox medicine. *Complementary Therapy in Medicine*, **1**, 120–6.

Goodman, J. (1997). Complementary medicine in the medical curriculum. *Journal of the Royal Society of Medicine*, **89**, 178 (and others: 90, 238–40, 299–300, 356–7).

MacLennan, A.H., Wilson, D.H. & Tatlor, A.W. (1996). Medicine in Australia. *Lancet*, **347**, 569–73.

Meade, T.W., Dyer, S., Browne, W. & Frank, A.O. (1995). Randomized comparison of chiropractic and hospital outpatient management for low back pain: Results from extended follow-up. *British Medical Journal*, 311, 349–51.

Patel, M., Gutzwiller, F., Paccaud, F. & Marrazi, A. (1989). A meta-analysis of acupuncture for chronic pain. *International Journal of Epidemiology*, 18, 900–4.

Rampes, H., Sharples, F., Maragh, S. & Fisher, P. (1997). Introducing complementary medicine into the medical curriculum. *Journal of the Royal Society of Medicine*, 90, 19–22.

Reilly, D., Taylor, M.A., Beattie, N.G.M., Campbell, J.H., McSharry, C., Aitchison, T.C., Carter, R. & Stevenson, R.D. (1994). Is evidence for homeopathy reproducible? *Lancet*, 344, 1601–6.

Resch, K-L. & Ernst, E. (1996). Research methodologies in complementary medicine: making sure it works. In E. Ernst (ed.) *Complementary Medicine: an Objective Appraisal*. Oxford: Butterworth-Heinemann.

Shekelle, P.G., Adams, A.H., Chassin, M.R., Hurwitz, E.L, & Brook, R.H. (1992). Spinal manipulation for low back pain. *Annals of Internal Medicine*, 117, 59–08.

Skrabanek, P. (1986). Demarcation of the absurd. *Lancet*, 1, 960–1.

Üstün, T.B. & Sartorius, N. (eds.) (1995). *Mental Illness in General Health Care: an International Study*. Geneva: WHO; Chichester: Wiley.

Vickers, A.J. (1996). Can acupuncture have specific effects on health? A systematic review of acupuncture anti-emesis trials. *Journal of the Royal Society of Medicine*, 89, 303–11.

Which? (1995). *Healthy choice*. Consumers Association of UK.

Which? (1996). *The User's Guide to Complementary Medicine*. Consumers Association of UK.

Part III

Unmet need: people with specific disorders

Introduction

Gavin Andrews

This is a good section, no more generalizing, 'just let me tell you how it is with the people I treat'. Sadly we have no contribution from psychogeriatricians and Dr Patel is the only representative of the developing world. We sought for people who would tell us how to serve multitudes with very small budgets. We asked too much. A doctor in a poor country needs someone to take over the clinical load and to provide research and secretarial assistance if they are to have time to prepare material for a book like this. We refer readers to Goldberg & Thornicroft (1998) for they managed to get papers from 11 countries, not all affluent by any means, that describe services in 11 cities.

It is pleasing therefore that the first chapter in this section is by Thornicroft and his group on the unmet need of people with schizophrenia (Chapter 13). Their definitions bear remembering: need is what people could benefit from; demand is what people ask for; and supply is what is provided. They distinguish between need at the personal and service-delivery levels, and they give many examples using different instruments and different studies. The Häfner and Maurer chapter (Chapter 14) takes quite a different approach to reducing unmet need: identify people before their first psychotic break and supply them with the best treatment. If you read nothing else in their chapter you should read their conclusions. Wilhelm and Lin (Chapter 15) also see prevention as vital to the management of depression. Their concern is with secondary and tertiary prevention – educating people who have had an episode of depression about the relapsing nature of the condition – and minimizing the vulnerability to relapse. They also emphasize one of the more disturbing findings of the long-term follow-up of the Stirling County study – that even after recovery, the quality of life for previously depressed people leaves a lot to be desired. They suggest that strategies to improve quality of life and prevent relapse are cheap, likely to be cost-effective and, best of all, are simple and easily taught. The Beautrais et al. study (Chapter 16) of suicide survivors also stresses secondary prevention and makes it clear that unless one does this properly there will be little opportunity for tertiary prevention.

Chapters 17 and 18, one from Germany and one from Australia, come to identical conclusions. Wittchen (Chapter 17) reports the results of a commu-nity survey of young people with anxiety disorders. Hunt (Chapter 18) reports on a parallel group of adults identified in a community survey. She reports on adults who sought, but dropped out of, treatment for anxiety.

Wittchen points out that, despite proven treatments being available, German adolescents with anxiety disorders seldom receive them. The Australian adults in Hunt's survey report exactly the same phenomenon: proven treatments were not delivered. Hunt identified a group of people who dropped out of or refused treatment in a specialized anxiety disorders program. She followed them for two years and showed that, despite continuing treatment from their regular doctor, their condition did not change, whereas most of those who received the proven treatment were well. A cynic might argue that for the anxiety disorders 'treatment as usual' too often equals 'disease as usual'. Wittchen laments that this mismatch between diagnosis and treatment represents a waste of personnel and financial resources, but the real worry is whether treatment for mental disorders generally is effective, that is, in practice is efficacious.

Hall and Teesson (Chapter 19) write about alcohol-use disorders. They think that the prevalences identified by the surveys do not represent the magnitude of the clinical problem because many of the cases identified by the survey remit spontaneously. They argue for public education to prevent the occurrence of the disorder and of self-help programs to encourage quitting. They are more conservative about the success of the formal programs and recommend centers specializing in alcohol-use or mental disorders to remain alert for comorbid conditions from each other's patch, as they make treatment so difficult. Chapter 20, by Anthony, reiterates that need defines a potential to benefit. In opioid dependence opioid therapy is effective at stabilizing the disorder. If we do not have a cure, is there an alternative? Anthony argues that we have to begin at the very beginning, before people take their first drug, not because the drug is so addictive but because early drug users are evangelistic and influence too many others.

Hickie et al. (Chapter 21) raise the issue that many mental health staff would like to ignore, that somatoform disorders are poorly recognized and equally poorly treated. They argue that these disorders are debilitating and costly to the service providers, and that we must provide education and training about these disorders and support for clinicians who treat such patients. In effect this position underlines the conclusions for this section. In new fields such as neurasthenia, there is no established treatment base and one has to just teach and support clinicians who manage such patients until the results of regular treatment are known. In mature fields such as schizophrenia, depression, anxiety disorders and substance-use disorders, one needs lateral strategies to make a dent in the residual unmet need.

Reference

Goldberg, D. & Thornicroft, G. (1998). *Mental Health in our Future Cities* (Maudsley Monograph 42). London: Psychology Press.

13

The unmet needs of people suffering from schizophrenia

Graham Thornicroft, Sonia Johnson, Morven Leese, and
Mike Slade

Increasing importance is being attached to the needs of those who suffer from
schizophrenia. This new orientation marks a wider public mood that emphasizes the active role of the recipients of health services as consumers, and also
raises a series of important consequent questions. How can needs be defined
and by whom? How can they be measured and compared? What importance
should be given to both met and unmet needs when assessing individual
patients, and when planning and evaluating the mental health services as a
whole? How should the needs of those suffering from schizophrenia be
prioritized in relation to the needs of other diagnostic groups?

These questions form the context of this chapter. Here we examine in turn
these two levels of need: individual and service. In the first section of the
chapter, we shall describe three methods of assessing individual patient's
needs (the Needs for Care Assessment, the Camberwell Assessment of Need,
and the Cardinal Needs Schedule), and we shall give details of one study in
South London which has used this approach to assess unmet *individual*
needs. In the second section we turn to service-level (or *population*) needs,
and describe four methods appropriate to this level. We then offer one
example to highlight this method of needs assessment which draws upon a
recent detailed review of the needs for mental health services throughout
London. Finally we return to one of the most central and intriguing issues:
who should define these needs?

Defining need, demand, supply and utilization

Need

Despite the ubiquitous current concern to base services upon assessed needs,
there is no consensus on how needs should be defined (Holloway, 1994), and
who should define them (Ellis, 1993; Slade, 1994). Individual needs, for
example, may be defined at the levels of impairment, disability, or in terms of
interventions. The fact that a need is defined does not mean that it can be

met. For example, needs may remain unmet because other problems take priority, because an effective method is not available, or because the person in need refuses treatment.

Various definitions of need have been suggested, which can be categorized into needs for improved health, needs for services, and needs for action by mental health staff (Brewin, 1992). The Community Care Act suggests that needs are, 'the requirements of individuals to enable them to achieve, maintain or restore an acceptable level of social independence or quality of life' (Department of Health and Social Services Inspectorate, 1991, p.10), which defines need as relating to improved health and social functioning. In this definition two types of need can be present: met needs (difficulties that are ameliorated through help received), and unmet needs (where a serious problem currently exists, whether or not any help is being given). In this chapter Stevens & Gabbay's (1991) working definition of need will be used, that is, 'the ability to benefit in some way from health (and social) care'.

A need may exist, as defined by a professional, even if the intervention is refused by a patient. Furthermore, a needs assessment is not intended to endorse the status quo. It is important to define need in terms of the care/agent/setting required, not those already in place. At the same time, a proper needs assessment process should not lead to the imposition of an expert solution upon patients. A professionally defined need may remain unmet, and have to be replaced by one acceptable to the patient.

Another approach to defining need has been suggested by health economists. First, they suggest that need refers both to the capacity to benefit from an intervention and the amount of expenditure required to reduce the capacity to benefit to zero – it is therefore a product of benefit and cost-effectiveness (Culyer & Wagstaff, 1992). Second, they suggest that diagnosis-related groups are notably irrelevant to mental health services (McCrone & Strathdee, 1994); and, third, that empirical data guide definitions of operational needs (Beecham, Knapp & Fenyo, 1993). The specification of an intervention, if accepted by the user, leads to the choice of a case manager to provide the care (Mangen & Brewin, 1991). In addition, it is important to distinguish need from demand, supply and utilization. Stevens & Gabbay (1991) define need, demand, and supply in the following way:

Need = what people benefit from
Demand = what people ask for
Supply = what is provided

Demand

A demand for care exists when an individual expresses a wish to receive it. Some demands are expressed in an unsophisticated form; for example, 'something needs to be done'. The user should negotiate which interventions should be provided for particular problems. This would include an explanation of the options. The process should not be directed purely by experts or professionals.

Supply

Supply (or provision) includes interventions, agents, and settings, whether or not they are used. Care coordination entails providing such a pattern of service after initial assessment, and then updating the assessment regularly to assess outcomes and to modify the care if needs remain unmet. Overprovision is provision without need. Underprovision is need without provision (unmet need).

Utilization

Utilization occurs when an individual actually receives care; for example, an in-patient admission. Need may not be expressed as demand; demand is not necessarily followed by provision or, if it is, by utilization; and there can be demand, provision and utilization without real underlying need for the particular service used.

Individual-level needs assessments

Measuring individual needs

In a reasonable planning framework, the needs of all patients would be comprehensively assessed, and the aggregated data would be used to plan the services. In practice this is seldom possible, but systematic assessment, review, and evaluation over months and years of contact should allow teams to work with their users to evolve services more appropriate to their needs (Brewin, Wing, Mangen, Brugha & MacCarthy, 1987). Patients who suffer from severe mental illness have a range of needs that goes far beyond the purely medical, such as those described in the US National Institute of Mental Health (1987) document *'Towards a Model for a Comprehensive Community-Based Mental Health System'*.

Individual needs assessments for homeless mentally ill people, for example, exemplify these issues. In a study by Herman, Struening & Barrow (1993), homeless people were asked if they needed 'help with nerves and emotional problems', and were independently rated by the interviewer as to need. A quarter (24%) of the interviewees reported no need for mental health services when the interviewer rated them as having a need. By contrast, Mavis,

Humphreys & Stöffelmayr (1993) report a study of homeless people seeking help for substance abuse, who were asked about specific areas of need. Two subgroups were identified: 78% were the 'economic homeless', with substantial employment and financial problems, and 22% were the 'multiproblem homeless', with substantial problems in physical health, alcohol/drug use, mental health, family and social life.

The issue of how best to construct an individual needs assessment measure has taxed both researchers and clinicians, not least because their requirements differ. An ideal assessment tool for use in a routine clinic setting would be one that is brief, easily learned, takes little time to administer, does not require the use of additional personnel, is valid and reliable in different settings and across gender and cultures, and, above all, can be used as an integral part of routine clinical work, rather than as a time-consuming extra. Macdonald (1991) suggests that in addition they should be sensitive to change, their potential inter-rater and test-rater reliability should be high, and they should logically inform clinical management (Hillier, Zaudig & Mobour, 1991). The decision of which measure to use will depend on whether the approach is to focus on particular diagnostic or care groups, and on the balance to be struck between economy of time and inclusiveness of the ratings, which can include a range of areas of clinical and social functioning. We next examine three measures that address individual needs.

MRC Needs for Care Assessment

The MRC Needs for Care Assessment (Brewin, 1992) is based on the following formal definition of need for care:

1. Need is present when (i) a patient's functioning (social disablement) falls below or threatens to fall below some minimum specified level, and (ii) this is due to a remediable, or potentially remediable, cause.

2. A need (as defined above) is met when it has attracted some, at least partly effective, item of care, and when there are no other items of care of greater potential effectiveness.

3. A need (as defined above) is unmet when it has attracted only partly effective or no items of care and when there are other items of care of greater potential effectiveness.

Substantial data have now been presented on individual needs assessments using this instrument (Brewin, Veltro, Wing, MacCarthy & Brugha, 1990; Brewin et al., 1988; Pryce et al., 1993; Van Haaster, Lesage, Cyr & Toupin, 1994) along with a detailed critique of this approach (Brewin & Wing, 1993; Hogg & Marshall, 1992).

Camberwell Assessment of Need

A shorter and more clinically orientated instrument is the Camberwell

Assessment of Need (CAN), which has been recently published by the PRiSM team at the Institute of Psychiatry. It is intended for both research and clinical use, especially in relation to the requirements of the British NHS and Community Care Act (House of Commons, 1990) to undertake needs assessments of people with mental health problems, and it includes both patient and staff views, considering a comprehensive range of health and social needs, and assessing need separately from interventions. The areas assessed by the CAN include:

- Accommodation
- Occupation
- Specific psychotic symptoms
- Psychological distress
- Information about condition and treatment
- Nonprescribed drugs
- Food and meals
- Household skills
- Self care and presentation
- Safety to self
- Safety to others
- Money
- Childcare
- Physical health
- Alcohol
- Basic education
- Company
- Telephone
- Public transport
- Welfare benefits

The psychometric properties of the scale have now been established both in terms of validity (face, consensual, content, criterion and construct) and reliability (Phelan et al., 1995) and the results are acceptable. It was striking that in a pilot survey of severely disabled psychiatric patients in South London, the mean number of problems identified by staff was 7.5 (95% confidence interval, CI, 6.7–8.4), and by patients was 7.9 (6.8–8.9). When examined in detail, however, the degree of agreement between staff and patients over individual items was rather poor, rejecting the hypothesis that staff and patients rate problems similarly (Slade, Phelan, Thornicroft & Parkman, 1996). The CAN is now being introduced to field trials in routine clinical settings and is being translated into 14 European languages.

Cardinal Needs Schedule

A third formal approach to individual needs assessment is that of Marshall

(1994), who is developing the Cardinal Needs Schedule. This is a modification of the MRC Needs for Care approach, and identifies cardinal problems as those which satisfy three criteria:

1. The 'cooperation criterion' (the patient is willing to accept help for the problem).
2. The 'carer stress criterion' (the problem causes considerable anxiety, frustration or inconvenience to people caring for the patient).
3. The 'severity criterion' (the problem endangers the health or safety of the patient, or the safety of other people).

To rate this schedule, data are collected using the Manchester Scale for mental state assessment, the REHAB scale and a specially developed questionnaire to give additional information. A computerized version (Autoneed) has also been developed. Patients' views are rated using the client opinion interview and carer ratings obtained from the carer stress interview. Marshall is undertaking both inter-rater and test-retest reliability studies.

Example of measuring individual needs – the PRiSM Psychosis Study

The PRiSM study is a five-year prospective evaluation of the outcomes of two different types of community mental health service provision for people with psychotic illnesses in two similar sectors in South London with a combined population of 80,285. In one sector (Nunhead) an intensive community-based service was introduced, whereas in the other (Norwood) the standard service continued. The methodology is described in detail by Slade, Phelan & Thornicroft (1998). A case-identification exercise was first carried out to establish the annual prevalence of all psychotic disorders for the index year, and cases were identified by combining data from a number of hospital and community sources. The sources of information were psychiatric hospital case records, local social service teams, general practice records, local sheltered accommodation, voluntary, private and self-help care providers, clergy, services for the homeless, and prisons. Cases were included on the basis of address of residence, even if no treatment was received in the index year.

For all possible cases information in case notes and other available records was screened. Possible cases were identified as those who had a clinical diagnosis at any time in their lives of any psychotic disorder, and they were rated using OPCRIT (Operational Criteria Checklist) version 3.2, a standardized procedure to produce operationalized research diagnoses, including the ICD-10, DSM-IIIR and research diagnostic criteria. Any respondent who had a diagnostic output from the OPCRIT of an affective or nonaffective functional psychotic disorder was included as a definite case.

This case-finding procedure identified an epidemiologically representative population of 566 psychotic individuals, from whom a random sample of 320

Table 13.1. Individual met and unmet needs: changes over time in intensive and standard sectors

Sector		Time 1 mean	Time 2 mean	Change	95% CI	P^c
Nunhead[a] (intensive)	CAN met needs	4.05	4.45	0.40	−0.31 to 1.10	0.26
	CAN unmet needs	1.23	1.90	0.68	0.20 to 1.15	0.0006
Norwood[b] (standard)	CAN met needs	4.51	3.73	−0.78	−0.17 to −1.39	0.01
	CAN unmet needs	1.57	1.86	0.29	-0.25 to 0.83	0.29

[a] $n = 62$ time 1 minus time 2 pairs.
[b] $n = 63$ time 1 minus time 2 pairs
[c] Paired t-test.
CAN, Camberwell Assessment of Need.

was chosen for interview. This sample was to was to be interviewed twice: first at 'time 1', when the services received were similar, and second two years later at 'time 2', by which time the impact of the different services subsequently received would be apparent. Eighteen individuals for whom no definite psychotic diagnosis could be established using research criteria were omitted from the analysis of this sample. Individual need was assessed using the Camberwell Assessment of Need (CAN), and we summarize in Table 13.1 the overall results of the user (patient) ratings of need from the 22 CAN domains. The results show that psychotic individuals, half of whom were schizophrenic, had an average of seven major needs, of which three-quarters were met and one-quarter unmet. The results also show that at time 2 the intensive sector (Nunhead) met more needs and identified more unmet needs than at time 1, suggesting that community mental health services improve needs assessment.

Population-level needs assessments

A comprehensive method for developing appropriate local services should be based on systematically assessing the needs of the population of individuals identified as mentally ill within the service's catchment area. Individual levels of need would then be collated from a case register or similar information source, and services developed in relation to the identified unmet needs of the population (Wing, 1989). Often there are no, or only poor-quality, direct data on service needs, and indicators or proxy variables may have to be used.

There are a number of alternative methods for assessing local needs for services, each with their own limitations (Shapiro, Skinner, Kramer, Steinwachs & Regier, 1985). First, estimates of need may be based on epidemiological estimates of the national prevalence of mental disorders that may cause individuals to contact the psychiatric services. Second, calculations of services needed locally may be derived from data on service utilization rates found nationally (Goldberg & Huxley, 1980, 1992; Goldman, 1981). Third, local levels of provision may simply be compared with national levels of provision. This method is not strictly based on needs, but it allows a rough comparison between the development of local services and the national picture. The suitability of the service provision for the local needs should be assessed by the numbers of places provided in a variety of services. The location of services should make them accessible to all, and should consider demographic variations in catchment areas, which may produce particularly high levels of need in certain areas. Fourth, a deprivation-weighted approach may be used. This adjusts estimates of service need according to current knowledge of the relationships between mental health disorders and age, sex, ethnic group, marital status, economic status, and other social variables (Thornicroft, 1991).

In this chapter, each of the above methods is explained and illustrated using the example of Planningham, a fictional catchment area.

Method 1. Using epidemiological rates of the prevalence of psychiatric disorder

The work of Goldberg & Huxley (1980, 1992) may be used as the basis of an approach which considers data on service utilization and findings from epidemiological population surveys. It has been established that in any year one-quarter (25%) of the adult population will suffer from a mental illness of at least moderate severity. Of this number, very few are referred to mental health services (1.7%) and less than half of these are admitted (0.6% of the population at risk).

An estimate of local morbidity may be derived from community studies of levels of psychiatric morbidity carried out elsewhere in the UK. Table 13.2 shows the expected numbers of people with psychiatric disorders in our fictional District, Planningham, based on the figures for expected morbidity summarized in the 'Health of the Nation' (Department of Health, 1994).

Epidemiological data provide an overall estimate of needs in the community. They do not indicate which forms of service are needed: most people with depression or anxiety do not need referral to specialist services. However, for schizophrenia and other psychoses these data are more useful, as it may be assumed that most patients with these severe mental illnesses will need some form of long-term contact with psychiatric services.

Table 13.2. Estimates of psychiatric morbidity in Planningham (population 250,000) based on national prevalence data

	Estimated prevalence/ 500,000 population	Estimated numbers for Planningham
Schizophrenia	1,000–2,500	500–1,250
Affective psychosis	500–2,500	250–1,250
Depression	10,000–5,000	5,000–12,500
Anxiety	8,000–30,000	4,000–15,000

Source: Department of Health, 1994.

Returning to our fictional district, Planningham's community services accommodate 200 people on Community Psychiatric Nurses' caseloads, 150 people in day centers, and 100 people in sheltered work placements. This might cause concern when considered in relation to epidemiological data. If the estimate that there are 1750 people with psychotic illnesses in the district is accurate, local community services do not currently have the capacity to provide for more than a minority of these people.

Method 2. Estimating service need from national patterns of service use

The work of Goldberg & Huxley (1980, 1992) may be used to compare local service use with national and international data on service utilization. Table 13.3 shows the expected Planningham levels of morbidity and of service use, based on Goldberg and Huxley's calculations of the proportion of the population using services at various levels. These figures include the elderly and younger adults.

Referring to the figures for Planningham, the number of people admitted at least once to a psychiatric hospital (1500) is high compared with these estimates of service use. However, the information considered so far gives no grounds for choosing between the various possible reasons for this discrepancy, including higher than average levels of need, greater than usual willingness to admit, and shortage of services providing alternatives to admission.

Wing's (1992) national figures for patients with mental disorders in contact with services per 250,000 in 1990/1 are given in Table 13.4. These figures include people with dementia. Again, expected levels of provision for the population of Planningham may be derived, and are also shown in Table 13.4.

Planningham has large numbers of acute admissions compared with rates predicted from national figures (2820 actual admissions compared with 1095 predicted). The number of out-patient contacts, on the other hand, is smaller than expected (6500 actual attendances compared with 8586 predicted). This pattern could be explained in various ways. One important possibility is that

Table 13.3. National and Planningham expected morbidity and service use

Level of service	1-year prevalence for population at risk (%)	Expected levels for Planningham (pop. 250,000)
Adults suffering from mental illness/distress	26–31.5	65,000–78,750
Consulting primary care	23	57,500
Identified by doctors as having mental illness/distress	10.2	25,500
Seen by specialist mental health services	2.4	6,000
Admitted to psychiatric hospital	0.6	1,500

Source: Goldberg and Huxley, 1992.

Table 13.4. National figures for service use and expected Planningham values

Type of contact	National figures for 1990/1 per 250,000 population	Expected for Planningham
No. of patients attending GP per annum	64,250	64,250
No. of patients attending outpatient per annum	2,858	2,858
Total no. of outpatient attendances per annum	8,586	8,586
No. of inpatients on one day, stay < 1 year	135	135
No. of acute admissions per annum	1,095	1,095
No. of inpatients on one day, stay 1–5 years	93	93
No. of in-patients on one day, stay > 5 years	70	70
No. in Local Authority residential care on one day	18	18
No. in Local Authority long-term day places on one day	63	63

Source: Wing 1992.

the out-patient service is underresourced, so that it cannot respond swiftly to referrals. Alternatively, patients may find the out-patient service geographically inaccessible or psychologically unwelcoming, or local professionals may have limited awareness of how to make referrals to it. Such difficulties may compromise the ability of the out-patient service to avert in-patient admissions.

An important disadvantage of national service-use data is that they are often based on incomplete or inaccurate returns, especially where they refer to community services (Glover, 1991). A good alternative may be to use data from studies in areas such as Salford, UK, where detailed case registers recording all service contacts have been kept (Fryers & Wooff, 1989; Wing, 1989).

Service utilization data do not of course allow for a normative assessment of the services that the health authority *should* have. However, planners may find it helpful to use them to get some idea of whether numbers of contacts for particular components of their local services are relatively large or small compared with services elsewhere.

Method 3. What are desirable levels of service provision?

The disadvantage of comparing local services with national data is that national average service use cannot be assumed to represent ideal levels of service provision. It is also unwise to assume that the current balance between service components such as acute beds, residential services outside hospital, day-care services and community services is the best possible. The development of ways for determining optimal levels of service provision is still in its infancy, but a number of writers have contributed to the debate. In the UK, the House of Commons *Second Report from the Social Services Committee, Session 1984–85, Community Care* (1985) noted that, 'a smaller number of in-patient beds is now thought necessary for general psychiatric services', and a Royal College of Psychiatrists working party has specified this number as 44 acute beds for a population of 100,000 (Hirsch, 1988).

Wing (1992) also used the expert estimate method to provide figures for targets for day-care provision by mental health services, and for total numbers in contact with any mental health services, again taking account of the prevalence of severe mental illness in the community. These figures include elderly people who have functional mental illnesses. Figures based on his calculations for the full range of provision for the mental health service are shown in Table 13.5.

Method 4. The deprivation-weighted population approach to needs assessment

The calculations of expected levels of morbidity and service utilization in Planningham have not considered its particular population characteristics. This is unsatisfactory, as there is strong evidence that social and demographic factors are closely associated with rates of psychiatric disorder.

The association between psychiatric disorders and social class (particularly for schizophrenia) is one of the most consistent findings in psychiatric epidemiology. The Jarman combined index of social deprivation has been shown to be highly correlated with psychiatric admission rates for Health Districts in the South East Thames Region (Hirsch, 1988; Jarman, 1983, 1984; Jarman & Hirsch, 1992; Thornicroft, 1991).

Strathdee & Thornicroft (1992) set out targets for service provision based on a Delphi method of summarizing expert opinion in Great Britain and on

Table 3.5. Estimated need of day/residential places needed for 250,000 population

Form of provision	Places per 250,000
Total in contact with specialist services	572–1716
NHS specialist residential care with night staff	82–246
Other residential	115–345
Specialist day care (4+ half days a week)	183–548*
Other active contact with specialist team (excluding those in above categories)	250–750

Source: Wing 1992.
* Including people in nonNHS residential care, of whom half are assumed to require day care.

likely prevalences of mental illness nationally, weighted by social deprivation values for the local population. These targets assume that services should be community based as far as possible, with community residential places and day-care taking the place of institutional care. Naturally, none of these suggested levels of provision should be taken in isolation – if one component of the mental health services is underdeveloped, this is likely to lead to a higher demand for the other elements in the system. Wing (1992) has made similar estimates of targets for general adult residential services. Third, based upon a detailed survey of the actual provision and adequacy of in-patient and residential services in London (Johnson et al., 1997), Ramsay, Johnson, Brooks, Thornicroft & Glover (1997) proposed the 1996 PRiSM values for expected levels of service. These three sets of estimates are shown in Table 13.6 in relation to the actual levels of provision, so that the scale of unmet need can be simply calculated as the difference between expected and actual provision.

In interpreting these estimates, it must be noted that it is crucial to look at all the elements in local services together. If the acute-bed provision were considered in isolation, it might be judged to be unnecessarily high. However, if considered in relation to the low levels of community provision, it becomes apparent that reliance on in-patient beds and high admission rates may well be a consequence of undeveloped community facilities. It thus seems unlikely that numbers of acute beds could reasonably be reduced without considerable further development of community services.

Specific local modifying factors

Weighting according to overall deprivation levels is a helpful beginning in planning epidemiologically based services. However, various other local

Table 13.6. Estimated need and actual provision general adult mental health services (aged 15-64 only) (in-patient and residential care), places per 250,000 population

	Estimated need			Actual level of provision		
	Wing 1992 (range)	Strathdee & Thornicroft 1992 (range)	PRiSM 1996 (range)	Outer London (overall)	Inner London (overall)	London (range)
Medium secure unit	1–10	1–10	5–30	4	26	0–58
Intensive care unit/ local secure unit	5–15	5–10	5–20	8	16	0–40
Acute ward	50–150	50–150	5–175	73	110	32–165
24-hour nurse-staffed units/ hostel wards/staff awake at night	25–75	40–150	12–50	50	38	0–158
24-hour nonnurse-staffed hostels/night staff sleep in	40–110	40–150	50–300	104	175	29–287
Day-staffed hostels	25–75	30–120	15–60	17	50	17–292
Lower support accommodation	n/a	48–100	30–120	43	115	17–292

Note: PRiSM, 1996, estimated need levels based upon: London actual values, and an expected variation of need from the least to the most deprived parts of England, for most categories of service, with a far greater variation in medium secure beds, and NHS Executive (1996) guidance for an average of 25 places for 24-hour nurse-staffed accommodation per 250,000; all estimates given assume that each category of service exists in the given appropriate range of volume; the Wing, 1992 figures include old age assessment places, and Strathdee & Thornicroft, 1992, figures apply only to general adult services for those aged 16–65.

demographic factors should also be considered in tailoring the overall approach to local conditions. These will be outlined in the following section.

Ethnicity

Ethnicity has a major influence on the services used and required. Afro-Caribbeans are an important group, as several studies indicate that they are at greater risk than their Caucasian neighbors of being admitted to psychiatric hospital (Davies, Thornicroft, Leese, Higgenbotham & Phelan, 1996) or of being diagnosed as suffering from schizophrenia (Harrison, Owens, Holton, Neilson & Boot, 1988; King, Coker, Leavey, Hoare & Johnson-Sabine, 1994). It has not been clearly established whether Asians have a higher rate of admission for psychosis (Thomas, Stone, Osborne, Thomas & Fisher, 1993), although King et al. (1994) argue that elevated rates of psychosis may be general among all immigrant groups. However, it has also been found that, despite identical rates of consultation in general practice, Asians are less likely than the Caucasian population to be referred to the psychiatric services, and that psychological disorders in this group may be more likely to go unrecognized (Brewin, 1980), perhaps reflecting linguistic and cultural barriers to service delivery.

Homelessness

Recent research in the UK suggests that probably between 30% and 50% of the homeless in hostels, night shelters and on the street are mentally ill, mostly psychotic (Marshall, 1989; Scott, 1993; Timms & Fry, 1989). Conventional psychiatric services often fail to contact or engage the homeless mentally ill, meaning that specific services are needed. For example, clinics could be provided in places where the homeless tend to congregate or assertive outreach work carried out on the streets.

Unemployment

Another characteristic of Planningham with specific significance for mental health service provision is a high unemployment rate. High levels of unemployment and suicide rates are correlated in several Western countries (Platt, Micciolo & Tansella, 1992; Pritchard, 1992), and becoming unemployed is associated with a general decline in mental health (Warr & Jackson, 1987). Thus, this demographic characteristic may suggest an increased need for mental health services.

Age structure

The age structure of the population may also serve as a pointer for service needs. Over-representation of people aged 20–29 may indicate a population at greater risk of developing psychotic disorders. Thus, there may be a slightly greater need than nationally for general adult services, and a slightly lower one for services for the elderly mentally ill.

Example of population-level needs assessment

In 1996 a consortium of research teams undertook a detailed survey of in-patient and residential mental health surveys in each London borough, conducted in the first half of 1996. Information was collected from Local Authorities and from NHS provider Trusts. We compare here a summary of the results with the expected levels.

An improved understanding of the relationships between sociodemographic factors and service utilization has allowed quantitative indices of need based on the demographic attributes of areas to be developed over the past five years. One of these, the MINI (Mental Illness Needs Index), estimates the likely level of facilities required for a geographical area by calculating where the area lies within the range of need levels for districts within England and applies this to published estimates of the range of necessary provision of various sorts of facility. The definitions used for each category of in-patient and residential care used in the MINI are shown below (from Glover, 1996):

Acute beds. Acute beds or crisis beds for adults with serious mental illness requiring short-term admission to hospital. Occasionally, these can be located in community facilities quite separate from hospitals.

Local secure beds. Low security beds; for example, on an intensive care unit (ICU), special care unit or locked ward.

Regional secure beds. Medium security beds in a regional secure unit.

Respite beds. Short-term beds for adults with chronic illness in hospital or community facilities.

Continuing care beds and hostel ward beds. Beds for adults with serious mental illness needing 24-hour care long term, on or very close to a hospital estate.

Twenty-four-hour staffed residential places. A highly staffed hostel or residential home whose staff are either on full duty at night, or sleep in residence. Staff may or may not be qualified.

Day-staffed residential places. A day-staffed hostel or residential home whose staff attend regularly for fixed hours, four to seven days a week.

Unstaffed hostel/group places. Minimally supported hostels or residential homes with visiting staff. Included in this category are any supported, self-contained flats with one or several staff on call in separate accommodation.

Table 13.7. Difference between actual and predicted levels of service provision in Inner London–Strathdee & Thornicroft, 1992, version of MINI

Borough	Difference between actual and predicted for:				
	Acute beds	Intensive care beds	Medium secure beds	24-hour-staff beds	Day-staffed, respite and lower-staffed beds
Camden	*−36.3*	*−0.1*	*not known*	*not known*	not known
City of London	+0.3	+0.4	+0.8	+9.5	*−0.9*
Greenwich	*−7.9*	*−3.3*	+3.8	+40.9	*−80.2*
Hackney	+2.4	+22.2	+35.3	*−11.9*	*−88.0*
Hammersmith & Fulham	+1.0	+5.8	*not known*	+19.5	*−118.8*
Islington	*−37.0*	*−0.1*	*not known*	+131.5	*−116.1*
Kensington & Chelsea	+10.2	+1.6	*not known*	+25.4	*−16.0*
Lambeth	*−38.8*	+12.5	+22.9	+161.9	+1.4
Lewisham	*−34.1*	*−0.6*	+12.6	+18.4	*−74.3*
Southwark	*−20.9*	+9.6	+13.7	+72.5	*−60.3*
Towers Hamlets	+10.2	+0.2	*not known*	+23.3	*−63.5*
Wandsworth	*−51.2*	*−4.5*	+13.9	+16.8	*−154.0*
Westminster	*−34.5*	+7.8	*not known*	+147.3	*−89.5*
Net difference	*−236.6*	+51.5	+103	+655.1	*−860.2*

Source: Johnson et al., 1997.

MINI, Mental Illness Needs Index.

Note: Positive figures indicate that actual provision is greater than predicted by MINI, negative ones that MINI suggests a deficit. All apparent deficits appear in italics.

Table 13.7 summarizes the information we obtained on expected and current provision of in-patient and residential services in Inner London. Despite our caution about the quality of data available from health and social services, these data are good enough to indicate overall patterns of service provision in London.

Conclusion

The central theme of this chapter is that it is feasible to use currently available information for each local area as the basis for a rational approach to planning mental health services. There is evidence that current mental health services, at least throughout England and Wales, are often not distributed in relation to need, however estimated. It is thus important to develop and apply simple pragmatic approaches to the assessment of local population needs. However, more finely tuned planning of services in each local area will require investment in a database that can be used to monitor service performance and continue to provide relevant information to underpin future planning cycles.

A further issue warrants careful consideration: who should define needs? For example, guidelines for needs assessment under the British *National Health Service and Community Care Act* (House of Commons, 1990) state that 'all users should be encouraged to participate to the limit of their capacity. Where it is impossible to reconcile different perceptions, these differences should be acknowledged and recorded'. Furthermore, so long as they are competent, the, 'user's views should carry the most weight.' (Department of Health Social Services Inspectorate, 1991, pp. 51–3). This emphasis indicates the need to measure the views of the user, and well-validated measures have been developed to assess the user's perspective on (among others) levels of need, satisfaction with services, social network and quality of life. There are other perspectives on need (Slade, 1994). In particular, the staff's assessment of need can and does differ from the user's (Carter, Crosby, Geertshuis & Startup, 1996; Slade et al., 1996). In our view it is likely that important areas of future research will address how and why patients and staff assess needs differently, and how this affects treatment compliance and the course and outcome of schizophrenia.

References

Beecham, J., Knapp, M. & Fenyo, A. (1993). Costs, needs and outcomes in community mental health care. In A. Netten & J. Beecham (eds.), *Costing Community Care: Theory and Practice.* United Kingdom: Ashgate Publishing Company.

Brewin, C. (1980). Explaining the lower rates of psychiatric treatment among Asian immigrants to the UK: a preliminary study. *Social Psychiatry*, 15, 17–19.

Brewin, C. (1992). Measuring individual needs for care and services. In G. Thornicroft, C.R. Brewin, & J. Wing (eds.), *Measuring Mental Health Needs*. London: Gaskell/Royal College of Psychiatrists.

Brewin, C. & Wing, J. (1993). The MRC Needs for Care Assessment: Progress and controversies. *Psychological Medicine*, 23, 837–41.

Brewin, C.R., Veltro, F., Wing, J., MacCarthy, B. & Brugha, T.S. (1990). The assessment of psychiatric disability in the community: a comparison of clinical, staff, and family interviews. *British Journal of Psychiatry*, 157, 671–4.

Brewin, C.R., Wing, J.K., Mangen, S.P., Brugha, T.S. & MacCarthy, B. (1987). Principles and practice of measuring needs in the long-term mentally ill: the MRC needs for care assessment. *Psychological Medicine*, 17, 971–82.

Brewin, C.R., Wing, J., Mangen, S., Brugha, T.S., MacCarthy, B. & Lesage, A. (1988). Needs for care among the long-term mentally ill: a report from the Camberwell High Contact Survey. *Psychological Medicine*, 18, 457–68.

Carter, M., Crosby, C., Geertshuis, S. & Startup, M. (1996). Developing reliability in client-centred mental health needs assessment. *Journal of Mental Health*, 5, 233–43.

Culyer, A. & Wagstaff, A. (1992). *Need, Equity and Equality in Health and Health Care*. York: Centre for Health Economics, Health Economics Consortium, University of York.

Davies, S., Thornicroft, G., Leese, M., Higginbotham, A. & Phelan, M. (1996). Ethnic differences in risk of compulsory admission among representative cases of psychosis in London. *British Medical Journal*, 312, 533–7.

Department of Health (1994). *The Health of the Nation* (2nd edition). London: HMSO.

Department of Health and Social Services Inspectorate (1991). *Care Management and Assessment: Practitioner's Guide*. London: HMSO.

Ellis, K. (1993). *Squaring the Circle: User and Carer Participation in Needs Assessment*. York: Joseph Rowntree Foundation.

Fryers, T. & Wooff, K. (1989). A decade of mental health care in an English urban community. Patterns and trends in Salford 1976–1987. In J.K. Wing (ed.), *Contributions to Health Services Planning and Research*. London: Gaskell.

Glover, G. (1991). The official data available on mental health. In R. Jenkins & S. Griffiths (eds.), *Indicators for Mental Health in the Population*. London: HMSO.

Glover, G. (1996). Mental Illness Needs Index (MINI). In G. Thornicroft & G. Strathdee (eds.), *Commissioning Mental Health Services*. London: HMSO.

Goldberg, D. & Huxley, P. (1980). *Mental Illness in the Community*. London: Tavistock.

Goldberg, D. & Huxley, P. (1992). *Common Mental Disorders. A Bio-Social Model*. London: Routledge.

Goldman, H. (1981). Defining and counting the chronically mentally ill. *Hospital and Community Psychiatry*, 32, 21–7.

Harrison, G., Owens, D., Holton, A., Neilson, D. & Boot, D. (1988). A prospective study of severe mental disorder in Afro-Caribbean patients. *Psychological Medicine*, 18, 643–57.

Herman, D., Struening, E. & Barrow, S. (1993). Self-assessed need for mental health services among homeless adults. *Hospital Community Psychiatry,* **44,**1181–2.

Hillier, W., Zaudig, M. & Mobour, W. (1991). Development of diagnostic checklists for use in routine clinical care. *Archives of General Psychiatry,* **47,** 782–4.

Hirsch, S. (1988). *Psychiatric Beds and Resources: Factors Influencing Bed Use and Service Planning.* London: Gaskell (Royal College of Psychiatrists).

Hogg, L. & Marshall, M. (1992). Can we measure need in the homeless mentally ill? Using the MRC Needs for Care Assessment in hostels for the homeless. *Psychological Medicine,* **22,** 1027–34.

Holloway, F. (1994). Need in community psychiatry: a consensus is required. *Psychiatric Bulletin,* **18,** 321–3.

House of Commons (1985). *Second Report from the Social Services Committee, Session 1984–85, Community Care.* London: HMSO.

House of Commons (1990). *The National Health Service and Community Care Act.* London: HMSO.

Jarman, B. (1983). Identification of underprivileged areas. *British Medical Journal,* **286,** 1705–9.

Jarman, B. (1984). Underprivileged areas: validation and distribution of scores. *British Medical Journal,* **289,** 1587–92.

Jarman, B. & Hirsch, S. (1992). Statistical models to predict district psychiatric morbidity. In G. Thornicroft, C. Brewin, & J.K. Wing (eds.), *Measuring Mental Health Needs,* Chapter 4. London: Gaskell/Royal College of Psychiatrists.

Johnson, S., Ramsay, R., Thornicroft, G., Brooks, L., Lelliot, P., Peck, E., Smith, H., Chisholm, D., Audini, B., Knapp, M. & Goldberg, D. (1997). *London's Mental Health.* London: Kings Fund.

King, M., Coker, E., Leavey, G., Hoare, A. & Johnson-Sabine, E. (1994). Incidence of psychotic illness in London: comparison of ethnic groups. *British Medical Journal,* **304,** 1115–19.

Macdonald, A. (1991). How can we measure mental health? In R. Jenkins & S. Griffiths (eds.), *Indicators for Mental Health in the Population.* London: HMSO.

Mangen, S. & Brewin, C.R. (1991). The measurement of need. In P.E. Bebbington (ed.), *Social Psychiatry. Theory, Methodology and Practice.* London: Transaction Publishers, pp. 162–82.

Marshall, M. (1989). Collected and neglected: are Oxford hostels filling up with disabled psychiatric patients. *British Medical Journal,* **299,** 706–9.

Marshall, M. (1994). How should we measure need? *Philosophy, Psychiatry & Psychology,* **1,** 27–36.

Mavis, B., Humphreys, K. & Stöffelmayr, B. (1993). Treatment needs and outcomes of two subtypes of homeless persons who abuse substances. *Hospital Community Psychiatry,* **44,** 1185–7.

McCrone, P. & Strathdee, G. (1994). Needs not diagnosis: towards a more rational approach to community mental health resourcing in Great Britain. *International Journal of Social Psychiatry,* **40,** 79–86.

National Institute of Mental Health (1987). *Towards a Model for a Comprehensive Community-Based Mental Health System.* Washington D.C.: NIMH.

Phelan, M., Slade, M., Thornicroft, G., Dunn, D., Holloway, F., Wyles, T., Strathdee,

G., Loftus, L., McCrone, P. & Hayward, P. (1995). The Camberwell Assessment of Need (CAN): the validity and reliability of an instrument to assess the needs of people with severe mental illness. *British Journal of Psychiatry*, **167**, 589–95.

Platt, S., Micciolo, R. & Tansella, M. (1992). Suicide and unemployment in Italy: description, analysis and interpretation of recent trends. *Social Science and Medicine*, **34**, 1191–201.

Pritchard, C. (1992). Is there a link between suicide in young men and unemployment? A comparison of the UK with other European Community countries. *British Journal of Psychiatry*, **160**, 750–6.

Pryce, I., Griffiths, R., Gentry, R., Hughes, I., Montaguss, L., Watkins, S., Champney-Smith, J. & McLackland, B. (1993). How important is the assessment of social skills in a long-stay psychiatric in-patients? *British Journal of Psychiatry*, **163**, 498–502.

Ramsay, R., Johnson, S., Brooks, L., Thornicroft, G. & Glover, G. (1997). Levels of in-patient and residential provision throughout London. In S. Johnson, R. Ramsay, G. Thornicroft, L. Brooks, P. Lelliot, E. Peck, H. Smith, D. Chisholm, B. Audini, M. Knapp, & D. Goldberg (eds.), *London's Mental Health*. London: Kings Fund.

Scott, J. (1993). Homelessness and mental illness. *British Journal of Psychiatry*, **162**, 314–24.

Shapiro, S., Skinner, E.A., Kramer, M., Steinwachs, D.M. & Regier, D.A. (1985). Measuring need for mental health services in a general population. *Medical Care*, **23**, 1033–43.

Slade, M. (1994). Needs assessment: who needs to assess? *British Journal of Psychiatry*, **165**, 287–92.

Slade, M., Phelan, M. & Thornicroft, G. (1998). A comparison of needs assessed by staff and by an epidemiologically representative sample of patients with psychosis. *Psychological Medicine*, **28**, 543–50.

Slade, M., Phelan, M., Thornicroft, G. & Parkman, S. (1996). The Camberwell Assessment of Need (CAN): comparison of assessments by staff and patients of the needs of the severely mentally ill. *Social Psychiatry and Psychiatric Epidemiology*, **31**, 109–13.

Stevens, A. & Gabbay, J. (1991). Needs assessment, needs assessment. *Health Trends*, **23**, 20–3.

Strathdee, G. & Thornicroft, G. (1992). Community sectors for needs-led mental health services. In G. Thornicroft, C. Brewin, & J.K. Wing (eds.), *Measuring Mental Health Needs*, Chapter 8. London: Gaskell/Royal College of Psychiatrists.

Thomas, C.S., Stone, K., Osborn, M., Thomas, P.F. & Fisher, M. (1993). Psychiatric morbidity and compulsory admission among UK born Europeans, Afro-Caribbeans and Asians in central Manchester. *British Journal of Psychiatry*, **163**, 91–9.

Thornicroft, G. (1991). Social deprivation and rates of treated mental disorder. *British Journal of Psychiatry*, **158**, 475–84.

Timms, P. & Fry, A. (1989). Homelessness and mental illness. *Health Trends*, **21**, 70–1.

Van Haaster, I., Lesage, A., Cyr, M. & Toupin, J. (1994). Problems and needs for care of patients suffering from severe mental illness. *Social Psychiatry and Psychiatric Epidemiology*, **29**, 141–8.

Warr, P. & Jackson, P. (1987). Adapting to the unemployed role: a longitudinal investigation. *Social Science and Medicine*, **25**, 1219–24.

Wing, J. (ed.) (1989). *Health Services Planning and Research. Contributions from Psychiatric Case Registers.* London: Gaskell Press.

Wing, J.K. (1992). *Epidemiologically-based-needs-assessments. Review of research on psychiatric disorders.* London: Department of Health.

14

The early course of schizophrenia: new concepts for early intervention

Heinz Häfner and Kurt Maurer

In schizophrenia, the first contact with mental health services is frequently preceded by a lengthy, mostly untreated prephase. We have retrospectively studied a population-based sample of 232 first episodes of broadly defined schizophrenia, using a semi-structured interview (interview for the retrospective assessment of the onset of schizophrenia, IRAOS) from first admission to the first sign of the disorder. A representative subsample (n=115) was followed prospectively over six occasions until five years after first admission. Three-quarters of the cases began with a prodromal phase, lasting five years on average. This was followed by a psychotic prephase of about one year with an exponential increase in all symptoms until the climax of the first episode.

The ten most frequent initial signs were predominantly negative and affective symptoms, including indicators of functional impairment. Depressive symptoms following the first psychotic symptom showed a significant correlation with the score of positive symptoms in the first psychotic episode. A lack of early depressive symptoms is a significant prediction of affective flattening and a weaker prediction of anhedonia over the five years after first admission.

Social disability occurred as early as two to four years before first admission. Compared with age- and sex-matched controls from the general population, the patients at onset of illness did not differ significantly from their healthy peers in terms of social status, but already showed considerable social deficits. These emerged in the prodromal phase, long before first admission. In early-onset cases, the expected social ascent was impeded, whereas in late-onset cases there was considerable downward drift from a higher status at onset. Social status, measured by financial autonomy five years after first admission, was predicted by the socioeconomic status when the first symptoms of psychosis became apparent, and by socially negative illness behavior (i.e., becoming withdrawn, autistic) of young men, indicated by eight PSE items.

Early intervention must consider the risk of false-positive cases. In our view it should proceed stepwise: (1) functional impairment and social handicap can and must be treated independently of any diagnosis; (2) depressive symptoms can be treated either with serotonin reuptake inhibitors, involving

Table 14.1. Duration of the prephase of schizophrenia from onset – first sign, first psychotic symptom – until first contact or first admission: selected studies

Author	n	Duration from 1st sign (in (years)	Duration from 1st psychotic symptom (in years)
Gross, 1969 (Germany)	290	3.5	
Lindelius, 1970 (Sweden)	237		4.1[a]
Huber, Gross & Schüttler, 1979 (Germany)	502	3.3	
Lewine, 1980 (USA)	97		1.9
Loebel et al., 1992 (USA)	70	2.9	1.0
Beiser, Erikson, Flemming & Iacono, 1993 (Canada)	70	2.1	1.1
Häfner et al., 1995 (Germany)	232	5.0[b]	1.1
McGorry, Edwards, Mihalopoulos, Harrigan & Jackson, 1996 (Australia)	200	8.8	3.7

[a] Duration from first psychotic symptoms or marked personality changes indicative of mental illness.
[b] Prodromal phase until appearance of first psychotic symptom only.

a low risk of side-effects, or cognitive-behavioral therapy independently of a diagnosis; (3) because of their possible side-effects, antipsychotic drugs should be given only after clear-cut positive symptoms have appeared. The risk of stigma must be weighed before finally assigning a diagnosis of schizophrenia.

By the early course of schizophrenia we mean the period from onset until the climax of the first psychotic episode. The few studies assessing the duration of the early period of illness from the first sign of the disorder until the first contact with mental health services give estimates ranging from two to almost nine years (see Table 14.1).

Various factors account for the differences in these study results: some of the samples studied were not representative, the assessment techniques used were mostly nonstandardized, and the onset of the prodromal phase was variably defined, more so than the psychotic episode. Further factors influencing the duration of the early illness are the time taken for the patient to first contact the mental health services and, therefore, the patients' help-seeking behavior and availability of mental health services. For these reasons we decided to conduct a systematic investigation, by recruiting a population-based sample of first-episode cases and developing a semi-standardized interview – IRAOS – for retrospectively assessing the onset and early course of schizophrenia. We focused on four questions: (1) when and with what symptoms does schizophrenia start? (2) how does the disorder develop before the first episode? (3) when and how does schizophrenia lead to social consequences? and (4) what are the implications for early intervention?

Methods

We analyzed the population-based Age, Beginning and Course (ABC) schizophrenia study, which is based on a sample of 232 first episodes of a broad diagnosis of schizophrenia (ICD 295, 297, 298.3/4) (84% of 276 first admissions from a German population of about 1.5 million). For a detailed description of the sample see Häfner, Maurer, Löffler & Riecher-Rössler (1993). Symptoms, functional impairment, and social disability were rated by the Present State Examination (PSE) (Wing, Cooper & Sartorius, 1974); the Scale for the Assessment of Negative Symptoms (SANS) (Andreasen, 1983); the Psychological Impairments Rating Schedule (PIRS) (Biehl, Maurer, Jablensky, Cooper & Tomov, 1989); and the Disability Assessment Schedule (DAS) (Jung, Krumm, Biehl, Maurer & Bauer-Schubart, 1989; World Health Organization, 1988) immediately upon first admission. Onset and early course were assessed by the IRAOS (Häfner et al., 1992), mainly after remission of psychotic symptoms, within three to five weeks of first admission.

Results

The few studies assessing the duration of the early period of illness give estimates ranging from two to almost nine years (Table 14.1). A precise assessment requires identification of the symptoms that mark the onset of schizophrenia (Maurer & Häfner, 1995). At onset, 73% of our sample exhibited nonspecific or negative symptoms, only 7% positive symptoms and the remainder both categories. Sixty-eight percent had a chronic, 18% an acute and 15% a subacute type of onset. There were no differences between men and women. Table 14.2 gives the ten most frequent early signs of schizophrenia cited by the patients. No positive symptoms were noted, and most were negative and affective symptoms. The only difference between men and women was that the women were more likely ($p < 0.05$) to worry.

Figure 14.1 gives the mean ages for men and women at the first sign of schizophrenia, the first negative and the positive symptoms, the climax of the first episode, and the first admission. The early course of this disorder is similar for men and women, as indicated by the parallel sequence of these milestones. However, the men are significantly younger than the women at each stage.

This impression is confirmed by the cumulative number of symptoms

Table 14.2. The ten most frequent early signs of schizophrenia (independent of the course) cited by the patients

	Total (n = 232) %	Men (n = 108) %	Women (n = 124) %	p
Restlessness	19	15	22	
Depression	19	15	22	
Anxiety	18	17	19	
Trouble with thinking and concentration	16	19	14	
Worrying	15	9	20	*
Lack of self-confidence	13	10	15	
Lack of energy, slowness	12	8	15	
Poor work performance	11	12	10	
Social withdrawal, distrust	10	8	12	
Social withdrawal, communication	10	8	12	

Source: Häfner et al., 1995.
Note: Based on closed questions, multiple counting possible. All items tested for sex differences.
* $p < 0.05$.

(Figure 14.2): the sum scores per year, and in the last year per month, increase exponentially, with negative and nonspecific symptoms appearing early, and positive symptoms later and more rapidly.

When the duration (in years) of the early period of illness is depicted as the percentage of cases, the distribution is heavily skewed to the left, with 28% of the patients having a duration of one year or less (Figure 14.3).

We went on to analyze how the main initial symptoms, that is depression and negative symptoms, developed after the onset of schizophrenia. We found that no fewer than 81% of the patients had suffered from a depressed mood for at least two weeks before their first admission. In this IRAOS-based retrospective assessment, depressive mood was operationalized by the following items: (1) have you ever been very depressed or low spirited? (2) have there been times when you thought that life was not worth living? (3) have you ever been unable to enjoy yourself in any way? (4) have there been times when you lost even your special interests? A continued persistence of depressed mood was reported by 39%, recurrent episodes by 34% and only one episode by 8%.

A subgroup of 57 people with schizophrenia in Mannheim were compared with 57 healthy controls drawn from the city's population register on four IRAOS items: depressed mood, feelings of guilt, lack of self-confidence, and attempted suicide. People suffering from schizophrenia suffered from signifi-

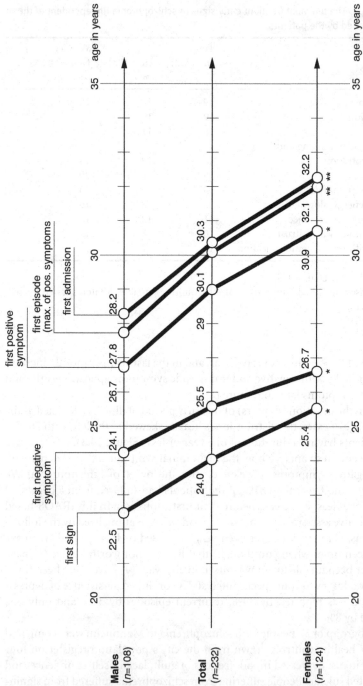

Figure 14.1 The mean ages for men and women at the first sign of schizophrenia, the first negative and the first positive symptoms, the climax of the first episode, and the first admission. (n=232); *p < 0.05; **p < 0.001.

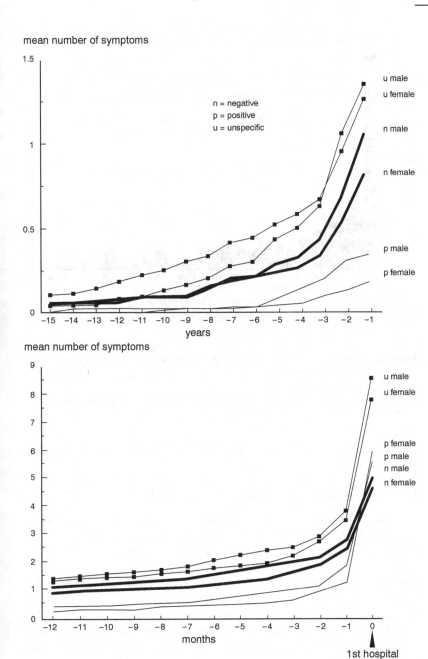

Figure 14.2 Cumulative numbers of positive, negative and nonspecific symptoms of the onset of schizophrenia until first hospital admission for schizophrenia (n=108 males, =124 females).

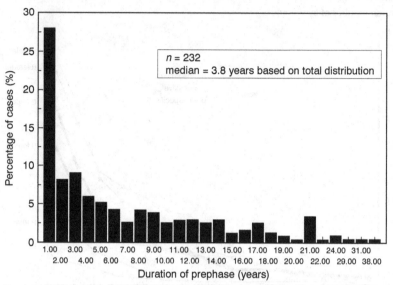

Figure 14.3 The duration of the prephase (from the first sign to first admission) of schizophrenia in years, according to the percentage of cases.

Table 14.3. Comparison of four depressive IRAOS items between patients and controls – lifetime prevalence by age at first admission of patients – continuously present or recurrent symptoms only

IRAOS item	Schizophrenia (n=57) %	Controls (n=57) %	χ^2 tests
Depressive mood (6)	70.2	19.3	***
Feelings of guilt (10)	33.3	10.5	**
Lack of self-confidence (8)	59.4	12.3	***
Suicide attempt (7)	12.3	8.8	n.s.

Note: IRAOS, interview for the retrospective assessment of the onset of schizophrenia. n.s.; not significant. **: $p < 0.01$, *** $p < 0.001$.

cantly more of these depressive symptoms compared with controls (Table 14.3). An important finding was an approximately 50% higher risk for attempted suicide in early schizophrenia. Although this was not statistically significant, due to the rareness of these events, it draws attention to the high prevalence of depressive symptoms in people with schizophrenia before neuroleptic medication.

Table 14.4. Depression in early schizophrenia and the course of negative symptoms (SANS scores) over five years after first admission

No D, D before P, D = P, and D after P, compared by oneway analysis of variance	First admission	Time after first admission				
		6 months	1 year	2 years	3 years	5 years
Affective flattening (18)	n.s.	**	**	*	n.s.	○
Alogia (13)	n.s.	n.s.	n.s.	n.s.	n.s.	○
Abulia/apathy (17)	n.s.	n.s.	n.s.	n.s.	n.s.	n.s.
Anhedonia/asociality (22)	n.s.	*	○	n.s.	n.s.	n.s.
Attention (25)	n.s.	n.s.	n.s.	n.s.	n.s.	n.s.
SANS total score	○	*	*	n.s.	n.s.	n.s.

Note: no significant differences in any of the CATEGO scores over time. D, depressed mood; P, first psychotic symptom; SANS, Scale for the Assessment of Negative Symptoms; n.s; not significant. ○ $p < 0.10$, *:$p < 0.05$, ** $p < 0.01$.

Depressive symptoms as predictors

We studied the prognostic implications of depressive symptoms for the first psychotic episode. For this purpose, we divided our sample into four subgroups: (1) no episode of depressed mood; (2) depressed mood before the first episode; (3) depressed mood at the same time as the first episode; and (4) depressed mood after the first psychotic symptom. Patients with no symptoms of depression in early schizophrenia had a significantly lower CATEGO (the PSE scoring system) total, and lower scores for specific (SNR) and nonspecific symptoms of neurosis (NSN). In contrast, patients who became depressed after the first positive symptoms of schizophrenia had significantly elevated scores for nonspecific symptoms of neurosis and CATEGO total scores. Depression emerging after the onset of positive symptoms seems to be an indication of the severity of the first psychotic episode.

The four types of onset of depression in early schizophrenia do not predict the main CATEGO symptom scores beyond the first episode in the five years after first admission. The lack of depression in the prephase predicted the occurrence of only a few negative symptoms: anhedonia until one year and, above all, increased affective flattening until two years after first admission and to a lesser extent at the five-year follow-up (Table 14.4).

A two-way analysis of variance with repeated measurements confirmed this result, showing that time significantly affected all CATEGO scores including the positive symptom score, but without any interaction. The only main effect depression had was on affective flattening, without a time effect and with no interaction (Figure 14.4).

As the mean values for the three subgroups with depression converged at the five-year follow-up, a *t*-test revealed a highly significant difference (with-

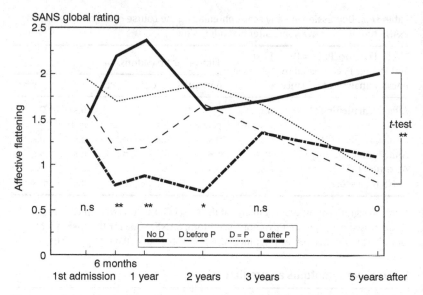

Figure 14.4 Depression in the early course, and the course of affective flattening (SANS global rating) over five years. SANS, Scale for the Assessment of Negative Symptoms; n.s., not significant; No D, no depression; D before P, depression before the first positive symptom; D=P, depression concurrent with the first positive symptom; D after P, depression develops after the first positive symptom. **p < 0.01, * < 0.05, ○ p < 0.1.

out early depression: mean = 2.0; with early depression: mean = 0.9; $p < 0.01$). This inverse relationship implies that early depression and affective flattening are negatively correlated, with point biserial correlation coefficients of –0.33 and –0.34 at the six-month and one-year follow-ups and of –0.31 five years after first admission. These correlations were significant at the 1% level.

Figure 14.5 illustrates the overlap between depressive and negative symptoms. This was pronounced in the first episode (50%), close to 20% after that and clearly reduced at the five-year follow-up. Both syndromes were significantly correlated with each other, with coefficients ranging from 0.4 to 0.6.

Maurer & Häfner (1996) demonstrated higher correlations of items within both syndromes than between the syndromes. A fairly stable depression factor could be identified for the entire period of illness studied, but the factor for negative symptoms was more stable. Depression and negative symptoms apparently represent two overlapping, but substantially distinguishable, syndromes in schizophrenia.

When does schizophrenia lead to social disability? After analyzing the affective component of the initial symptoms, we continued by finding out when negative symptoms produce social disability (Häfner, 1996). We were surprised to find that many DAS items (e.g., parental role in 6% and

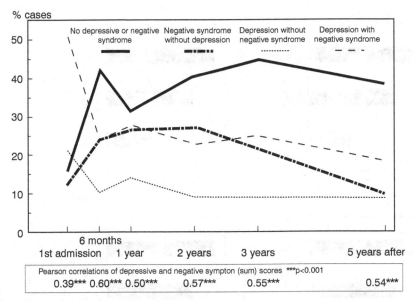

Figure 14.5 Cases with negative[1] and/or depressive[2] syndrome over five years after first admission. [1]Negative syndrome: at least two SANS global scores ≥ 2. [2]Depressive syndrome: at least two CATEGO syndromes ≥ 2.

underactivity in 64% of cases) occurred as early as two to four years before first admission. Consequently, there is a high risk of adverse social effects even in the prodromal phase.

How do the social consequences come about? We tested the two classic hypotheses: (1) impeded social development, or the nonstarter hypothesis; and (2) social decline from an achieved social status, the so-called social-drift hypothesis. More than two-thirds of those with schizophrenia fell ill before the age of 30, which is in the main period of social ascent in life. To test the effect of age on the level of social development at the onset of schizophrenia, we divided our sample into three age groups: under 21, 21–35, and over 35. Assessing the extent to which the patients had taken up six key social roles, we found, as expected, a highly significant association between age and the percentage of patients fulfilling the social roles tested (Figure 14.6).

The next stage was an attempt to gain an objective picture of the social course of schizophrenia. We compared the performance in the same six key roles at exactly the same age between the subsample of 57 patients and 57 age- and sex-matched healthy controls. Despite equal levels of social development at the beginning, the patients remained at the levels they had achieved by the onset, while the age-matched controls moved continuously upwards. The most pronounced difference emerged with marriage and stable partnership (Figure 14.7). Patients and controls had almost the same initial values, but

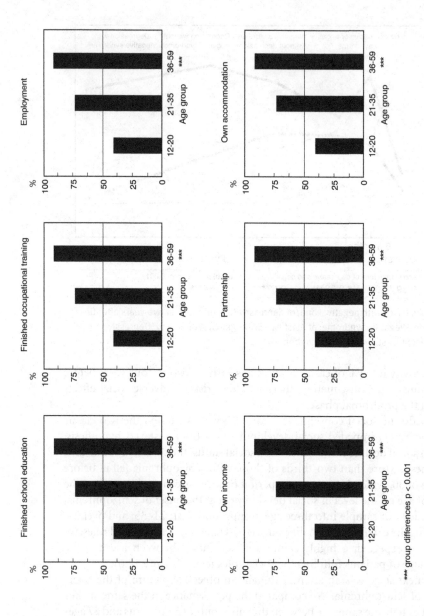

Figure 14.6 The stage of social development by performance of six key roles at the onset of schizophrenia (first sign) by age. Data are from the ABC Schizophrenia Study first-episode sample (n=232).

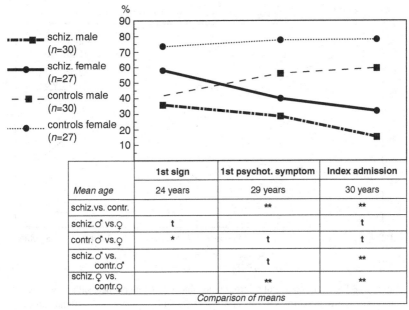

	1st sign	1st psychot. symptom	Index admission
Mean age	24 years	29 years	30 years
schiz.vs. contr.		**	**
schiz.♂ vs.♀	t		t
contr. ♂ vs.♀	*	t	t
schiz.♂ vs. contr.♂		t	**
schiz. ♀ vs. contr.♀		**	**
		Comparison of means	

** = $p \leq 0.01$ * = $p \leq 0.05$ t = $p \leq 0.10$

Figure 14.7 The social course of schizophrenia: marriage and stable partnership.
**p ≤ 0.01, *p ≤ 0.05, ᵗp ≤ 0.10. Data are taken from Häfner, 1996.

the percentage of married men and women with schizophrenia declined continuously, but increased for the controls. The maximum social disadvantage in schizophrenia apparently emerges before the climax of the first episode or first admission.

Further social outcome was studied in our population-based subsample of 115 first-episode cases over five years by using financial independence as an indicator of the objective social status (Häfner, Hambrecht, Löffler, Munk-Jørgensen & Riecher-Rössler, 1998). Except for a slight variation, the percentage of individuals who earned their own living did not increase over the 11 years from onset until five years after first admission. Women retained their slightly better social statuses because of their greater age at onset. Five years after first admission, 58% of the men and 35% of the women with schizophrenia continued to be financially dependent. Analysis of early-, medium-, and late-onset patients showed that the early-onset group ascended slightly but not significantly from their initially low levels (Figure 14.8). The late-onset group experienced a steep social drift from their high status at onset, but nevertheless had a slightly better five-year outcome than the early-onset group, whose social status possibly continues to be determined by their initially low levels of social development throughout their lives. Being young at the onset of schizophrenia, coupled with a low level of social development

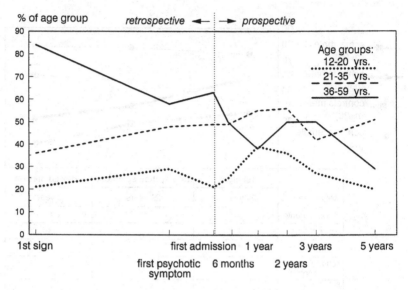

Figure 14.8 The social course of schizophrenia: financial independence, with autonomy due to one's own or partners income. Data are taken from the ABC Schizophrenia Study, (n=115). Source: Häfner et al., 1997.

probably influences the social course of the illness, which agrees with the nonstarter hypothesis. In contrast, if the schizophrenia starts when the patient is older and has a comparatively high level of social development, they usually experience a social decline.

The illness appears to stabilize after the first episode remits, regardless of gender, although women have slightly better CATEGO scores than men. This stability of the illness coincides with the results of the methodologically sound long-term studies on the course of schizophrenia, e.g., the WHO disability study from Groningen (Wiersma, Nienhuis, Giel, de Jong & Slooff, 1996), Nottingham (Mason, Harrison, Glazebrook, Medley & Croudace, 1996), and Mannheim (an der Heiden et al., 1995, 1996).

Conclusions

The early course of schizophrenia, from the first prodromal sign until the climax of the first psychotic episode, seems to be a decisive period in the total course of the illness. Early detection and early intervention are therefore necessary and meaningful. The main initial symptoms, i.e., depressive, negative and positive symptoms, are targets for effective therapy. The first two can be treated long before a diagnosis of schizophrenia can be established. Before assigning a reliable diagnosis, positive symptoms should be treated with great caution to avoid false-positive cases with the attendant risk of social stigmatization and the side-effects of neuroleptic medication.

References

an der Heiden, W., Krumm, B., Müller, S., Weber, I., Biehl, H. & Schäfer, M. (1995). Mannheimer Langzeitstudie der Schizophrenie. *Nervenarzt*, **66**, 820–7.

an der Heiden, W., Krumm, B., Müller, S., Weber, I., Biehl, H. & Schäfer, M. (1996). Eine prospektive studie zum langzeitverlauf schizophrener psychosen: Ergebnisse der 14-jahres-katamnese. *Zeitschrift für Medizinische Psychologie*, 5, 66–75.

Andreasen, N.C. (1983). *The Scale for the Assessment of Negative Symptoms (SANS)*. Iowa City: University of Iowa.

Beiser, M., Erickson, D., Flemming, J.A.E. & Iacono, W.G. (1993). Establishing the onset of psychotic illness. *American Journal of Psychiatry*, 150, 1349–54.

Biehl, H., Maurer, K., Jablensky, A., Cooper, J.E. & Tomov, T. (1989). The WHO Psychological Impairments Rating Schedule (WHO/PIRS). I. Introducing a new instrument for rating observed behaviour and the rationale of the psychological impairment concept. *British Journal of Psychiatry*, 155 [Suppl. 7], 68–70.

Gross, G. (1969). Prodrome und Vorpostensyndrome schizophrener Erkrankungen. In G. Huber (ed.), *Schizophrenie und Zyklothymie. Ergebnisse und Probleme*, pp. 177–87. Stuttgart: Thieme.

Häfner, H. (1996). The epidemiology of onset and early course of schizophrenia. In H. Häfner & E.M. Wolpert (eds.), *New Research in Psychiatry*, pp. 33–61. Bern: Hogrefe & Huber Publishers.

Häfner, H., Hambrecht, M., Löffler, W., Munk-Jørgensen, P. & Riecher-Rössler, A. (1998). Is schizophrenia a disorder of all ages? A comparison of first episodes and early course over the life-cycle. *Psychological Medicine*, **28**, 351–65.

Häfner, H., Maurer, K., Löffler, W., Bustamante, S., an der Heiden, W., Riecher-Rössler, A. & Nowotny, B. (1995). Onset and early course of schizophrenia. In H. Häfner & W.F. Gattaz (eds.), *Search for the Causes of Schizophrenia*, pp. 43–66, Volume III. Berlin: Springer-Verlag.

Häfner, H., Maurer, K., Löffler, W. & Riecher-Rössler, A. (1993). The influence of age and sex on the onset and early course of schizophrenia. *British Journal of Psychiatry*, **162**, 80–6.

Häfner, H., Riecher-Rössler, A., Hambrecht, M., Maurer, K., Meissner, S., Schmidtke, A., Fätkenheuer, B., Löffler, W. & an der Heiden, W. (1992). IRAOS: an instrument for the assessment of onset and early course of schizophrenia. *Schizophrenia Research*, **6**, 209–23.

Huber, G., Gross, G. & Schüttler, R. (1979). *Schizophrenie. Eine verlaufs - und sozialpsychiatrische Langzeitstudie*. Berlin: Springer-Verlag.

Jung, E., Krumm, B., Biehl, H., Maurer, K. & Bauer-Schubart, C. (1989). *DAS-M: Mannheimer Skala zur Einschätzung Sozialer Behinderung*. Weinheim: Beltz.

Lewine, R.J. (1980). Sex differences in age of symptom onset and first hospitalization in schizophrenia. *American Journal of Orthopsychiatry*, **50**, 316–22.

Lindelius, R. (1970). A study of schizophrenia. *Acta Psychiatrica Scandinavica, Supplementum* 216.

Loebel, A.D., Lieberman, J.A., Alvir, J.M.J., Mayerhoff, D.I., Geisler, S.H. & Szymanski, S.R. (1992). Duration of psychosis and outcome in first-episode schizophrenia. *American Journal of Psychiatry*, 149, 1183–8.

Mason, P., Harrison, G., Glazebrook, C., Medley, I. & Croudace, T. (1996). The course of schizophrenia over 13 years. A report from the International Study on Schizophrenia (ISoS) coordinated by the World Health Organization. *British Journal of Psychiatry*, 169, 580–6.

Maurer, K. & Häfner, H. (1995). Methodological aspects of onset assessment in schizophrenia. *Schizophrenia Research*, 15, 265–76.

Maurer, K. & Häfner, H. (1996). Depression and negative symptoms: overlapping or distinguishable syndromes of schizophrenia? Paper presented at the AEP conference in Cambridge, April 11–13, 1996.

McGorry, P.D., Edwards, J., Mihalopoulos, C., Harrigan, S.M. & Jackson, J.H. (1996). EPPIC: an evolving system of early detection and optimal management. *Schizophrenia Research*, 22, 305–26.

Wiersma, D., Nienhuis, F.J., Giel, R., de Jong, A. & Slooff, C.J. (1996). Assessment of the need for care 15 years after onset of a Dutch cohort of patients with schizophrenia, and an international comparison. *Social Psychiatry and Psychiatric Epidemiology*, 31, 114–21.

Wing, J.K., Cooper, J.E. & Sartorius, N. (1974). *Measurement and Classification of Psychiatric Symptoms: An Instruction Manual for the PSE and CATEGO program*. London: Cambridge University Press.

World Health Organization (1988). *Psychiatric Disability Assessment Schedule* (WHO/DAS). Geneva: WHO.

15

Unmet need in depression: varying perspectives on need

Kay Wilhelm and Elizabeth Lin

Summary

Unmet need is examined from the perspectives of various stakeholders, including clinicians in primary and specialist care, depressed people and their families, fundholders and health planners, and society in general. The various perspectives lead to a number of needs which may conflict with one another, but not necessarily so. Areas of unmet need include: increasing the importance of depression in preventive programs; increasing education about the relapsing nature of depression, identifying underlying vulnerability to relapse and the importance of conveying such information in user-friendly formats; translating this information into practical programs that improve prevention, detection, and management; and identifying areas where there are unanswered questions requiring further research. Strategies aimed at increasing the quality of life and reducing risk factors for depression also improve health in general, are relatively cheap and are acceptable to the general public. Thus, they simultaneously address a number of crucial economic and social concerns.

Varying perspectives on need

Major depression is a common illness with a significant morbidity (Goering, Lin, Campbell, Boyle & Offord, 1996; Kessler, McGonagle, Schwartz, Blazer & Nelson, 1993; Regier et al., 1988). A depressive episode is associated with increased morbidity and mortality from a range of medical and other psychiatric disorders (Fawcett, 1993; Livingston Bruce, Leaf, Rozal, Florio & Hoff, 1994), and an increased functional and economic burden for depressed individuals, the health budget and society (Bushnell & Bowie, 1995; Murphy et al., 1991; Simon, Von Korff & Barlow, 1995). The significance of depression also recently received considerable public attention following the World Bank report (Murray & Lopez, 1996) that the toll, measured by disability-adjusted life years (DALYs), is currently fourth behind respiratory diseases, diarrheal diseases, and perinatal conditions. It was predicted that by 2020 depression will rank second behind ischemic heart disease and ahead of morbidity from motor vehicle accidents. On the other hand, in a recent consensus statement concerning treatment for depression, the National Depressive and Manic Depressive Association in USA (Hirschfield et al., 1997) identified *undertreatment of depression* as a key issue. The authors draw attention to the findings that depression leads to longstanding distress and suffering, suicide, occupational impairment and impaired interpersonal relationships, and that safe, cost-effective treatments are available and underutilized.

The focus for health care has been widened to include definitions and determinants of outcomes and the cost-effectiveness of defined interventions. While much of this has been driven by the economics of health care, it has also led to clearer definitions of clinical effectiveness and 'need'. Bebbington, Marsden & Brewin (1997) defined 'need for treatment' as states where there are changes (or potential changes) in function following effective intervention. This definition is readily adaptable to embrace preventive as well as treatment issues. It is important to bear in mind that perceptions of these changes in function will vary according to who defines them. The first step is to decide whether the needs implied by these perceptions are appropriate, in line with current knowledge, and have achievable outcomes. 'Unmet need' is a corollary of this process. We will outline the issues and areas of concern from the perspective of five groups of 'stakeholders' – clinicians in primary care; clinicians in secondary and tertiary care; depressed individuals and their families; the general community; and the fundholders.

Depression and the provision of primary care

Epidemiological and clinical reports (Fawcett, 1993; Goldberg, Bridges, Duncan-Jones & Grayson, 1988; Tiemens, Ormel & Simon, 1996; Wells, Burnam, Rogers, Hays & Camp, 1992) state that a high proportion of those suffering from depression go untreated. Education campaigns have been directed at increasing public awareness of the illness (Macaskill, Macaskill & Nicol, 1997; O'Hara, Gorman & Wright, 1996; Regier et al., 1988). The role of the family doctor has also received a lot of attention since a majority of those with untreated depression do consult general practitioners (Bebbington et al., 1997; Goldberg et al., 1988; Tiemens et al., 1996), and there has been a focus on increasing the 'hit rate' of recognition and case finding. The Dutch group (Tiemens et al., 1996) make the point that increased recognition is only valuable if general practitioners are given the resources to deal with the cases they discover.

Bebbington et al. (1997) reported that 10% of patients presenting in general practice have a current psychiatric problem and that the greatest 'unmet need' is for treatment of mixed anxiety and depression. In terms of treatment needs, they considered that general practitioners (primary physicians) could treat most depression, provided they had adequate education and support. There has been less emphasis in primary care on preventing the physical and psychosocial morbidity that can follow a depressive episode, because it is assumed that those with depression 'bounce back' after successful treatment.

Primary care is affected by a number of problems to do with treatment and awareness of depression. First, in many countries, family physicians are being called upon to screen for increasing numbers of conditions, and to make cost-effective use of their time in offering first-line treatment. The time required for education, new administrative demands and the required paperwork erodes that available for recognition and treatment. Second, public education programs tend to depict depression as a unitary illness requiring a single treatment, rather than making it clear that different interventions are needed for the acute phase and to prevent recurrence and relapse. Such interventions must be multimodal to deal with the patient's psychological, social, and biological problems. Such a multimodal approach may be provided by other staff according to a coordinated management plan. Third, depression is often portrayed as occurring in discrete episodes, usually precipitated by a psychosocial event, with the unwritten assumption that resolution of the psychosocial stressors, with or without antidepressants, is enough to bring the episode to a close. It is only recently that there has been more emphasis on preventing relapse or recurrence with specific interventions. This 'episode concept' of depression also ignores the importance of chronic forms of depression such as dysthymia, characterological depression, and subsyndromal depression (Akiskal et al., 1980; Sherbourne et al., 1994). Patients whose depression is persistent, resistant to treatment or characterized by frequent relapses need clearly identified referral pathways to specialist treatment.

Sufferers, their families and the general community need better access to clear and comprehensive information about mental illness. The patient's social network, general practitioners, and other health professionals need to learn more about the fluctuating course of depression and factors contributing to relapse (including the potential effects of personality and inherent vulnerability).

If general practitioners and other primary care workers are to be encouraged to treat depression more effectively, the clinical guidelines must be presented clearly in a 'user-friendly' way. The Primary Mental Health Toolkit from the National Primary Care Facilitation Programme in the UK (1997) and the Clinical Practice Guidelines from the United States Department of Health and Human Services (1993) are examples of what is possible. Such material should identify interventions that are relevant to various stages of depressive disorders, i.e., first onset, relapse prevention, treatment for further episodes. At the same time, there should be greater access to cost-effective, time-limited nondrug treatments, which are probably most cost-effective in primary care. These may stand alone or complement and enhance the action of antidepressant medication. Interventions also need to reflect the patient's social network.

Depression and the provision of specialist care

Parker & Hadzi-Pavlovic (1996) emphasize that many patients with depression seen at specialist centers do not have just a mood disorder, but also a disorder of neurocognitive and motor function. This is particularly the case for the melancholic subtype of depression. It tends to occur in patients who are older and have a family history of depression or bipolar disorder – groups which tend to come to the attention of secondary and tertiary services. Recent developments in neuroimaging and neurocognitive testing have provided evidence of brain pathology in some patients with a later-onset melancholic depression. Changes include cortical atrophy in frontal, parietal, and temporal regions as well as decreased basal ganglia volume, which correlate with underlying cerebrovascular disease (Alexopoulos et al., 1997; Hickie, Hickie, Scott & Wilhelm, 1996). The cortical and subcortical changes, and associated disruption of frontal-subcortical neural networks, are consistent with disorders of cognition, volition, and mood. The 'vascular depression' hypothesis has important implications for late-onset depression, in terms of preventing cerebrovascular disease, and for treatment which may be determined by the site of the lesion (Alexopoulos et al., 1997). This will become increasingly important as populations age and the morbidity profile changes towards even more chronic illness.

Some interesting work has also been done on the nature of nonmelancholic depression, particularly in relation to underlying personality vulnerability. Joyce's group (Mulder & Joyce, 1997) used a dimensional personality questionnaire (Cloninger, Svrakic & Przybeck, 1993) to consider the association of psychological constructs underlying depression with possible neurotransmitter correlates.

Two longitudinal cohort studies of young adults (Merikangas & Angst, 1994; Wilhelm, Parker & Hadzi-Pavlovic, 1997) identified patterns of depression that appear to have different treatment implications. Early onset seems to be related to a greater number of anxiety disorders and greater experience of inherent vulnerability. There have also been attempts to differentiate between the frequency of relapse, the time to recovery, and the duration of episodes that have different associated risk factors. The Sydney cohort showed that the frequency of episodes of major depression up to the age of 40 was predicted by neuroticism and by reports of maternal over-protection and poor paternal care during the first 16 years of life, the age of onset of depression, and the number of anxiety disorders reported over the individual's lifetime to date (Wilhelm, Parker, Dewhurst-Savellis & Asghari, in press).

Long-term follow-up studies (Keller et al., 1984; Kiloh, Andrews & Neilson, 1988; Lee & Murray, 1988; Merikangas & Angst, 1994) highlight the potential for relapse following a first episode of depression. Depression as a lifelong disorder is being better understood. There are a number of clinical guidelines relating to both pharmacological and psychotherapeutic treatment (United States Department of Health and Human Services, 1993), and growing confidence in indications of when combinations of the two are more effective than either alone (Akiskal, 1992; Thase et al., 1997).

We still require information on the comparative costs and outcomes of treating (and not treating) individuals with depression, and on when more extensive treatment interventions are warranted. We also need more data on when and how to stop treatment (as opposed to the current emphasis on starting treatment), as well as information about when various maintenance therapies (pharmacological and psychological) are required.

Depressed individuals and their families

There is considerable evidence that lay and professional perspectives often differ on what constitutes illness and effective treatment. In an epidemiological survey of household residents in Ontario, Canada (Goering et al., 1996), nearly half of the respondents meeting diagnostic criteria for major depression felt that they had no mental health problems. Furthermore, while these respondents had the same expectations as the rest of the sample about the abstract benefits of receiving professional help, they reported that they personally would be reluctant and uncomfortable about seeking such help, even if they felt that they had a serious mental health problem. Areas for further research include investigating how individuals determine the severity of their own psychological distress and then the need to seek help.

In a study of consumer attitudes to treatment, Jorm et al. (1997) found a moderate degree of recognition of depression within the community, with some agreement that active treatment (rather than 'letting time heal') was required. However, public understanding of psychiatric syndromes and their treatments needs to be improved, as many treatments considered standard by mental health professionals, including antidepressants and electroconvulsive treatment, were more often than not rated harmful by the public.

A depressed person often places a burden on other family members. In some families, there is an aggregation of members with depression and several family members may be depressed at the same time. Several groups (Beardslee et al., 1997; Epstein, Keitner, Bishop & Miller, 1988; Falloon, Hole, Mulroy, Norris & Pembleton, 1988) have taught cognitive-behavioral or problem-solving strategies to the families of depressed people. They show that this is associated with decreased relapse rates (Epstein et al., 1988; Falloon et al., 1988) and long-term benefits (Beardslee et al., 1997), which reflect the importance of including some families in the recovery process.

There is a need to give families who are known to be vulnerable to depression information about, and strategies to deal with, situations that are likely to produce or exacerbate depression (Keitner, Ryan, Miller & Zlotnick, 1997). Families that could be said to be particularly at risk include pregnant women and their offspring, especially if they are also using nicotine, alcohol, cocaine or narcotics; families with one or more chronically unemployed men; migrant families transposed to a different culture, possibly with their own unresolved traumas; families with a high depressive loading; and families with a member with a severe personality disorder, where episodes of depression may be short-lived but very intense. These families are likely to require extra support and may benefit from specific targeted interventions to provide appropriate coping strategies.

The public, and primary care providers need to know more about the current range and applicability of treatments, and resources should be channeled to those who are likely to have recurrent episodes of depression. Innovative interventions to support patients and their families are needed; for example, Cox (1990) identified support networks in African villages and used this to devise a program of volunteers to support British women with postnatal depression.

Depression and its relevance to the general community

Depression has a high economic and social cost. It is associated with in-creased numbers of days off work, lowered productivity, increased risk of medical morbidity, and death (Bushnell & Bowie, 1995). It makes a signifi-cant contribution to burden, measured by DALYs, as noted in the World Bank's recent report (Murray & Lopez, 1996). The same report states that disability produced by depression constitutes 10.7% of the years lived with a disability due to any disease, mental or physical.

The World Bank study also notes the importance of tobacco as a cause of morbidity and mortality, and predicts that tobacco will become the greatest contributing risk factor to mortality in the early twenty-first century. There are high rates of usage amongst those with depression (Glassman, 1993), and complex interactions between smoking and depression, with particular relevance to pregnant women (Wilhelm, 1997) and women in socially disadvantaged groups (Graham, 1995). They include the findings that adolescents start smoking during periods of dysphoria (Patton et al., 1997) and that depressed people may increase the amount they smoke (Glassman, 1993). Recent data indicate that those who are nicotine dependent, have a history of depression, and decide to stop smoking may have an increased risk of relapsed depression (Borelli et al., 1996).

Klerman (1985) highlights the rising rates of depression in young people, particularly in young men, closing the gap between males and females. There is also increasing awareness of the relationship with substance abuse, particularly in the young (Patton et al., 1997). Youth suicide is a major area of interest in a number of countries, including Australia and Canada, where there are unacceptably high rates particularly among marginalized subpopulations (Gotowiec & Beiser, 1994; Raphael, 1993a,b; Sakinofsky & Leenaars, 1997). There is also concern over the high rates of suicide in young men in rural communities of Australia (Krupinski, Tiller, Burrows & Hallenstein, 1994). It is not clear how relevant models of adult depression are to young people. The usefulness of antidepressant therapy for the young is unclear, and it may be that a more holistic approach, embracing stress management, improving self-esteem and social skills, and increasing activity, efficacy and creativity, would be more effective for preventing depression and other illnesses such as anxiety disorders and substance abuse.

We must investigate when and where it would be most effective to implement intervention programs aimed at preventing depression, anxiety, and substance abuse in the young.

Depression and its relevance to fundholders and health planners

Lastly, issues concerning treatment priorities for planners and fundholders become more important in times of increased budgetary accountability. As depression tends to overlap with other psychiatric disorders and is linked with many medical disorders, one of the most important issues for fundholders is to find an effective way of evaluating the treatment of depression independently of the other illnesses that may occur at the same time. This has been a focus of interest for the managed health care organizations in the USA, who recognize the importance of depression as a predictor of significantly increased need for health care and greater health-related costs (Henk, Katzelnick, Kobak, Greist & Jefferson, 1996). The increased costs are just as important in the case of those with dysthymia and subthreshold depressive symptoms (Wells et al., 1992). It is recognized that treating depression is cost-effective because of the hidden costs of non treatment. The newer and more expensive antidepressants appear to be cost-effective. The improved side-effect profile means that they are taken rather than left in the medicine cabinet (Jonsson & Bebbington, 1995).

Conclusions

Improved appreciation of the true amount of disability attributed to repeated episodes of depression has greatly changed our perceptions of the disorder. There is better appreciation of the biological vulnerability and personality traits that underpin recurrent depression, and the need to view depression as a potentially lifelong disorder. We are also beginning to realize that preventive interventions may need to start at an early age. We need to identify those who will not have further episodes of depression, for whom simple interventions may be sufficient. We have stated the need for a public health approach to depression. Strategies aimed at increasing the quality of life and reducing risk factors for depression also improve health in general (particularly in relation to cardiovascular and cerebrovascular disease) and are relatively cheap and acceptable to the general public. Thus, they simultaneously address a number of crucial economic and social concerns.

There are many different groups concerned with mental health, all of whom have their own particular perspectives of depression. This may lead to conflicts of interest and need. The working definition (Bebbington et al., 1997) of unmet need was defined in the context of areas of dysfunction for which there are potential remedies or interventions. We have proposed four areas to tackle unmet need:

1. Adding depression to the public health agenda and to the preventive health campaigns which already exist in many countries.
2. Giving the different groups concerned with mental health existing information in a manner that is less directed to professionals and is more 'user-friendly'.
3. Translating this information into practical programs that will improve prevention, detection, and management by both the providers of health care and the individuals whose lives are affected by this disease.
4. Identifying areas where there are unanswered questions requiring further research.

References

Akiskal, H. (1992). Psychopharmacological and psychotherapeutic strategies in intermittent and chronic affective conditions. In S.A. Montgomery & F. Rouillon (eds.), *Long-Term Treatment of Depression*. Chichester: John Wiley & Sons.

Akiskal, H., Rosenthal, T., Haykal, R., Lemmi, H., Rosenthal, R. & Scott-Strauss, A. (1980). Characterological depressions: clinical and sleep EEG findings separating 'subaffective dysthmias' from 'character spectrum disorders'. *Archives of General Psychiatry*, **37**, 777–83.

Alexopoulos, G., Meyers, B., Young, R., Campbell, S., Silbersweig, D. & Charlson, M. (1997). 'Vascular depression' hypothesis. *Archives of General Psychiatry*, **54**, 915–22.

Beardslee, W., Salt, P., Versage, E., Gladstone, T., Wright, E. & Rothberg, P. (1997). Sustained change in parents receiving preventive interventions for families. *American Journal of Psychiatry*, **154**, 510–15.

Bebbington, P.E., Marsden, L. & Brewin, C.R. (1997). The need for psychiatric treatment in the general population: the Camberwell Needs for Care survey. *Psychological Medicine*, **27**, 821–34.

Borelli, B., Niaura, R., Keuthen, N., Goldstein, M., DePue, J., Murphy, C. & Abrams, D. (1996). Development of major depressive disorder during smoking-cessation treatment. *Journal of Clinical Psychiatry*, **57**, 534–8.

Bushnell, J.A. & Bowie, R.D. (1995). Costs of depression. In P.R. Joyce, S.E. Romans, P.M. Ellis, & T.S. Silverstone (eds.), *Affective Disorders*. Christchurch: University of Otago.

Cloninger, C.D., Svrakic, D.M. & Przybeck, T.R. (1993). A psychobiological model of temperament and character. *Archives of General Psychiatry*, **50**, 975–90.

Cox, J.C. (1990). Childbirth as a life event: sociocultural aspects of postnatal depression. *Acta Scandanavia Psychiatrica*, **79**, 75–83.

Epstein, N., Keitner, G., Bishop, D. & Miller, I. (1988). Combined use of pharmacological and family therapy. In J. Clarkin, G. Haas, & I. Glick (eds.), *Affective Disorders and the Family: Assessment and Treatment*. New York: Guildford Press.

Falloon, I., Hole, V., Mulroy, L., Norris, L. & Pembleton, T. (1988). Behavioural family therapy. In J. Clarkin, G. Haas, & I. Glick (eds.), *Affective Disorders and the Family: Assessment and Treatment*. New York: Guildford Press.

Fawcett, J. (1993). The morbidity and mortality of clinical depression. *International Clinical Psychopharmacology*, **8**, 217–20.

Glassman, A.H. (1993). Cigarette smoking: implications for psychiatric illness. *American Journal of Psychiatry*, **150**, 546–53.

Goering, P., Lin, E., Campbell, D., Boyle, M.H. & Offord, D.R. (1996). Psychiatric disability in Ontario. *Canadian Journal of Psychiatry*, **41**, 564–71.

Goldberg, D., Bridges, K., Duncan-Jones, P. & Grayson, D. (1988). Detecting anxiety and depression in general medical settings. *British Medical Journal*, **297**, 897–9.

Gotowiec, A. & Beiser, M. (1994). Aboriginal children's mental health: unique challenges. *Canada's Mental Health*, **41**, 7–11.

Graham, H. (1995). Women, smoking and disadvantage. In K. Slama (ed.), *Tobacco and Health*. New York: Plenum Press.

Henk, H., Katzelnick, D., Kobak, K., Greist, J. & Jefferson, J. (1996). Medical costs attributed to depression among patients with a history of high medical expenses in a health maintenance organization. *Archives of General Psychiatry*, 53, 899–904.

Hickie, I., Hickie, C., Scott, E. & Wilhelm, K. (1996). Magnetic resonance imaging in primary and secondary depression. In G. Parker & D. Hadzi-Pavlovic (eds.), *Melancholia: A Disorder of Movement and Mood*. New York: Cambridge University Press.

Hirschfield, R., Keller, M., Panico, S., Arons, B., Barlow, D., Davidoff, F., Endicott, J., Froom, J., Goldstein, M., Gorman, J., Guthrie, D., Marek, R., Maurer, T., Meyer, R., Phillips, K., Ross, J., Schwenk, T., Sharfstein, S., Thase, M. & Wyatt, R. (1997). The National Depressive and Manic-Depressive Association consensus statement on the undertreatment of depression. *Journal of the American Medical Association*, 277, 333–40.

Jonsson, B. & Beddington, P. (1995). What price depression? The cost of depression and cost-effectiveness of pharmacological treatment. In P.R. Joyce, S.E. Romans, P.M. Ellis, & T.S. Silverstone (eds.), *Affective Disorders*. Christchurch: University of Otago.

Jorm, A.F., Korten, A.E., Jacomb, P.A., Christensen, H., Rodgers B. & Pollitt, P. (1997). 'Mental health literacy': a survey of the public's ability to recognise mental disorders and their beliefs about the effectiveness of treatment. *Medical Journal of Australia*, 166, 182–6.

Keitner, G., Ryan, C., Miller, I. & Zlotnick, C. (1997). Psychosocial factors and the long-term course of major depression. *Journal of Affective Disorders*, 44, 57–67.

Keller, M., Klerman, G., Lavori, P., Coryell, W., Endicott, J. & Taylor, J. (1984). Long-term outcome of episodes of major depression: clinical and public health significance. *Journal of the American Medical Association*, 252, 788–92.

Kessler, R., McGonagle, K., Schwartz, M., Blazer, D. & Nelson, C. (1993). Sex and depression in the National Comorbidity Survey I: Lifetime, prevalence, chronicity, and recurrence. *Journal of Affective Disorders*, 29, 85–96.

Kiloh, L., Andrews, G. & Neilson, M. (1988). The long-term outcome of depressive illness. *British Journal of Psychiatry*, 153, 752–7.

Klerman, G.L. (1985). The current age of youthful melancholia: evidence of increase in depression among adolescents and young adults. *British Journal of Psychiatry*, 152, 4–14.

Krupinski, J., Tiller, J., Burrows, G. & Hallenstein, H. (1994). Youth suicide in Victoria: a retrospective study. *The Medical Journal of Australia*, 160, 113–16.

Lee, A. & Murray, R. (1988). The long-term outcome of Maudsley depressives. *British Journal of Psychiatry*, 153, 741–51.

Livingston Bruce, M., Leaf, P., Rozal, G., Florio, L. & Hoff, R. (1994). Psychiatric status and 9-year mortality data in the New Haven epidemiological catchment area study. *American Journal of Psychiatry*, 151, 716–21.

Macaskill, A., Macaskill, N. & Nicol, A. (1997). The Defeat Depression Campaign. A mid-point evaluation of its impact on general practitioners. *Psychiatric Bulletin*, 21, 148–50.

Merikangas, K. & Angst, J. (1994). Heterogeneity of depression: classification of depression subtypes by longitudinal course. *British Journal of Psychiatry*, 164,

342–8.

Mulder, R. & Joyce, P. (1997). Temperament and the structure of personality disorder symptoms. *Psychological Medicine*, **27**, 99–106.

Murphy, J.M., Olivier, D.C., Monson, R.R., Sobol, A.M., Federman, E.B. & Leighton, A.H. (1991). Depression and anxiety in elation to social status. *Archives of General Psychiatry*, **48**, 223–9.

Murray, C.J. & Lopez, A.D. (1996). *The Global Burden of Disease.* Geneva: World Health Organization.

National Primary Care Facilitation Programme (1997). *The Primary Mental Health Toolkit.* London: Royal College of General Practitioners.

O'Hara, M.W., Gorman, L.L. & Wright, E.J. (1996). Description and evaluation of the Iowa depression awareness, recognition, and treatment program. *American Journal of Psychiatry*, **153**, 645–9.

Parker, G. & Hadzi-Pavlovic, D. (1996). *Melancholia: A Disorder of Movement and Mood.* Cambridge: Cambridge University Press.

Patton, G., Harris, R., Carlin, J., Hibbert, M., Coffey, C., Schwartz, M. & Bowes, G. (1997). Adolescent suicidal behaviours: a population-based study of risk. *Psychological Medicine*, **27**, 715–24.

Raphael, B. (1993a). Depression and related syndromes. In *Scope for Prevention in Mental Health.* Canberra: Australian Government Publishing Service.

Raphael, B. (1993b). Target areas for preventative mental health. In *Scope for Prevention in Mental Health.* Canberra: Australian Government Publishing Service.

Regier, D.A., Hirschfeld, R.M.A., Goodwin, F.K., Burke, J.D., Lazar, J.B. & Judd, L.L. (1988). The NIMH depression awareness, recognition, and treatment program: structure, aims, and scientific basis. *American Journal of Psychiatry*, **145**, 1351–7.

Sakinofsky, I. & Leenaars, A. (1997). Suicide in Canada with special reference to the difference between Canada and the United States. *Suicide and Life-Threatening Behavior*, **27**, 112–26.

Sherbourne, C., Wells, K., Hays, R., Rogers, W., Burnam, A. & Judd, L. (1994). Subthreshold depression and depressive disorder: clinical characteristics of general medical and mental health speciality outpatients. *American Journal of Psychiatry*, **151**, 1777–84.

Simon, G., Von Korff, M. & Barlow, W. (1995). Health care costs of primary care patients with recognized depression. *Archives of General Psychiatry*, **52**, 850–6.

Thase, M.E., Greenhouse, J.B., Frank, E., Reynolds, C.F., Pilkonis, P.A., Hurley, K., Grochocinski, V. & Kupfer, D.J. (1997). Treatment of major depression with psychotherapy or psychotherapy-pharmacotherapy combinations. *Archives of General Psychiatry*, **54**, 1009–15.

Tiemens, B.G., Ormel, J. & Simon, G.E. (1996). Occurrence, recognition, and outcome of psychological disorders in primary care. *American Journal of Psychiatry*, **153**, 636–44.

United States Department of Health and Human Services. (1993). *Depression in Primary Care: Treatment of Major Depression* (Volume 2). Rockville: US Department of Health.

Wells, K.B., Burnam, M.A., Rogers, W., Hays, R. & Camp, P. (1992). The course of depression in adult outpatients. *Archives of General Psychiatry*, **49**, 788–94.

Wilhelm K. (1997). Smoking, pregnancy and depression. *Journal of CNS Disorders in Primary Care*, **1**, 5–7.

Wilhelm, K., Parker, G., Dewhurst-Savellis, J. & Asghari, A. (in press). Psychological predictors of single and recurrent major depression episodes. *Journal of Affective Disorders*.

Wilhelm, K., Parker, G. & Hadzi-Pavlovic, D. (1997). Fifteen years on: evolving ideas on researching sex differences in depression. *Psychological Medicine*, **27**, 875–83.

16

Unmet need following serious suicide attempt: follow-up of 302 individuals for 30 months

Annette Beautrais, Peter Joyce, and Roger Mulder

Summary

A consecutive sample of 302 individuals who had made medically serious suicide attempts was followed for two and a half years after the index attempt, with personal interviews at six, 18, and 30 months. During the follow-up period, mortality and psychiatric morbidity were high and measures of psychosocial functioning indicated a range of long-term adverse outcomes. Within 30 months of the index suicide attempt, 19 (6.7%) people died, 51.7% made at least one further suicide attempt, and 44.4% were admitted at least once to a psychiatric hospital or residential drug treatment center. There was evidence of enduring psychiatric morbidity: 46.1% of the sample met DSM-III-R criteria for major depression at the time of at least one of the three follow-up interviews. In addition, 40.1% of the sample met DSM-III-R criteria for substance-use disorder during the follow-up period. Those who made serious suicide attempts experienced high and enduring levels of a range of difficulties during the 30 months after such attempts: 58.7% reported relationship problems; 29.5% faced legal charges; 8.9% had at least one term of imprisonment; and 72.8% were social welfare beneficiaries at the time of at least one of the three follow-up interviews. It is concluded that those who make medically serious suicide attempts are a group at high and enduring risk for a range of adverse outcomes. The needs for care for this group which are implied by these outcomes are examined.

Introduction

Suicidal behavior is a significant medical, public health and mental health problem in New Zealand, just as it is in many countries (Diekstra & Gulbinat, 1993; La Vecchia, Lucchina & Levi, 1994; New Zealand Health Information Service, 1997; World Health Organization, 1992). In New Zealand, suicide is the second leading cause of death from all sources (after motor vehicle accidents) for males aged 15–44 years and for females aged 15–24 years (New Zealand Health Information Service, 1995). Furthermore, international comparisons suggest that New Zealand has one of the highest rates of suicide for young males aged 15–24 years in industrialized countries (World Health Organization, 1994, 1995).

Suicide attempts with a nonfatal outcome are also a significant public health problem (Schmidtke et al., 1996). Estimates suggest that there are approximately 30 to 50 suicide attempts of varying degrees of severity for every completed suicide (Kosky, 1987). While many of these attempts are minor and do not come to medical attention, there are a large number of nonfatal suicide attempts for which hospital admission and/or emergency department and psychiatric crisis team care are required.

Those who attempt suicide present as emergencies and are heavy consumers of acute primary and secondary health services (Platt et al., 1992). Those who have made suicide attempts are at high risk of making further nonfatal suicide attempts and of suicide (see, for example, Cullberg, Wasserman & Stefansson, 1988; Ekeberg, Ellingsen & Jacobsen, 1994; Greer & Lee, 1967; Hawton & Fagg, 1988; Morgan, Barton, Pottle, Pocock & Burns-Cox, 1976; Nordentoft et al., 1993; Öjehagen, Danielsson & Träskman-Bendz, 1992; Pokorny, 1966; Suokas and Lönnqvist, 1991). The clear majority of those who make medically serious suicide attempts will be suffering from diagnosable psychiatric disorders at the time of the attempt (Beautrais, Joyce & Mulder, 1996) and will require professional inpatient and/or outpatient psychiatric care following the suicide attempt.

Suicide and serious suicide attempts are seemingly preventable major sources of morbidity and mortality. Despite this, relatively few studies have attempted to follow the natural history of samples of individuals who have made medically serious suicide attempts. A review of the literature suggests that many of the follow-up studies of attempted suicide have consisted of certification studies, in which medical and coroner's files have been searched to identify individuals who had died within the follow-up period, to ascertain the proportion of the original sample who had subsequently died by suicide. Worldwide, there appear to be relatively few studies that have attempted to follow-up samples of individuals who have made a serious suicide attempt with personal interviews to evaluate outcome in broader terms than merely the assessment of the subsequent risk of suicide.

Against this background, the aims of this analysis are to report the results of a longitudinal study of a consecutive sample of 302 individuals who had made medically serious suicide attempts and who were then followed-up for a period of 30 months subsequent to these attempts. The aim of this analysis is to document the history of this cohort in the following areas of functioning: (1) rates of mortality, suicide and nonfatal suicide attempt; (2) history of psychiatric morbidity; and (3) rates of a series of selected measures of psychosocial functioning including relationship problems, social welfare benefit receipt, criminality and imprisonment.

Method

Overview

The data were gathered during the course of the Canterbury Suicide Project which consists of: (1) a case–control study of suicide (202 cases), medically serious suicide attempts (302 cases) and 1028 randomly selected controls; and (2) a five-year follow-up study of the 302 individuals from the case–control study who made medically serious suicide attempts. This chapter presents preliminary and descriptive findings from the first 30 months of the follow-up study.

Sample

The cases were a consecutive series of 302 individuals aged 13–88 years who made medically serious suicide attempts from 1 September 1991 to 31 May 1994 in Christchurch (New Zealand), a mixed urban/rural region with a population of 430,000. Medically serious suicide attempts were defined as those for which hospital admission for more than 24 hours was required and which, during admission, met specified criteria for severity. In total, 317 individuals made serious suicide attempts during the study period and 302 of these participated in the study, giving a response rate of 95.3%. The study design has been described previously (Beautrais et al., 1996).

Outcome

Each individual in the study was contacted and assessed at six, 18, and 30 months after the index suicide attempt. A semi-structured interview was conducted personally by trained, experienced interviewers. Information was obtained on the following outcomes: mortality, including suicide; further (nonfatal) suicide attempt; psychiatric morbidity; psychiatric hospital admission; relationship problems; social welfare benefit status; legal charges; and imprisonment.

Findings and conclusions

This study has followed, prospectively, a consecutive sample of 302 individuals who made medically serious suicide attempts with personal interviews at six, 18, and 30 months after the index suicide attempt. High response rates were maintained throughout the follow-up study: 90.5–94.7% of individuals alive and eligible to be interviewed were assessed at each of the three follow-up dates. In addition to determining mortality rates during the follow-up period, this preliminary analysis examined a range of outcomes including psychiatric morbidity, further suicidal behavior and psychosocial functioning.

This analysis suggests that the profile of the subsequent life history of those who had made serious suicide attempts was that of a group with the following characteristics: (1) they were at high risk of death from suicide, motor vehicle accidents, and natural causes; (2) they were at high risk of further suicide attempt behavior; (3) subsequent to the index serious suicide attempt they had high and enduring rates of psychiatric morbidity and psychiatric hospitalization; and (4) they were a group characterized by severe lifestyle difficulties including relationship problems, beneficiary status, criminality, and imprisonment.

The cumulative mortality rate after two and half years was 6.6% (19 deaths), with mortality occurring from both suicide and other causes. The mortality rate in the first year following the index suicide attempt was 3.6%, with six individuals (2%) dying by suicide within the first year of follow-up. These findings are consistent with those of a large number of previous studies which have indicated elevated risks of mortality from both suicide and other causes subsequent to an index suicide attempt (Buglass & Horton, 1974; Cullberg et al., 1988; Dahlgren, 1977; Ekeberg, Ellingsen & Jacobsen, 1991, 1994; Ettlinger, 1975; Hawton & Fagg, 1988; Kessel & McCulloch, 1966; Nielsen, Wang & Bille-Brahe, 1990; Nordentoft et al., 1993; Öjehagen et al., 1992; Paerregaard, 1975; Rosen, 1976; Rygnestad, 1988; Suokas & Lönnqvist, 1991; Tuckman & Youngman, 1963). While comparisons between different studies are complicated by the differing composition of samples, varying periods of follow-up, and differences in the medical severity of the index suicide attempt, the results of the present study are broadly consistent with upper limit estimates from these studies which have suggested that between 1% and 2% of those who attempt suicide die in the first year after the index attempt. The results of the present study are somewhat higher than those reported by several of these studies, which suggest a 1% suicide rate in the first year following a suicide attempt. This discrepancy probably reflects the fact that the present sample consisted of patients who had made medically serious suicide attempts, rather than those making both medically serious and less serious attempts.

A series of studies suggest that both the mortality rate and the suicide rate for those who have attempted suicide remains high beyond the first year following an attempt. In particular, two 10-year follow-up studies have indicated especially high rates of mortality and suicide. A study by Ekeberg et al. (1994) reported a mortality rate of 22% and a suicide rate of 4.9%, and a study by Nordentoft et al. (1993) found a mortality rate of 31% and a suicide rate of 11% after ten years. The results of the present study, which suggest a mortality rate of 6.6% and a suicide rate of 3.8% after 30 months of follow-up, are consistent with the high mortality and suicide rates suggested in these two previous studies.

The present analysis also indicates that deaths from causes other than suicide are high. This finding is consistent with the results of a series of previous studies (Ekeberg et al., 1994; Hawton & Fagg, 1988; Nordentoft et al., 1993; Pederson, Teftt & Babigian, 1975). It is notable that three individuals in the present study died during the follow-up period in single-vehicle motor accidents. It has been suggested that single-vehicle accidents may represent a source of 'hidden' or unacknowledged suicides which contribute to an underestimation of suicides (Grossman, Soderberg & Rivara, 1993; Morild, 1994; Peck & Warner, 1995). If the three single-vehicle accident deaths which occurred in our study were to be included in our total of suicides, then there would be a total of 14 suicides, representing an upper limit estimate of cumulative mortality from suicide within 30 months of a serious suicide attempt of 5%.

The high rates of mortality and suicide in the present study, compared with previous studies, are likely to reflect the fact that our sample consisted of individuals who had all made medically serious suicide attempts. These findings confirm the results of previous studies which suggest that individuals who make serious suicide attempts have a higher risk of subsequent suicide than those who make less serious attempts (Rosen, 1976; Suokas & Lönnqvist, 1991), and indicate that they are a group which needs carefully planned and long-term psychiatric follow-up and aftercare in efforts to reduce risk of subsequent death.

Those making serious suicide attempts are also at high risk of further (nonfatal) suicide attempts and psychiatric hospitalization, and have high levels of continuing psychiatric morbidity. Within the follow-up period more than half the individuals in the present study (51.7%) made at least one further suicide attempt. This observation is consistent with a number of studies that have established relatively high rates of repeated suicide attempts amongst those who have tried previously, with annual rates of further suicide attempts ranging from 9.7% to 27%, with a subsequent mean per annum suicide attempt rate of 16.8% (Adam, Valentine, Scarr & Streiner, 1983; Brent et al., 1993; Greer & Bagley, 1971; Johnsson Fridell, Öjehagen & Träskman-Bendz, 1996; Morgan et al., 1976; Nielsen et al., 1990; Nordstrom, Samuelsson, & Asberg, 1995; Öjehagen et al., 1992; Stern, Mulley & Thibault, 1984; Suleiman, Moussa & El-islam, 1989).

Rates of psychiatric morbidity were high throughout the follow-up period of the present study with almost half of the sample (46.1%) meeting DSM-

III-R (American Psychiatric Association, 1987) criteria for current major depression at the time of at least one of the three follow-up interviews. In addition, 44.4% met criteria for substance-use disorder (including alcohol, cannabis and other drug-use disorders) during the follow-up period. These results are consistent with those previously reported; for example, Adam et al. (1983) showed significantly and consistently elevated rates of psychiatric symptomatology in a group of suicide attempters followed-up over 18–24 months and compared with a control series. High rates of psychiatric morbidity were reflected in elevated rates of psychiatric hospital admission: within the 30-month follow-up period almost half (44%) of the sample were admitted at least once to a psychiatric hospital.

The results of the present study clearly suggest the importance of monitoring the subsequent mental health of this population and examining the extent to which psychiatric morbidity tends to resolve or deteriorate with time elapsed from the index suicide attempt. The high levels of major depression and substance-use disorders observed in our study, together with high rates of further suicide attempt behavior and high rates of hospital admission, suggest that those who make serious suicide attempts are a population with chronic severe psychiatric morbidity which is currently undertreated. Both in terms of suicide prevention and effective treatment, they are a group who clearly need well-planned and long-term treatment and aftercare programs.

Those making serious suicide attempts are a population at high risk of a range of poor or adverse psychosocial outcomes in the period following such attempts. These include relationship difficulties, with more than half (58.9%) of the individuals reporting relationship problems during the follow-up period. Since interpersonal conflict is the most common precipitant for suicidal behavior (Beautrais, Joyce & Mulder, 1997; Brent et al., 1993; Hawton, Cole, O'Grady & Osborn, 1982; Shaffer, 1974), it is important that follow-up care after serious suicide attempts includes adequate care and treatment to optimize interpersonal functioning and minimize the opportunity for subsequent relationship problems to precipitate further suicidal behavior.

Almost three-quarters of the sample were receiving social welfare benefits at the time of at least one of the three follow-up interviews. This finding suggests that those making serious suicide attempts are a population of relatively poor, low-income individuals in the community who are likely to have enduring financial and other problems as a consequence of their relatively long-term dependence on social welfare, and highlights the need for strengthening social work and related services for this population.

It appears that the high incidence of criminality found amongst individuals in the present study has not been previously reported. In the 30 months following a serious suicide attempt, one-third (29.5%) of the present sample faced legal charges (at least once) and almost one in ten (8.9%) were imprisoned at least once. Since a number of studies have found antisocial behaviors to be a major risk factor for suicidal behavior (Beautrais et al., 1996; Brent et al., 1988; Fergusson & Lynskey, 1995; Lesage et al., 1994; Marttunen, Aro, Henriksson & Lönnqvist, 1991; Shaffer et al., 1996), and strong associations have been reported between legal or disciplinary problems and risk of suicide among adolescents (Beautrais, 1996; Brent et al., 1993), it is perhaps not surprising to find high levels of criminality and imprisonment in this sample. Since up to 10% of those making serious suicide attempts may be imprisoned after such attempts, the provision of care for these individuals may become the responsibility of forensic psychiatric services. In addition, since legal problems and the threat of imprisonment may precipitate further suicidal behavior, those providing care to this population need to be aware of, and alert to, this possibility. It is also possible that a period of imprisonment may provide a window of opportunity to offer treatment to these individuals.

The risk of poor outcome shows little diminution with time elapsed from the index suicide attempt. While the risk of mortality appears to diminish with time elapsed since the index suicide attempt, those making serious suicide attempts tend to remain at high risk for a series of long-term and severe outcomes up to at least 30 months following the attempt, with, for example, almost half the sample receiving social welfare benefits two and half years after index suicide attempts, and 15.3% facing legal charges in the period from 18 to 30 months after the index attempt.

In conclusion, these findings suggest that there is highly consistent evidence from a series of outcome measures that the population of individuals making medically serious suicide attempts is at high risk of a range of adverse experiences and outcomes in the 30 months immediately subsequent to such attempts. Three lines of evidence support this conclusion:

1. Mortality rates in the follow-up period were high, with death arising from suicide, single-vehicle motor accidents, and natural causes.
2. Rates of further (nonfatal) suicidal behavior, hospital admission and psychiatric morbidity were high throughout the follow-up period.
3. After the index suicide attempt there were high rates of a series of selected psychosocial outcomes, including interpersonal and relationship problems, social welfare beneficiary status, legal charges, and imprisonment.

Implications

The results of this study suggest that the outcome following serious suicide attempts is often considerably bleak, characterized not only by continuing psychiatric illness, hospitalization and further suicidal behavior, but also by long-term and severe psychosocial problems and by lives which begin to reflect deprivation of care.

These results suggest the need for substantial improvements in the care of individuals who have made serious suicide attempts. In 1967 Greer and Lee, reporting on the progress of individuals who had made potentially lethal suicide attempts commented, '(There is) a striking contrast between the efficient, modern techniques of resuscitation which saved the lives of these patients, and the inadequate psychiatric and social services available for their after-care'. Thirty years later it would appear that this conclusion is still pertinent and that strong efforts have not yet been made to improve the delivery to this population of the psychiatric and social work care they so obviously need. It appears that current services are failing to recognize and meet the needs for treatment and care of patients who have made serious suicide attempts during the period following such attempts. These observations imply that the following improvements are needed in the delivery of care to those making medically serious suicide attempts:

1. Well-designed, appropriate, intensive and innovative follow-up and aftercare programs. For example, the characteristics of this population are such that consideration may need to be given to delivering much of this care on a domiciliary basis rather than using existing structures, which are usually heavily dependent on clinic-based services.

2. Social supports and services to address the lifestyle problems that are often comorbid with serious suicidal behavior and which include social welfare beneficiary status, relationship problems, criminality, and imprisonment.

3. Well-designed and, ideally, randomized field trials to evaluate the efficacy of various intervention approaches in dealing with the enduring psychiatric and lifestyle problems faced by this population.

References

Adam, K.S., Valentine, J., Scarr, G. & Streiner, D. (1983). Follow-up of attempted suicide in Christchurch. *Australian and New Zealand Journal of Psychiatry*, **17**, 18–26.

American Psychiatric Association (1987). *Diagnostic and Statistical Manual of Mental Disorders* (3rd edition, revised). Washington, DC: American Psychiatric Association.

Beautrais, A.L. (1996). Serious suicide attempts in young people: a case control study. Unpublished doctoral dissertation, University of Otago, New Zealand

Beautrais, A.L., Joyce, P.R. & Mulder, R.T. (1996). Prevalence and comorbidity of mental disorders in persons making serious suicide attempts: a case–control study. *American Journal of Psychiatry*, **153**, 1009–14.

Beautrais, A.L., Joyce, P.R. & Mulder, R.T. (1997). Precipitating factors and life events in serious suicide attempts among youth aged 13 through 24 years. *Journal of the American Academy of Child and Adolescent Psychiatry*, **36**, 1543–51.

Brent, D.A., Perper, J.A., Goldstein, C.E., Kolko, D.J., Allan, M.J., Allman, C.J. & Zelenak, J.P. (1988). Risk factors for adolescent suicide, a comparison of adolescent suicide victims and suicidal inpatients. *Archives of General Psychiatry*, **45**, 581–8.

Brent, D.A., Perper, J.A., Moritz, G., Allman, C., Friend, A., Roth, C., Schweers, J., Balach, L. & Baugher, M. (1993). Psychiatric risk factors for adolescent suicide: a case-control study. *Journal of the American Academy of Child and Adolescent Psychiatry*, **32**, 521–9.

Buglass, D. & Horton, J. (1974). A scale for predicting subsequent suicidal behaviour. *British Journal of Psychiatry*, **124**, 573–8.

Cullberg, J., Wasserman, D. & Stefansson, C.-G. (1988). Who commits suicide after a suicide attempt? An 8 to 10 year follow-up in a suburban catchment area. *Acta Psychiatrica Scandinavica*, **77**, 598–603.

Dahlgren, K.G. (1977). Attempted suicides – 35 years afterward. *Suicide and Life-Threatening Behaviour*, **7**, 75–9.

Diekstra, R.F.W. & Gulbinat, W. (1993). The epidemiology of suicidal behaviour: a review of three continents. *World Health Statistics Quarterly*, **46**, 52–68.

Ekeberg, O., Ellingsen, O. & Jacobsen, D. (1991). Suicide and other causes of death in a five-year follow-up of patients treated for self-poisoning in Oslo. *Acta Psychiatrica Scandinavica*, **83**, 432–7.

Ekeberg, O., Ellingsen, O. & Jacobsen, D. (1994). Mortality and causes of death in a 10-year follow-up of patients treated for self-poisoning in Oslo. *Suicide and Life-Threatening Behaviour*, **124**, 398–405.

Ettlinger, R (1975). Evaluation of suicide prevention after attempted suicide. *Acta Psychiatrica Scandinavica, Supplement*, 260, 1–135.

Fergusson, D.M. & Lynskey, M.T. (1995). Suicide attempts and suicidal ideation in a birth cohort of 16 year old New Zealanders. *Journal of the American Academy of Child and Adolescent Psychiatry*, **34**, 1308–17.

Greer, S. & Bagley, C. (1971). Effect of psychiatric intervention in attempted suicide: a controlled study. *British Medical Journal*, 1, 310–12.

Greer, S. & Lee, H.A. (1967). Subsequent progress of potentially lethal attempted suicides. *Acta Psychiatrica Scandinavica*, **43**, 361–71.

Grossman, D.C., Soderberg, R. & Rivara, F.P. (1993). Prior injury and motor vehicle crash as risk factors for youth suicide. *Epidemiology*, **4**, 115–19.

Hawton, K. & Fagg, J. (1988). Suicide, and other causes of death, following attempted suicide. *British Journal of Psychiatry*, **152**, 359–66.

Hawton, K., Cole, D., O'Grady, J. & Osborn, M. (1982). Motivational aspects of deliberate self-poisoning in adolescents. *British Journal of Psychiatry*, **141**, 286–91.

Johnsson Fridell, E., Öjehagen, A. & Träskman-Bendz, L. (1996). A five year follow-up study of suicide attempts. *Acta Psychiatrica Scandinavica*, **93**, 151–7.

Kessel, N. & McCulloch, W. (1966). Repeated acts of self-poisoning and self-injury. *Proceedings of the Royal Society of Medicine*, **59**, 89–92.

Kosky, R. (1987). Is suicide increasing among Australian youth? *The Medical Journal of Australia*, **147**, 164–6.

La Vecchia, C., Lucchini, F. & Levi, F. (1994). Worldwide trends in suicide mortality: 1955–1989. *Acta Psychiatrica Scandinavica*, **90**, 53–64.

Lesage, A.D., Boyer, R., Grunberg, F., Vanier, C., Morissette, R., Ménard-Buteau, C. & Loyer, M. (1994). Suicide and mental disorders: a case–control study of young men. *American Journal of Psychiatry*, **151**, 1063–8.

Marttunen, M.J., Aro, H.M., Henriksson, M.M. & Lönnqvist, J.K. (1991). Mental disorders in adolescent suicide. *Archives of General Psychiatry*, **48**, 834–9.

Morgan, H.G., Barton, J., Pottle, S., Pocock, H. & Burns-Cox, C.J. (1976). Deliberate self-harm: a follow-up study of 279 patients. *British Journal of Psychiatry*, **128**, 361–8.

Morild, I. (1994). Traffic accidents in Western Norway. A study from the county of Hordland 1986 to 1990. *Forensic Science International*, **64**, 9–20.

New Zealand Health Information Service (1995). *Mortality and Demographic Data (1993)*. Wellington: Ministry of Health.

New Zealand Health Information Service (1997). *Suicide Trends in New Zealand 1974–94*. Wellington: Ministry of Health.

Nielsen, B., Wang, A.G. & Bille-Brahe, U. (1990). Attempted suicide in Denmark. IV. A five-year follow-up. *Acta Psychiatrica Scandinavica*, **81**, 250–4.

Nordentoft, M., Breum, L., Munck, L.K., Nordestgaard, A.G., Hunding, A. & Laursen Bjaeldager, P.A. (1993). High mortality by natural and unnatural causes: a 10-year follow-up study of patients admitted to a poisoning centre after suicide attempts. *British Medical Journal*, **306**, 1637–40.

Nordstrom, P., Samuelsson, M. & Asberg, M. (1995). Survival analysis of suicide risk after attempted suicide. *Acta Psychiatrica Scandinavica*, **91**, 336–40.

Öjehagen, A., Danielsson, M. & Träskman-Bendz, L. (1992). Deliberate self-poisoning: treatment follow-up of repeaters and non-repeaters. *Acta Psychiatrica Scandinavica*, **85**, 370–5.

Paerregaard, G. (1975). Suicide among attempted suicides: a 10-year follow-up. *Suicide*, **5**, 140–4.

Peck, D.L. & Warner, K. (1995). Accident or suicide? Single vehicle car accidents and the intent hypothesis. *Adolescence*, **30**, 463–72.

Pederson, A.M., Tefft, M.A., Babigian, H.M. (1975). Risk of mortality of suicide attempters compared with psychiatric and general populations. *Suicide*, **5**, 145–57.

Platt, S., Bille-Brahe, U., Kerkhof, A., Schmidtke, A., Bjerke, T., Crepet, P., De Leo, D., Haring, C., Lönnqvist, J., Michel, K., Philippe, A., Pommereau, X., Querejeta, I., Salander-Renberg, E., Temesvary, B., Wasserman, D. & Sampaio-Faria, J. (1992). Parasuicide in Europe: the WHO/EURO multicentre study on parasuicide. I. Introduction and preliminary analysis for 1989. *Acta Psychiatrica Scandinavica*, **85**, 97–104.

Pokorny, A.D. (1966). A follow-up study of 618 suicidal patients. *American Journal of Psychiatry*, **122**, 1109–16.

Rosen, D.H. (1976). The serious suicide attempt: epidemiological and follow-up study of 886 patients. *American Journal of Psychiatry*, **127**, 764–70.

Rygnestad, T. (1988). A prospective 5-year follow-up study of self-poisoned patients. *Acta Psychiatrica Scandinavica*, **77**, 328–31.

Schmidtke, A., Bille-Brahe, U., De Leo, D., Kerkhof, A., Bjerke, T., Crepet, P., Haring,

C., Hawton, K., Lönnqvist, J., Michel, K., Pommereau, X., Querejeta, I., Phillipe, I., Salander-Renberg, E., Temesvary, B., Wasserman, D., Fricke, S., Weinacker, B. & Sampaio-Faria, J.G. (1996). Attempted suicide in Europe: rates, trends and sociodemographic characteristics of suicide attempters during the period 1989–1992. Results of the WHO/EURO Multicentre Study on Parasuicide. *Acta Psychiatrica Scandinavica*, **93**, 327–38.

Shaffer, D. (1974). Suicide in childhood and early adolescence. *Journal of Child Psychology and Psychiatry*, **15**, 275–91.

Shaffer, D., Gould, M.S., Fisher, P., Trautman, P., Moreau, D., Kleinman, M. & Flory, M. (1996). Psychiatric diagnosis in child and adolescent suicide. *Archives of General Psychiatry*, **53**, 339–48.

Stern, T.A., Mulley, A.G. & Thibault, G.E. (1984). Life-threatening drug overdose: precipitants and prognosis. *Journal of the American Medical Association*, **251**, 1983–5.

Suleiman, M.A., Moussa, M.A. & El-islam, M.F. (1989). The profile of parasuicide repeaters in Kuwait. *International Journal of Social Psychiatry*, **35**, 146–55.

Suokas, J. & Lönnqvist, J. (1991). Outcome of attempted suicide and psychiatric consultation: risk factors and suicide mortality during a five-year follow-up. *Acta Psychiatrica Scandinavica*, **84**, 545–9.

Tuckman, J. & Youngman, W.F. (1963). Suicide risk among persons attempting suicide. *Public Health Reports*, **78**, 585–7.

World Health Organization (1992). *Health-for-all Targets. The Health Policy for Europe*. Summary of the updated edition, September 1991. Copenhagen: World Health Organization, EUR ICP/HSC 013.

World Health Organization (1994). *World Health Statistics Annual*. Geneva: World Health Organization.

World Health Organization (1995). *World Health Statistics Annual*. Geneva: World Health Organization.

17

Met and unmet need for interventions in community cases with anxiety disorders

Hans-Ulrich Wittchen

Requirements for population-based needs assessment in anxiety disorders

The basic prerequisites for a population-based evaluation of need for anxiety disorder treatment in developed health care systems are: (1) clearly specified disorders and/or related disabilities for which (2) effective and (3) acceptable interventions/treatments are available and (4) can be provided (Häfner, 1979; Wittchen, 1988).

It is generally agreed that these basic requirements are widely met for most forms of anxiety disorder. First, explicit diagnostic criteria, operationalized diagnoses [DSM-III, American Psychiatric Association (APA), 1980; DSM-IV, APA, 1994; and ICD-10, World Health Organization (WHO), 1993] and diagnostic instruments [i.e., the Composite International Diagnostic Interview (CIDI, WHO, 1990)] allow mental health specialists and primary care doctors to recognize and diagnose most forms of anxiety disorder reliably (Wittchen, 1994).

The improved diagnostic techniques have led to better identification of the risk factors for first developing anxiety disorders, secondary psychosocial disability, and psychopathological complications (Kessler et al., 1994; Magee, Eaton, Wittchen, McGonagle & Kessler, 1996; Wittchen et al., 1995a,b,c). They have also allowed characterization of the disorder's natural course, which is usually persistent (Wittchen, 1991). Rice & Miller (1998) demonstrate the impact that anxiety disorders have on society, by revealing that more is spent, in direct and indirect costs, on anxiety disorders than on depressive or psychotic disorders.

Second, there are various highly effective pharmacological and psychological treatments for anxiety disorders, and their disadvantages and limitations have been described (Andrews, Crino, Hunt, Lampe & Page, 1994; Bond & Lader, 1996; Elkin, Pilkonis, Docherty & Sotsky, 1988; Fineberg & Drummond, 1995). Highly significant short-term improvements of anxiety disorders can be achieved with short-term anxiolytic drugs, long-term antidepressants (tricyclics as well as serotonin-reuptake inhibitors or SSRIs), and cognitive-behavioral and exposure types of psychological treatments; indeed the latter can produce long-term improvements (Clum, 1989; Lader & Bond, 1998; Michelson & Marchione, 1991). Third, these various forms of pharmacological and psychological treatments are acceptable and, fourth, available in developed countries, although one needs to acknowledge the marked variations between countries in treatment delivery and reimbursement.

Met and unmet needs for treatment of anxiety disorders in the community

In spite of this quite positive situation, general population studies in several countries (USA, Kessler et al., 1994, 1997; Canada, Offord et al., 1994; Germany, Wittchen, Nelson & Lachner, 1998*a*) show that only one-third of those affected by anxiety disorders receive any professional treatment, and even fewer receive specialist mental health treatment. Does this mean that the vast majority of people with anxiety disorders identified in the population require treatment and yet do not receive appropriate professional help and attention?

This conclusion can only be justified by equating the diagnosis of an anxiety disorder – as assessed in these population surveys – directly with specific professional treatment needs. Regier et al. (1998) questions the validity of this assumption for anxiety disorders. Unlike other mental disorders such as schizophrenia, where such an assumption might meet more professional consensus (Häfner, 1978, 1979), we know that at least some forms of anxiety disorder may have significant spontaneous remission rates, and that the severity of anxiety symptoms, related impairments and risk of complications may fluctuate (Wittchen, 1991). Furthermore, a significant proportion of people with anxiety disorders might not need formal drug or psychological therapy, but might improve significantly by using self-help manuals or low-impact psychoeducative measures. The substantial proportion of what is labeled the 'placebo' response in randomized trials, where the inactive ingredient consists only of information and comprehensive self-monitoring tools, provides further evidence for the value of such low-impact interventions (Bond & Lader, 1996).

Therefore, when determining the degree of unmet need in anxiety disorders in the population, several additional considerations might be necessary beyond merely establishing a reliable diagnosis and providing effective services. Unfortunately the available epidemiological studies do not provide such sufficiently detailed data (Regier et al., 1998). Almost all available general population studies lack sufficiently detailed information about symptom severity, persistence, and disorder-specific disabilities beyond the mere documentation of classificatory diagnostic issues. Neither do they provide detailed data about the *individual's self-perceived need* or *needs*, or information about intervention needs, as rated by clinicians or other mental health experts. The reasons for this deficit are twofold. First, evaluation of need in mental disorders is a complicated undertaking, and, possibly because of the lack of systematic studies in this area, there are currently no agreed strategies that can adequately assess the degree of met and unmet needs for anxiety treatments. Second, one simple (however clearly problematic) alternative, namely using clinicians to provide ratings for each individual's treatment needs, has only rarely been used, because such clinical appraisals are usually too expensive to be included in large-scale epidemiological studies. To conclude, our current knowledge about unmet needs for anxiety treatments in the population is poor.

A conceptual framework to evaluate needs

In light of these deficits, we recently added a need-evaluation and health-utilization module to a prospective community survey of 3021 adolescents and young adults (Early Developmental Stages of Psychopathology, EDSP). In designing this module, we referred to a conceptual framework of comprehensive need evaluation, developed several years ago in a seven-year follow-up study of former patients and a community sample (Münchener Follow-up Study, Wittchen, 1988; Wittchen & von Zerssen, 1987). This five-step model is described comprehensively elsewhere (Cording-Tömmel, Wittchen & von Zerssen, 1988; Wittchen, 1988), and is only briefly described here.

A five-step model of comprehensive need evaluation

Basic prerequisites (and examples of evaluative activities)

1. Reliable and valid case-definition and case-finding procedures, and specified professional consensus about appropriate interventions (explicit diagnostic criteria and instruments, e.g., CIDI).
2. Well-defined geographical area with detailed information about health/ mental health structure/service provision characteristics (e.g., catchment area or regional case register).
3. Appropriate assessment instruments for need and appropriate assessors/ clinicians (questionnaires, interviews, clinical ratings).
4. Preferably a prospective design (allow for a detailed process description).

Step 1: Identification of cases with the target disorder (what is a case?) – current and lifetime prevalence; symptom/disorder severity; psychosocial and other disabilities; risk factors for onset/persistence; comorbidity.

Step 2: What are the needs of cases? – subjective (patients') needs domains; expert-rated needs domains.
Step 3: Do cases get what they need? – how well are patients' needs met?; how well are expert-rated needs met?; are appropriate services provided?; what are the gaps between the fulfillment of patient- and expert-rated needs?; what factors influence these gaps?
Step 4: Do cases need what they get? – how suitable are the actual interventions?
Step 5: Summary evaluation. How many and what type of services and intervention strategies are needed? – how can the system be improved in terms of the number, mix, structure, type of services, and other provision characteristics?

There are three main characteristics/principles of this need-evaluation approach: (1) the orientation towards evaluating individual (patients') needs and outcomes over time; (2) conceptualizing of mental disorders as a process of stages and psychological, social, and medical patterns, each of which has its own requirements; and (3) the comprehensive nature of the evaluation process, i.e., it evaluates the patient, as well as the health care system available and responsible for the individual, and its care characteristics (Donabedian, 1966). Thus, basic requirements for applying this approach are twofold. First, a defined catchment area with detailed information about the availability of services, personnel, care characteristics, and types of treatments offered. Second, a personnel assessment of a sample of this community, with specific emphasis on diagnosing symptom severity, disabilities, use of and attitudes to the health services, and, most importantly, an experienced clinician must assess treatment needs. Ideally the design of such a community study would be prospective, to cover the 'process' element of the model. The model above lists the five steps of this approach along with the evaluative strategies linked to each of these operations.

Aims of the Munich Community Study

This chapter reports the preliminary findings of the baseline investigation of a random population sample of 3021 people, aged 14–24, conducted in the greater Munich area, Germany, in 1994. The primary goal of this longitudinal prospective study (three waves of interviews one to two years apart) is to study developmental patterns of early stages of psychopathology, focusing on anxiety, depressive and substance-use disorders. Referring to the above-mentioned five-step model this chapter addresses the question of met and unmet need for treatment by answering the following questions:

1. What is the 12-month and lifetime prevalence of DSM-IV anxiety disorders in community respondents aged 14–24?

2. How many cases with anxiety disorders reported using any type of professional help for their disorder, and how many expressed any subjective or perceived need for intervention?
3. For what proportion of the sample does the expert suggest specific types of drug and psychological intervention?
4. What kinds of services were provided for those with anxiety disorders, and do they need – according to the expert – what they get?

Methods of the Munich Community Study

The data were collected as part of the baseline investigation of the EDSP study funded by the German Ministry of Research and Technology. (For a full description see Wittchen, Perkonigg, Lachner & Nelson, 1998b; Wittchen & Pfister, 1997.) The results presented here are from the first wave of data collection which was conducted from January to July of 1995.

Sample

The sample was drawn from the 1994 Bavarian government registry of residents in metropolitan Munich, with all registrants 14–24 years old during the first half of 1995 eligible for selection. Munich is the capital of the state of Bavaria, with a population of 2.6 million inhabitants. A large proportion of the population is employed in educational (three large universities) and service settings (32%). The greater Munich area has many varied providers of care for general and mental health problems, covering inpatient and outpatient facilities (see below).

As the study is longitudinal, with special interest in the development of substance-use disorders, 14–15 year olds were sampled at twice the probability of people 16–21 years of age, and 22–24 year olds were sampled at half this probability. From the total of 4809 sampled individuals, 4263 were located and determined to be eligible for the study. Sampled individuals who were not included were disproportionately older, or could not be contacted because either they had moved outside the metropolitan Munich area since registering (8.8%), or could not be found at their listed address during the field work period (2.4%). From the 4263 individuals a total of 3021 interviews were completed resulting in a response rate of 71%. In addition, partial information (telephone interviews, short version of interview) was obtained from an additional 6.2%. These findings will not be reported here. Refusal to participate (18.2%) was the most frequent reason for not responding, followed by a reported lack of time (3.3%), failure to contact anyone in the identified household (3.1%), and failure to contact the sampled individual in an identified household (3.0%).

Demographically, nonresponse increased with age, especially among women, whose nonresponse rates were slightly higher than those of men. To account for the differences in sampling probabilities and nonresponse, the data have been adjusted by age, sex, and geographical location to match the distribution of the sampling frame.

Approximately one-third were currently attending or had attended gymnasium (secondary education between the ages of 11 and 19 which prepares students for entrance to university) and another third were at university. Eleven percent were attending lower school (Grund-/Hauptschule = mandatory basic school), and 18.4% Realschule (an intermediate type of advanced school between gymnasium and Hauptschule allowing qualification for specific university curricula). Consistent with the mandatory schooling laws, only 0.5% had left school without any qualification. Only 22.6% of all study participants were currently in the work force, and 4.9% were registered as unemployed. Most respondents were currently living with their parents; only a few were married. The vast majority of respondents were classified as middle class, with only 7.8% belonging to the lower social classes. (For a full description of the sample and sampling process see Wittchen et al., 1998*b*; Wittchen & Pfister, 1997.)

Diagnostic assessment

Psychopathological and diagnostic assessments were based on the computer-assisted personal interview (CAPI) version of the Munich Composite International Diagnostic Interview (M-CIDI, Wittchen et al., 1995*a,b,c;* Wittchen & Pfister, 1997). The M-CIDI is a modified version of the World Health Organization (WHO) CIDI, version 1.2 supplemented by questions to cover DSM-IV and ICD-10 criteria (Wittchen & Pfister, 1997; Wittchen et al., 1995*a,b,c*). The M-CIDI allows assessment of the symptoms, syndromes and diagnoses of 48 mental disorders (not counting various subtypes of main disorders), along with information about the onset, duration, and clinical and psychosocial severity. The CAPI version of the M-CIDI has a separate supplemental respondents' booklet that includes several scales and questionnaires that are important for the longitudinal component of our study, as well as cognitive aids to help and assist the respondent to date the onset and recency of symptoms, by answering complicated questions about their symptoms and identifying course patterns. Analysis of the diagnosis is based on the M-CIDI/DSM-IV diagnostic algorithms (Pfister & Wittchen, 1995). Diagnostic findings reported in this chapter are based on the M-CIDI/DSM-IV algorithms without using the DSM-IV hierarchy rules, unless otherwise stated in the text. It took a mean of 77 minutes to complete the CAPI M-CIDI, including questionnaires.

Reliability and validity of the M-CIDI

The psychometric properties of the M-CIDI have been investigated by studying various sites and samples (overview: Lachner et al., 1998; Wittchen, Perkonigg, Lachner & Nelson, 1998b; Wittchen & Pfister, 1997). Briefly, the main findings are as follows. The test–retest reliability (T–RT) of the computerized M-CIDI has been investigated by studying 73 community respondents aged 14–24 and 68 psychiatric outpatients (aged 17–54). The average time interval between the test and retest was 6.5 days. The T–RT reliability for lifetime DSM-IV diagnosis was acceptable to high for most disorders [kappa values ranging from 0.55 (obsessive compulsive disorder) to 0.83 (anorexia nervosa) (Wittchen & Pfister, 1997)] and particularly high (above 0.68) for all anxiety disorders (Lachner et al., 1998; Wittchen et al., 1998a).

Characteristics of the care system, assessment of need and use of the health services

This assessment module is specifically tailored to the characteristics of mental health care in Germany, taking into account the specific characteristics of the Munich area. Briefly, the German health care system is based on mandatory comprehensive health care insurance covering the whole population. It is comprehensive in the sense that it covers all mental health costs – inpatient and outpatient, as well as all kinds of drug and psychological services (short- and long-term psychoanalytical as well as behavioral treatments) – as long as they are provided by registered doctors or clinical psychologists. The reimbursement schedule is based on a fee-for-service regulation. For long-term psychotherapy (more than 25 sessions) a special peer review process is required before the treatment starts. There is a large number of all types of psychotherapists in the Munich area. Treatment is also available through counseling centers financed by other sources.

Variables relevant to the assessment of need and service utilization were assessed in three parts of the interview. Current (12-month) subjective need for intervention was assessed within the section on anxiety disorders. Whenever the respondent fulfilled criteria for at least one subthreshold anxiety disorder, subjective need referring to the anxiety disorder was assessed. In addition to questions asking whether the subject had consulted a doctor, another health professional or mental health specialist, each respondent was asked whether they had ever thought about professional help, and if yes, how frequently and when, and whether they thought they might currently need professional help (defined as that provided by doctors, psychologists, psychotherapists, counseling centers or any other of a total of 25 types of institutionalized professional help). If the latter question was endorsed this was defined as *individual need*. Actual use of services was assessed in a separate health service utilization module at the end of the interview, by using a response list. The respondent listed all institutions consulted and detailed the interventions received, and then their reasons for doing so, the length of time spent there, and the nature of the therapy (drug or psychological). These latter data were used to define the *actual use of health services* and formed the basis for the clinical experts' ratings of the *adequacy of treatment*.

Expert-rated needs were based on the ratings agreed between the clinicians involved, using all available information from the interview and question-naire. The clinician was free to ask and use any type of additional information to arrive at a rating, subsequently reviewed by a team of at least three other clinical interviewers. To arrive at this final rating for need, the clinicians were asked whether they considered the particular case as being in need of at least one of 14 interventions or treatment options listed. If yes, they were asked to indicate the type and mode of the suggested treatment in more detail (for example if counseling was indicated, by whom and with what focus, with or without self-help material and psychoeducation, etc.). The clinician was then asked to rate the importance of these interventions and to justify why it was necessary, according to: the degree of subjective suffering, the risk of psycho-pathological complications, and the risk of psychosocial complications in-cluding work productivity.

The results of the Munich Community Study

What proportion of the population is affected by anxiety disorders?

Table 17.1 reveals that about 26% of the EDSP population had been affected in their lifetime, at least once, by one or more of the five rigidly defined DSM-IV anxiety disorders listed. The 12-month rate was 17.7%. Specific phobias of various types (such as animal, situational, environmental) were by far the most common type of anxiety disorder in our sample aged 14–24, with a lifetime prevalence of 19.2% and a 12-month rate of 12.5%. Other frequent diagnoses were social phobia (lifetime 7.3%, 12 months 5.2%) with slightly less than one-third belonging to the generalized type of social phobia. As compared with other epidemiological studies covering a wider age range, such as the National Comorbidity Survey (NCS, age range included 15–55) the younger EDSP sample reveals slightly lower prevalence estimates for panic disorder (lifetime 1.6%), lower rates for agoraphobia (lifetime 2.6%) and generalized anxiety disorder (GAD, lifetime 0.8%). These differences might be explained by the stricter DSM-IV criteria used in the EDSP, and by differences in the age groups studied.

It is also noteworthy that about one-third of all cases with one anxiety disorder also fulfilled criteria for another anxiety disorder; furthermore, there

Table 17.1. Twelve-month and lifetime prevalence of DSM-IV anxiety disorders among 14–24 year olds in the EDSP

DSM-IV diagnoses	Lifetime			12-month		
	Nuw	Nw	%	Nuw	Nw	%
Any anxiety disorder	764	787	26.0	522	534	17.7
Panic disorder	42	49	1.6	30	35	1.2
Generalized anxiety disorder	20	24	0.8	12	16	0.5
Agoraphobia	78	79	2.6	45	43	4.4
Social phobia	201	219	7.3	146	158	5.2
Specific phobias	574	580	19.2	374	378	12.5

Note: Nuw, unweighted sample size; Nw, weighted sample size; %, weighted prevalence in %.

is considerable comorbidity within specific phobia, not dealt with in this chapter.

How many cases have used mental health services?

Figure 17.1 summarizes the proportion of 12-month cases in each diagnostic group that reported having used any type of professional mental health service at least once, irrespective of the type and duration. Health services are broadly defined and include psychiatrists, other doctors, psychologists, school psychology services as well as self-help groups and primary care doctors, as long as the latter provide some specifiable mental health intervention. Of all 12-month cases ($n = 136$) 25.6% reported having contacted at least one mental health service, 84 cases reported having used just one, 29 two, and the remaining cases three or more. Those with a 12-month diagnosis of panic disorder or GAD were most likely to receive mental health treatment, those with specific phobias were least likely (21.4%). Among providers, psychotherapists (51%) (mostly clinical psychologists) were most frequently mentioned, followed by primary care doctors (42%), counseling centers (31%), psychiatrists (19%), and school psychologist services (13%) (Figure 17.2). In addition, 26% reported at least one inpatient treatment episode because of their anxiety problems. Only 4% were in contact with self-help organizations.

The comparison with health services use rates obtained in the USA and Canada in Figure 17.1 (Kessler et al., 1997) reveals – in light of the availability of these services free of charge in Germany – surprisingly similar overall rates of mental health use in both countries. Except for higher utilization rates for GAD and social phobia in Germany, there are no differences between the diagnostic groups. The higher rates of utilization by those with GAD and

DSM-IV diagnoses

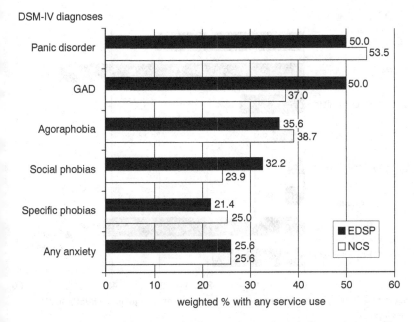

Figure 17.1 A summary of the proportion of 12-month cases in each diagnostic group (the EDSP and the NCS) that reported having used any type of professional mental health service at least once, irrespective of the type and duration. EDSP, Early Developmental Stages of Psychopathology from Germany; NCS, National Comorbidity Survey from the USA.

social phobia may reflect the effect of a public awareness campaign, which took place in the years preceding the study. However, in interpreting the similarities between the USA and Germany one should consider the different age groups of the two samples: the EDSP only covers ages 14–24, whereas the NCS covers 15–55 year olds.

What do anxiety cases need? Patient-rated individual needs and expert-rated needs for intervention

Figure 17.3 reports the proportion of 12-month cases rated by the clinician as being in need of treatment, the proportion of those reporting a self-perceived need and the proportion with either self- or expert-rated needs. Figure 17.3 indicates that not all cases with a 12-month anxiety disorder needed some kind of professional help, and low levels of self-perceived need were found for specific phobias (51.2%). Self-perceived needs were greatest for panic disorder and GAD. Expert-rated needs were lower than patient-rated needs, except for agoraphobia. Finally, there was less than perfect agreement between the expert opinion and the patients' self-perceived need for help.

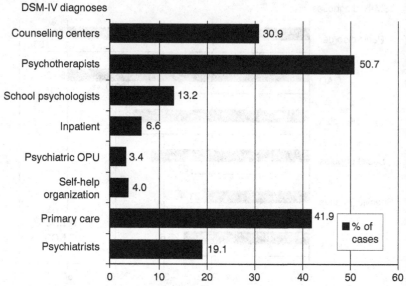

Figure 17.2 Types of services used among 12-month cases (n=136) in the EDSP sample of 14–24 year olds.

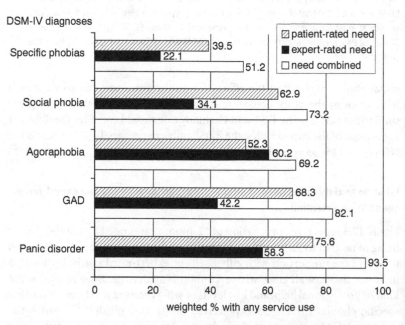

Figure 17.3 The proportion of anxiety cases in the EDSP, with subjective and expert-rated needs and actual service use.

DSM-IV diagnoses

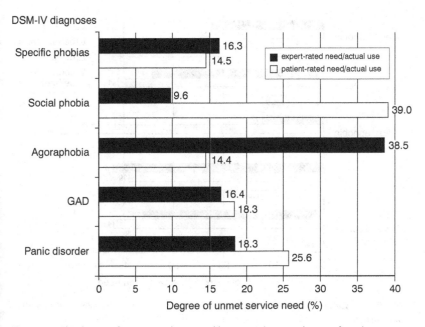

Figure 17.4 The degree of unmet need assessed by comparing actual rates of service use with patient- and expert-rated needs.

Figure 17.4 compares patient- and expert-rated needs with the actual use of mental services, irrespective of adequacy in terms of the time, duration, and frequency of care received. Taking this as a yardstick to determine the degree of unmet need from the patients' point of view reveals that the gap between use and perceived need is greatest for those suffering from social phobia (39%) and panic disorder (25.6%), and smallest for simple phobia and agoraphobia. Experts rated the greatest gaps for agoraphobia (38.5%), and the smallest gap for social phobia (9.6%). Overall, there was only moderate agreement between expert-rated need and actual use ($r = 0.48$), and between individual- and expert-rated need ($r = 0.59$). However, individual-rated needs correlated well with actual use ($r = 0.78$).

Figure 17.5 specifies the main types of interventions recommended by the expert for those rated to be in need. In interpreting these figures one needs to acknowledge that for many individuals more than one intervention was recommended. Those with panic disorder and GAD in particular were recommended many types of intervention. The types of interventions suggested varied according to the disorder. For specific phobias the most frequently suggested type of intervention (42% of those with expert-rated need) was disorder-specific counseling and the provision or encouragement of psychoeducative or self-help materials. This intervention was rarely mentioned as the only, or primary, intervention suitable for other disorders,

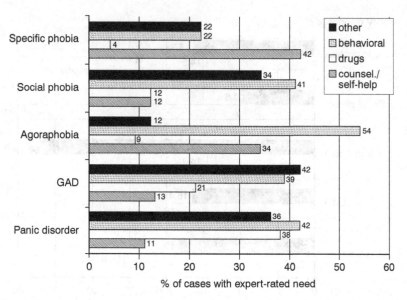

Figure 17.5 Types of interventions suggested by experts for 12-month cases, according to diagnosis.

except agoraphobia (34%). For agoraphobia the primary suggestions were cognitive-behavioral and exposure treatments, rarely drugs; whereas for GAD and panic disorder a considerable proportion were rated as needing drug treatment, either alone or combined with psychological treatments. Other forms of interventions were crisis intervention (particularly frequent in GAD and panic disorder and social phobia), and other forms of psychotherapy. The latter was relatively frequently indicated for GAD patients. In 9% of the cases no clear decision about treatment recommendations was reached.

Do anxiety cases need what they get?

In steps 4 and 5 (see p. 259), information about the actual services received by the patients and the experts' opinions are brought together to try and evaluate more specifically how well expert-rated needs are fulfilled. It is important to note that Table 17.2 labels any mental health service use as treatment, regardless of its appropriateness. Thus, even single consultations are included. Table 17.2 reports how the overall number of 522 12-month cases with a M-CIDI/DSM-IV anxiety disorder are distributed across the groups, along with information about special features in some of the groups.

According to this analysis 34% of all anxiety cases identified were rated by the expert as having no need for professional intervention and these cases did

Table 17.2. Summary expert evaluation: met and unmet needs among 522 cases with a 12-month anxiety disorder (prevalence 17.7%) taking into account expert-rated needs, treatment and care characteristics recommended and actual service use

Groups	12-month cases (n)	12-month cases (%)	Remarks
Group 1: no need/no treatment	175	34%	Among the 175 cases, 85 (mostly specific and social phobias) indicated a self-perceived need.
Group 2: no need/treatment	32	6%	Most (n=28) of these cases (all but three with phobias) had self-perceived needs; 4 were brought by parents
Group 3: need/no treatment	216	42%	Some of this group told their doctors, but no action was reported.
Group 4: need/treatment	88	17%	
adequate	(40)	(8%)	
inadequate	(48)	(9%)	Examples for inadequate treatments (n=48): too short/one contact only (22), completely inadequate drug or psychological intervention (19), long unspecific inpatient (14), unspecific counseling (12), (predominantly by primary care doctors).
Group 5: unclear	11	2%	includes cases where the expert does not agree about diagnosis, or has insufficient information
Total	522	100%	

not report any service use (group 1). However, nearly half of these cases – mostly with specific and social phobia – did express a self-perceived need for help. The second group consisted of people reporting service use, including extensive therapy, but the clinician did not see any reason for counseling or self-help material. These were mostly those with phobic disorders (agoraphobia, social and specific phobias) with a clear self-perceived need.

Group 3 – the largest group – describes the cases where some professional intervention was rated as indicated by the expert, but no service use or treatment was reported by the patient. Forty-six out of 216 individuals reported having told their family doctor or other doctors about their disorder, but no counseling or anxiety-specific consultation was given. This group was relatively evenly distributed across all types of anxiety disorders, with some emphasis on agoraphobia, GAD, and panic disorder.

Group 4, covering only 17% of all 12-month anxiety cases, includes most of the cases receiving clearly inadequate treatments. The major reasons for rating the treatment as grossly inadequate (multiple response categories) were: intervention/treatment too short (e.g., just one ten-minute session, only one or two sessions, antidepressant drugs taken for less than two weeks, long-term Gestalt or esoteric therapies with no recognizable anxiety-specific component, month-long inpatient treatment without any reasonable drug or psychological intervention, counseling with no specific help elements). Most of the group with inadequate interventions were seen by a primary care doctor.

Discussion

In this community study we tried to improve upon previous assessments of the degree of met and unmet needs of those with DSM-IV anxiety disorders. We used a comprehensive community-based needs evaluation model, applied in a comprehensive health and mental health system that offers almost any type of drug and psychological treatment free of charge, to focus on the assessment of self-perceived individual needs, actual use characteristics, expert-defined needs and final consensus appraisals. Before discussing the findings in more detail, limitations of the study should be mentioned.

We included only some of the anxiety disorders, and excluded obsessive-compulsive disorders and posttraumatic stress disorders. In comparing these EDSP findings with those from other countries, such as the USA or Canada, one should remember that the EDSP uses the somewhat stricter DSM-IV algorithms, whereas the other studies are based on DSM-III-R. Also this study is restricted to adolescents and young adults. At this point the need-evaluation findings are only based on the baseline 'snapshot' assessment and do not yet include the more detailed information that will become available in the second and third waves of this investigation. In terms of appraising expert-rated need, one should acknowledge the imperfect nature of such clinical assessment. A clinician's evaluation of need is heavily dependent on the evaluator's professional background and experience, their knowledge and attitudes towards such disorders. Although we tried to control for this by providing all clinical raters with official anxiety treatment consensus documents prior to the study, as well as by performing a consensus process at the end of the assessment, it is likely that systematic rating biases are still influencing the results of our study. However, since there is currently no general agreed assessment guide for evaluating needs, it was the best that could be done. Finally, the findings are preliminary, and lack sophistication in terms of controlling for possibly confounding variables for need, such as comorbidity with depressive disorders, social support, and the degree of disability. Disregarding these limitations our study nevertheless reveals important findings.

Does service availability count?

Even in a community with an extremely well organized, comprehensive and accessible mental health system infrastructure, the utilization rates remain as low as found in previous studies, such as those in the USA and Canada (Kessler et al., 1997; Magee et al., 1996). This finding was also evident in the Ontario-USA comparison reported recently (Katz et al., 1997), and indicates that we must continue to search for the reasons why those with anxiety disorders do not use the mental health services as much as they should. One could argue that our EDSP sample is too young to include the severe cases seen later in life. However, this speculation is not supported by our findings that the EDSP sample includes cases of significant clinical severity and disability, often with an illness history of several years.

Type of anxiety disorder matters

Our EDSP findings strongly suggest that the different anxiety disorders vary in terms of the services used, and the degree of self-perceived and expert-rated needs. GAD and panic disorder lead to help-seeking behavior in at least every second case, whereas only every fifth case with specific phobias reported any service use. Agoraphobia and social phobia lie somewhere in the middle. Similar diagnosis-specific differences were also evident for self-perceived and expert-rated needs. Although those in the EDSP with social phobia and GAD used the mental health services considerably more than their counterparts in the USA, our service-use data are generally consistent with those from the NCS (Katz et al., 1997). With regard to the between-country differences in utilization rates for social phobia and GAD, we suspect that the much stricter DSM-IV criteria in the EDSP may play an important role. Another reason for the higher treatment rates for social phobia might be a public awareness campaign that took place during the same year as our baseline investigation.

Moderate agreement between patient-rated and expert-rated needs

There is only moderate agreement between patient-rated and expert-rated needs, with a correlation coefficient, r, of 0.48. In contrast, the patient-rated need for intervention correlates well with service use ($r = 0.78$). This clearly indicates that self-perceived needs strongly affect actual service use, whether appropriate or not. Differences between self-perceived and expert-rated needs for intervention seem to vary in direction: for specific and social phobias, patients' needs are considerably greater than as judged by the expert. However, the situation is reversed for agoraphobia. One also needs to remember that the discrepancies between expert-rated and self-perceived needs are not always consistent within the disorder.

Unmet need for mental health service

In this study we examined unmet need from two perspectives: that of the patient and that of the professionals in mental health services. Both methods demonstrated that approximately 40% of patients required an intervention specifically for anxiety that was not provided, even when the widest possible definition of service provision was used. However, it is important to acknowledge that the patients' opinions did not always coincide with those of the clinicians in individual cases. For example, clinicians frequently rated agoraphobics as needing treatment, whereas the individuals frequently did not perceive this need themselves. In social phobia we found the reverse picture. The two interventions most frequently suggested by the experts were seldom provided in phobic disorders. These interventions are anxiety-specific counseling and psychoeducation on the basis of self-help manuals, and specialist psychiatrist or psychotherapist interventions (of either psychological or drug type). In light of previous findings and critical discussions (Regier et al., 1998), this finding of approximately 40% expert-defined unmet need in the population was not unexpected. However the poor correlation between expert and self-perceived need calls for a much more extensive search for potential reasons. Since self-perceived needs seem to be a stronger predictor for actual service utilization, this is important. The risk involved might be that those in most need do not get treatment. The significant number of cases in our study with no expert-defined need who were in treatment underlines the importance of this issue.

The problem of inappropriate treatment provision is significant

Our findings that few of those with an expert-rated need received some type of interventions were discouraging. Evidently, in our sample and catchment area, the most effective treatments are rarely provided at all, and, if they are, they are frequently provided inadequately. Only 8% of all 12-month cases were rated as receiving some form of adequate treatment. This discouraging picture in a catchment area with an extremely comprehensive care structure, including many clinical psychologists, other psychotherapists and psychiatrists, raises many critical questions. Are mental health providers not aware of the most effective anxiety treatments? Are they not trained to provide them? Is it not attractive enough to apply highly sophisticated antianxiety interventions under routine conditions (are the barriers financial, organizational or educational)? Although the study in its current stage is not able to answer any of these questions, they will be addressed at a later stage.

To conclude, our preliminary findings from the EDSP clearly indicate that there is a substantial number of people with anxiety disorders in the community in need of treatment who are not receiving any type of professional attention. We estimated this to be about 40% of people with all anxiety disorders active in the month prior to the study; this constitutes an untreated rate of 8% of 14–24 year olds in our population. There is a considerable proportion (15%) who either need therapy but receive grossly inadequate interventions or who have no expert-rated need and do get treatment. Assuming that scientifically proven treatment recommendations are correct, this points to a serious mismatch problem and possibly a waste of personnel and financial resources. There is clearly a need to develop more refined strategies for assessing need than those used in this study.

References

American Psychiatric Association (1980). *Diagnostic and Statistical Manual of Mental Disorders* (3rd edition). Washington, D.C.: American Psychiatric Association.

American Psychiatric Association (1994). *Diagnostic and Statistical Manual of Mental Disorders* (4th edition). Washington, D.C.: American Psychiatric Association.

Andrews, G., Crino, R., Hunt, C., Lampe, L. & Page, A. (1994). *The Treatment of Anxiety Disorders. Clinician's Guide and Patient Manuals.* New York: Cambridge University Press.

Bond, A.J. & Lader, M.H. (1996). *Understanding Drug Treatment in Mental Health Care.* Chichester: Wiley.

Clum, G.A. (1989). Psychological interventions vs. drugs in the treatment of panic. *Behavior Therapy*, **20**, 429–57.

Cording-Tömmel, C., Wittchen, H.-U. & von Zerssen, D. (1988). Evaluation des Verlaufs und outcomes affektiver Psychosen. Implikationen für eine patientenorientierte Bedarfsplanung. In P. Zweifel (ed.), *Neue Ansätze der Bedarfsforschung und neue Formen der Angebotsplanung im Gesundheitswesen. Beiträge zur Gesundheitsökonomie*, pp. 179–222. Gerlingen: Bleicher Verlag.

Donabedian, A. (1966). Evaluating the quality of medical care. *Milbank Memorial Fund Quarterly* (part 2).

Elkin, I., Pilkonis, P.A., Docherty, J.P. & Sotsky, S.M. (1988). Conceptual and methodological issues in comparative studies of psychotherapy and pharmacotherapy: II. Nature and timing of treatment effects. *American Journal of Psychiatry*, **145**, 1070–6.

Fineberg, N. & Drummond, L.M. (1995). Anxiety disorders: drug treatment or behavioral cognitive therapy? *CNS Drugs*, **3**, 448–66.

Häfner, H. (ed.) (1978). *Psychiatrische Epidemiology.* Berlin: Springer-Verlag.

Häfner, H. (ed.) (1979). *Estimating Needs for Mental Health Care. A Contribution of Epidemiology.* Berlin: Springer-Verlag.

Katz, S.J., Kessler, R.C., Frank, R.G., Leaf, P., Lin, E. & Edlund, M. (1997). The use of outpatient mental health services in the United States and Ontario: the impact of mental morbidity and perceived need for care. *American Journal of Public Health*, **87**, 1136–43.

Kessler, R.C., Frank, R.G., Edlund, M., Katz, S.J., Lin, E. & Leaf, P. (1997). Differences in the use of psychiatric outpatient services between the U.S. and Ontario. *New England Journal of Medicine*, **336**, 551–7.

Kessler, R.C., McGonagle, K.A., Zhao, S., Nelson, C.B., Hughes, M., Eshleman, S., Wittchen, H.-U. & Kendler, K. S. (1994). Lifetime and 12-month prevalence of DSM-III-R psychiatric disorders in the United States: results from the National Comorbidity Survey. *Archives of General Psychiatry*, **51**, 8–19.

Lachner, G., Wittchen, H.-U., Perkonigg, A., Holly, A., Schuster, P., Wunderlich, U., Türk, D., Garczynski, E. & Pfister, H. (1998). Structure, content and reliability of the Munich-Composite International Diagnostic Interview (M-CIDI). Substance use sections. *European Addiction Research*, **4**, 28–41.

Lader, M.H. & Bond, A.J. (1998). The interaction of pharmacological and psychological treatments of anxiety. *British Journal of Psychiatry*, **173**, 42–8.

Magee, W.J., Eaton, W.W., Wittchen, H.-U., McGonagle, K.A. & Kessler, R.C. (1996). Agoraphobia, simple phobia, and social phobia in the National Comorbidity Survey. *Archives of General Psychiatry*, **53**, 159–68.

Michelson, L.K. & Marchione, K. (1991). Behavioral, cognitive, and pharmacological treatments of panic disorder with agoraphobia: critique and synthesis. *Journal of Consulting and Clinical Psychology*, **59**, 100–14.

Offord, D., Boyle, M., Campbell, D., Cochrane, J., Goering, P., Lin, E., Rhodes, A. & Wong, M. (1994). *Ontario Health Survey 1990. Mental Health Supplement.* Toronto: Ministry of Health.

Pfister, H. & Wittchen, H.-U. (1995). *M-CIDI Computerprogramm.* Munich: Max-Planck-Institut für Psychiatrie, Klinisches Institut.

Regier, D.A., Kaelber, C.T., Rae, D.S., Farmer, M.E., Knauper, B., Kessler, R.C. & Norquist, G.S. (1998). Limitations of diagnostic criteria and assessment instruments for mental disorders: implications for research and policy. *Archives of General Psychiatry*, **55**, 109–15.

Rice, D.P. & Miller, L.S. (1998). Health economics and cost implications of anxiety and other mental disorders in the United States. *British Journal of Psychiatry*, **173**, 4–9.

Wittchen, H.-U. (1988). Follow-up investigations as a basis for need evaluation – an empirical approach to patient-oriented psychiatric need evaluation. In P. Zweifel (ed.), *Neue Ansätze der Bedarfsforschung und neue Formen der Angebotsplanung im Gesundheitswesen. Beiträge zur Gesundheitsökonomie*, pp. 115–77. Gerlingen: Bleicher Verlag.

Wittchen, H.-U. (1991). Der Langzeitverlauf unbehandelter Angststörungen: Wie häufig sind Spontanremissionen? *Verhaltenstherapie-Praxis, Forschung, Perspektiven*, 1, 273–82.

Wittchen, H.-U. (1994). Reliability and validity studies of the WHO-Composite International Diagnostic Interview (CIDI): a critical review. *Journal of Psychiatric Research*, 28, 57–84.

Wittchen, H.-U. & Pfister, H. (eds.) (1997). *DIA-X-Interviews: Manual für Screening-Verfahren und Interview; Interviewheft Längsschnittuntersuchung (DIA-X-Lifetime); Ergänzungsheft (DIA-X-Lifetime); Interviewheft Querschnittuntersuchung (DIA-X-12 Monate); Ergänzungsheft (DIA-X-12Monate); PC-Programm zur Durchführung des Interviews (Längs-und Querschnittuntersuchung); Auswertungsprogramm.* Frankfurt: Swets & Zeitlinger.

Wittchen, H.-U. & von Zerssen, D. (1987). *Verläufe behandelter und unbehandelter Depressionen und Angststörungen. Eine klinisch-psychiatrische und epidemiologische Verlaufsuntersuchung.* Berlin: Springer-Verlag.

Wittchen, H.-U., Beloch, E., Garczynski, E., Holly, A., Lachner, G., Perkonigg, A., Pfütze, E.-M., Schuster, P., Vodermaier, A., Vossen, A., Wunderlich, U. & Zieglgänsberger, S. (1995a). *Münchener Composite International Diagnostic Interview* (M-CIDI, Paper-pencil 2.2, 2/95). München: Max-Planck-Institut für Psychiatrie, Klinisches Institut (Eigendruck).

Wittchen, H.-U., Beloch, E., Garczynski, E., Holly, A., Lachner, G., Perkonigg, A., Pfütze, E.-M., Schuster, P., Vodermaier, A., Vossen, A., Wunderlich, U. & Zieglgänsberger, S. (1995b). *Manual zum Münchener Composite International Diagnostic Interview* (M-CIDI, Paper-Pencil 2.0, 1/95). München: Max-Planck-Institut für Psychiatrie, Klinisches Institut. (Eigendruck).

Wittchen, H.-U., Beloch, E., Garczynski, E., Holly, A., Lachner, G., Perkonigg, A., Pfütze, E.-M., Schuster, P., Vodermaier, A., Vossen, A., Wunderlich, U. & Zieglgänsberger, S. (1995c). *Listenheft zum Münchener Composite International Diagnostic Interview* (M-CIDI, Paper-Pencil 2.2, 2/95). München: Max-Planck-Institut für Psychiatrie, Klinisches Institut. (Eigendruck).

Wittchen, H.-U., Nelson, G.B. & Lachner, G. (1998a). Prevalence of mental disorders and psychosocial impairments in adolescents and young adults. *Psychological Medicine*, 28, 109–26.

Wittchen, H.-U., Perkonigg, A., Lachner, G. & Nelson, C.B. (1998b). The early developmental stages of psychopathology study (EDSP) – objectives and design. *European Addiction Research*, 4, 18–27.

World Health Organization (1990). *Composite International Diagnostic Interview* (CIDI). Geneva: World Health Organization, Division of Mental Health.

World Health Organization (1993). *International Statistical Classification of Diseases and Related Health Problems. Tenth Revision.* Geneva: World Health Organization.

Notes

The Early Developmental Stages of Psychopathology (EDSP) is a five-year prospective epidemiological study funded by the German Ministry of Research and Technology to investigate the prevalence of substance-use and other mental disorders, their early development and progression, and patterns of comorbidity. H.-U. Wittchen is the principal investigator. Scientific advisors are Dr. J. Angst (Zürich), Dr. W. Esser (Mannheim), Dr. C. Merikangas (New Haven), and Dr. R.C. Kessler (Boston). Collaborating sites and investigators are Dr. G. Bühringer (Institut für Therapieforschung, Munich) and Dr. John (Medizinische Hochschule, Lübeck). Staff members of the EDSP group are: E. Beloch, E. Garcsynski, A. Holly, A. Perkonnig, H. Pfister, V. Reed, P. Schuster, D. Türk, A. Vossen, and U. Wunderlich.

The complete M-CIDI interview package containing the lifetime and 12-months version with respondents booklets, manuals as well as the diagnostic programs are published in German (Wittchen & Pfister, 1997), but are also available in English by writing to the main author.

18

The unmet need for treatment in panic disorder and social phobia

Caroline Hunt

Summary

Effective treatment for anxiety disorders does exist and we have good evidence that symptoms and disability can be significantly reduced for the majority of patients who complete treatment. Furthermore, treatment protocols of randomized controlled trials and the associated patient improvement can be replicated in routine care, given the availability of clinicians with appropriate expertise. However, we can also present evidence that many patients who fail to receive such specialist treatment have a poor long-term outcome when treated in the community. This problem is a serious challenge for mental health services, for these services are unable to offer specialist treatment programs to the majority of individuals in the community who meet diagnostic criteria for an anxiety disorder. But does every individual who meets such criteria require specialist treatment? Data from a community survey and from patients attending a specialist anxiety disorders unit are presented in an attempt to answer the following questions: (1) does the level of disability associated with a diagnosis in the community match the level of disability of patients who reach specialist care?; (2) are different experiences of an anxiety disorder in the general population associated with different levels of disability?; and (3) if we are able to identify different levels of 'disorder' and disability, are these levels related to health service utilization and the perceived need for treatment? Answering these questions will provide the first step towards determining whether different levels of care might produce comparable outcomes in individuals with different levels of disorder and disability.

Introduction

Cognitive-behavioral treatments effectively reduce the panic, anxiety and associated avoidance behavior in panic disorder and agoraphobia, as well as the social anxiety and avoidance behavior in social phobia. Randomized controlled trials show that cognitive-behavioral treatment produces a better outcome than a credible placebo for patients with panic disorder with agoraphobia (Chambless, Foa, Groves & Goldstein, 1982; Marks et al., 1993), panic disorder without agoraphobia (Beck, Sokol, Clark, Berchick & Wright, 1992; Craske, Maidenberg & Bystritsky, 1995; Klosko, Barlow, Tassinari & Cerny, 1990), and social phobia (Heimberg, Dodge, Hope, Kennedy & Zollo, 1990). Furthermore, meta-analytic treatment reviews consistently support the efficacy of cognitive-behavioral therapy for these disorders (Chambless & Gillis, 1993; Feske & Chambless, 1995; Gould, Otto & Pollack, 1995; Taylor, 1996). Follow-up studies show that the patients continue to improve for a number of years after their treatment stops (Clark et al., 1994; Craske, Brown & Barlow, 1991; Heimberg, Salzman, Holt & Blendell, 1993; Scholing & Emmelkamp, 1996a,b).

An important issue is whether the treatment protocols of randomized controlled trials and the associated patient improvement can be replicated in routine care. A recent meta-analysis of past therapy outcome tentatively concluded that the effect sizes for more clinically representative studies were the same as those of the more experimental studies. However, these results were interpreted carefully, because few studies tested the therapy in clinical conditions. Hunt & Andrews (1998) recently studied a consecutive sample of patients treated at a specialist unit for anxiety disorders. They showed that cognitive-behavioral therapy in routine care is an effective treatment, as the patients significantly improved during the treatment itself and during the two-year follow-up, as assessed by measuring a number of variables. The cognitive-behavioral group treatment was delivered intensively by therapists experienced in using this treatment for anxiety disorders. The treatment was guided by published patient-treatment manuals (Andrews, Crino, Hunt, Lampe & Page, 1994). The follow-up data indicate that treatment effects are somewhat diluted compared to published randomized controlled trials of cognitive-behavioral therapy. Yet, they do show that this treatment can be delivered in routine care and can produce effects that are clinically significant and maintained over time.

However, health services do not provide this level of treatment for all patients in the community with an anxiety disorder. The evidence from epidemiological and clinical samples indicates that while the majority of sufferers seek treatment for their complaint, this nonspecialized treatment appears to have little impact on the course of their disorder. Wittchen (1988) reports that every individual with panic disorder who took part in the Munich Follow-up Study had received some form of treatment, usually in the form of medication from their general practitioner. Wittchen comments that despite the high rates of therapeutic contact, the majority of individuals in the sample did not appear to receive any specific or adequate help and their disorders remained persistent and chronic. Pollack et al. (1990) report in the Massachusetts General Hospital Naturalistic Study of the Longitudinal

Course of Panic Disorder that, despite 91% of the sample receiving pharmacotherapy for their disorder (77% benzodiazepines), brief periods of
remission were experienced by less than half the sample over the 2 years of
follow-up. Only 7% of the sample had received behavior therapy. Keller
(1992) comments on preliminary findings from the Harvard/Brown Anxiety
Disorders Research Project, in which 725 patients were gathered from five
sites across the USA. He states, 'despite that fact that almost all patients
received some type of somatotherapy during the follow-up period, it is
alarming to see that the intensity of treatment is far below levels shown to be
effective in randomized clinical trials' (p. 172A). More recently, Bandelow,
Sievert, Rothemeyer, Hajak & Ruther (1995) interviewed 100 patients with
panic disorder about their past treatment. In regard to pharmacological
treatments, 40% had received benzodiazepines, 32% tricyclic antidepressants, and 29% herbal remedies. In regard to psychological treatments, 43%
had received autogenic training, 33% psychodynamic therapy, and only 20%
cognitive-behavioral therapy. These studies suggest that the majority of
individuals with anxiety disorders do not receive either specific or adequate
professional treatment, and subsequently their disorders tend to persist
inappropriately. The aim of the following study was to determine whether the
long-term follow-up of patients who stop or refuse specialist treatment
reveals a similar time course. In other words, what becomes of those individuals with comparable disorders who are assessed at, but do not receive
treatment from, a specialist clinic?

Part I: A study of treatment dropout

Patients

Sixty-five of 189 consecutive patients who were offered treatment for panic
disorder or social phobia at a specialist clinic for anxiety disorders over a
6-month period either refused the offer of treatment ($n = 48$) or dropped out
before it was complete ($n = 17$). The 124 patients who were the focus of the
Hunt & Andrews (1998) study completed the intensive treatment programs
for panic disorder or social phobia over the same 6-month period and are
used as a comparison group. The mean age, sex and treatment diagnosis of
the patients in the three samples are listed in Table 18.1. All patients in the
sample fulfilled DSM-III-R diagnostic criteria for panic disorder or social
phobia, with or without agoraphobia, and had no other psychiatric disorder
requiring immediate treatment.

Procedure

All participants completed questionnaires at the initial intake interview. We

Table 18.1. Demographic characteristics of the three samples

Treatment diagnosis	Treated sample (n=124)	Drop-out sample (n=17)	Refusal sample (n=48)
Panic without agoraphobia	41	10	21
Panic with agoraphobia	43	3	11
Social phobia	40	4	16
Mean age (S.D.)	32.4 (9.6)	32.8 (10.3)	33.5 (9.6)
% Male	45.2	41.2	27.1

tried to contact each participant by telephone one to two years after the end of treatment, and asked them if they would be interviewed over the telephone and complete questionnaires, sent and returned through the mail. The questionnaires included the Symptom Checklist 90 Revised SCL-90-R (Derogatis, 1977), the Eysenck Personality Questionnaire (Eysenck & Eysenck, 1975), the Locus of Control of Behaviour Scale (Craig, Franklin & Andrews, 1984), and additional questions concerning the frequency of panic attacks, levels of avoidance of phobic situations, and the degree to which the panics and avoidance behavior interfered with their life or activities. In addition, participants were requested to rate the current status of their main problem identified at the initial assessment interview, determining how much it currently interfered with their life or activities (Main Problem Question, MPQ, Andrews et al., 1994).

Statistical analysis

Due to the small numbers in the 'refusal' and 'drop out' samples, there was insufficient power to detect large effects for most within-sample comparisons and therefore outcome is described for the combined diagnostic groups. A previous analysis failed to detect a significant difference in outcome between diagnostic groups of patients treated for panic disorder or social phobia (Hunt & Andrews, 1998). Ten variables assessing symptoms, disablement and traits were subjected to a principal components analysis so as to concisely describe the relationship between the measured variables, while taking into account the patterns of correlations between the variables. The ten variables were three factors of the SCL-90-R (anxiety, phobic anxiety, depression), neuroticism (a trait measure of emotionality from the EPQ), the Locus of Control of Behaviour Scale, frequency of panic attacks, mean rating of avoidance, rating of interference from panic attacks, rating of disablement from avoidance, and the MPQ. At each stage of the analysis, the data were screened for fit between the distribution of variables, and the assumptions of multivariate analysis and data transformations carried out where necessary

(Tabachnick & Fidell, 1989). The multivariate analysis of variance (MANOVA) method for repeated measures analysis, as outlined by O'Brien & Kister Kaiser (1985), allowed the analysis to be free of the sphericity assumptions that affect type 1 error rate and power in traditional repeated-measures designs (such as mixed-model ANOVAS). This method treats the analysis of the principal component variable as an overall test, which, if significant, can be followed by analyses of each variable of interest as follow-up tests.

Results

Of the 17 individuals who dropped out from treatment, 15 (88%) were located and nine (53%) agreed to be interviewed over the telephone and to complete the questionnaires by mail. Of the 48 individuals who refused the offer of treatment, 30 (63%) were located and 20 (42%) agreed to be interviewed. They were interviewed an average of 39 months following their initial assessment at the clinic. In regard to the comparison group of 124 patients who completed their course of treatment, 109 (88%) were located and 93 (75%) agreed to be interviewed. These patients were interviewed an average of 20 months following the conclusion of their treatment.

The principal components analysis extracted two factors which were subjected to oblique rotation and accounted for 55.9% and 10.1% of the variance in the scores, respectively. These two sets of factor scores were used for statistical analysis across the measurement occasions and diagnostic groups. To control the experiment-wise error rate at $\alpha = 0.05$ the decision-wise error rate was set at $\alpha/6 = 0.008$ on the basis of planned tests of three variable contrasts (pretreatment test, posttest and a pre–post difference variable) and two orthogonal group contrasts ('treated' sample versus 'the rest', 'drop out' versus 'refuser' samples). The two factor variables derived from the principal components analysis were analyzed independently.

The MANOVA approach produced a significant time effect for each factor (factor 1: $F = 18.56$, $df = 1$, $p = 0.000$; factor 2: $F = 19.72$, $df = 1$, $p = 0.000$), rejecting the null hypothesis that there was no difference between intake and follow-up scores across the three groups. The time by group interaction was also significant for both factors (factor 1: $F = 8.86$, $df = 2$, $p = 0.002$; factor 2: $F = 11.67$, $df = 2$, $p = 0.000$), suggesting that the three samples had different mean changes over time. Two interaction subeffects were tested which (1) compared the treated sample with the combined drop out and refuser samples; and (2) compared the drop out sample with the refuser sample. The results support a significant difference in change over time between the treated sample and those who either dropped out or refused treatment (factor 1: $F = 12.87$, $df = 1$, $p = 0.001$; factor 2: $F = 20.35$, $df = 1$, $p = 0.000$). The comparison between the drop out and refuser samples was not significant, suggesting that these two samples do not differ in their mean changes over time (factor 1: $F = 0.12$, $df = 1$, $p = 0.728$; factor 2: $F = 0.99$, $df = 1$, $p = 0.322$). Simple effects of the group contrasts were tested at intake and follow-up. In terms of the comparison between the treated sample and the combined drop out and refuser samples, there was no significant difference at intake (factor 1: $F = 0.57$, $df = 1$, $p = 0.452$; factor 2: $F = 0.05$, $df = 1$, $p = 0.829$), but a significant difference was found at follow-up (factor 1: $F = 15.54$, $df = 1$, $p = 0.000$; factor 2: $F = 16.9$, $df = 1$, $p = 0.000$). The drop out and refuser samples were not significantly different in either factor score at intake (factor 1: $F = 1.24$, $df = 1$, $p = 0.267$; factor 2: $F = 6.62$, $df = 1$, $p = 0.011$), or at follow-up (factor 1: $F = 0.04$, $df = 1$, $p = 0.841$; factor 2: $F = 0.00$, $df = 1$, $p = 0.949$).

Discussion of results

In summary, the sample of patients who refused or dropped out from specialist care remained significantly more symptomatic and disabled compared with patients, matched for symptom and disablement severity at the initial assessment, who received a full course of cognitive-behavioral therapy. This poor outcome occurred despite the fact that 66.7% of those who dropped out and 75% of those who refused treatment had subsequent ongoing contact with a health professional specifically for help with anxiety. It is likely that the level of treatment delivered in trials of treatment outcome or in specialist clinics is not being given in other settings. Routine care, as Keller (1992) and Bandelow et al. (1995) report, is simply not good enough; being seen does not equate with being treated effectively.

This problem is a serious challenge for mental health services, for it is unreasonable to expect that these services will offer specialist treatment programs to the majority of individuals in the community who meet diagnostic criteria for an anxiety disorder. But does every individual who meets such criteria require specialist treatment? Perhaps not all the patients who left specialist treatment or refused the offer of it needed that treatment. The 'undertreated' samples from the earlier analysis were combined into two groups based on their reports that they sought treatment for their anxiety disorder over the follow-up period ($n = 20$), or that they did not seek treatment ($n = 9$). The outcome at follow-up, based on measures of panic attacks, anxiety, avoidance and disablement, for these two samples indicates that those 'undertreated' individuals who chose not to seek further treatment during the follow-up had a mean outcome that was comparable to that of the 'fully treated' sample (Table 18.2). It is likely that those same individuals who did not seek treatment, either at the specialist clinic or during the follow-up period, chose wisely and did not need treatment for their anxiety disorder. On the other hand, the outcome for those individuals who sought further treatment remained poor. There is no evidence that the mental health care

Table 18.2. Comparison of people who dropped out of treatment, who either sought (n=20) or did not seek treatment (n=9) over the follow-up: measures at follow-up

	Number of panic attacks	SCL-90-R Anxiety factor scores	Avoidance scale scores	Main Problem Questionnaire scores
	mean (SD)	mean (SD)	mean (SD)	mean (SD)
Treatment sought	8.3 (18.5)	2.0 (0.1)	2.5 (2.2)	4.2 (1.9)
No treatment sought	2.5 (3.8)	1.1 (0.7)	0.8 (0.5)	2.7 (1.8)
'Fully treated' sample	1.9 (2.8)	0.8 (0.7)	0.8 (0.5)	3.0 (1.5)

SCL-90-R, Symptom Checklist 90 Revised.

provided in the community for individuals with these anxiety disorders changed their symptoms or associated level of disability.

In the light of data from those individuals who chose not to seek treatment for their anxiety disorder, health services may not need to provide specialist treatment programs for everyone in the community with an anxiety disorder. However, we still need to know how to determine who should receive specialist treatment, and the treatment needs of the remaining individuals with anxiety disorders. Treatment providers may be able to determine the level of care required by measuring disability. The measurement of disability is also important in burden in studies of mental disorders, where burden is underestimated if one only considers associated mortality. Appropriate methods for calculating the disability of mental disorders, taking into account the effect of concurrent comorbidity, are being developed, and it appears that the disability associated with mental disorders might be comparable to that associated with physical disorders (Andrews, Sanderson & Beard, 1998). Therefore, it might be possible to estimate the need for intensive or specialist treatment by measuring the level of disability associated with an individual's experience of a mental disorder.

Part II: Comparison of disability in specialist and community settings

Data from individuals with an anxiety disorder diagnosis from a community survey and from patients attending a specialist anxiety disorders clinic are used to try and determine whether the level of disability associated with a diagnosis in the community matches that of patients who reach specialist care.

The community sample was drawn from a survey of 1364 individuals who had originally been screened as being likely to meet criteria for a mental disorder from a random population sample of 10,000 individuals in a semi-rural Australian town. All individuals completed the Composite International Diagnostic Interview (CIDI-Auto, version 2.0) and a number of questionnaires including measures of disability and health utilization. The Mental Health Summary Scale from the SF-12 (Ware, Kosinski & Keller, 1996) was used to compare the disability of individuals from the community sample who met criteria for two anxiety disorders (panic disorder or social phobia, with or without agoraphobia), with that of patients with these two disorders who had attended the anxiety disorders clinic for treatment. Comorbidity, defined as the existence of additional Axis I anxiety or depressive disorders, was used as a covariate in the comparison, as clinic samples tend to have higher levels of comorbidity than community samples, and level of disability is significantly associated with comorbidity (Andrews, Sanderson & Beard, 1998). The data in Table 18.3 show that in both diagnostic groups, patients attending the specialist clinic were significantly more disabled than the community sample, even when comorbidity was held constant. These data support the argument that not all individuals with an anxiety disorder have the same level of disability, and, quite possibly, a number will have a lesser need for treatment, particularly treatment at a specialist level. But are those individuals who are significantly disabled by their disorder receiving adequate treatment?

Part III: Levels of disability and associated health service use in a community sample

Data from individuals with panic disorder or social phobia from a community survey were used to answer the following questions: (1) are different experiences of an anxiety disorder in the general population associated with different levels of disability, and (2) if we are able to identify different levels of disorder and disability, are these levels related to health service utilization?

The first question asks whether different experiences of an anxiety disorder in the general population are associated with different levels of disability. In other words, is it possible to identify patients with a high level of disability, and presumably a high level of need for treatment, by identifying factors associated with their disorder? A multiple regression analysis tested the association between disability (again using the Mental Health Summary Scale of the SF-12) and the presence of comorbid Axis I disorders, duration of disorder, level of avoidance, age, neuroticism, and the presence of a major depressive episode, using data from the 142 individuals with panic disorder or social phobia in the community sample. The comorbidity variable was entered as a first step and accounted for 35% of the variance in disability,

Table 18.3. Level of disability with Mental Health Summary Scale (SF-12) in patients who reach specialist care and in a community sample

	n	Level of disability
Panic disorder (with or without agoraphobia)		
Community sample	85	39.94
Specialist clinic sample	57	31.99

Note: $F = 16.508$, $df = 1$, $p = 0.000$

Social phobia		
Community sample	69	40.94
Specialist clinic sample	57	29.22

Note: $F = 38.985$, $df = 1$, $p = 0.000$

which was significant at $p = 0.0000$. The remaining five variables were entered as a second step, accounting for a further 12% of the variance in disability, this $R2$ change was also significant at $p = 0.001$. The variables of neuroticism and the presence of major depression were found to significantly contribute to the explained variance, at $p = 0.004$ and $p = 0.01$, respectively. These results replicate those of Hollifield et al. (1997) who, having assessed 62 patients with panic disorder and 61 primary care patients, found that major depression and neuroticism significantly contribute to variance in the SF-36 Mental Health Summary Scale. A diagnosis of panic disorder, chronic medical illness, gender, ethnicity, age, education, or place of residence did not significantly contribute to the variance in disability. These results indicate that marked neuroticism (or trait emotionality) and the presence of major depression may well be markers of higher levels of disability, and hence the need for more intensive or specialist intervention.

The second question considers the relationship between disability and use of mental health services, again using data from the 142 individuals with panic disorder or social phobia from the community sample. Of the total sample, 41.5% had seen a general practitioner for a mental health problem, 11.3% had seen a psychiatrist, and 9.2% had seen a psychologist in the prior 12 months. The sample was split into four levels of disability based on quartiles from US population norms of the SF-36 Mental Health Summary Scale (Ware, Kosinski & Keller, 1994). Table 18.4 shows, not surprisingly, that the disability scores for the sample are skewed towards higher levels of disability, with the majority of the sample being in the most disabled quartile. For many individuals, panic disorder and social phobia are indeed disabling. Interestingly, the mean disability score for the most disabled group matches the average level of disability previously found in the patients attending the

Table 18.4. Individuals from community sample with panic disorder or social phobia split into four levels of disability by the Mental Health Summary Scale (MHSS) (SF-12)

Percentile	n	Mean MHSS	SD
0–25	82	32.8	8.1
26–50	37	49.0	2.2
51–75	18	54.9	1.3
76–100	5	62.0	1.6

Note: lower MHSS scores mean greater disability.

Table 18.5. Relationship between level of disability and 'level of care' in community sample

	0–25	26–50	51–75	76–100
No mental health consultations	36	20	14	2
General practitioner consultations	25	12	4	2
Psychiatrist or psychologist consultations	21	5	0	1

Note: Overall chi square = 10.03, $df = 6$, $p = 0.12$.

specialist anxiety disorders clinic. This finding confirms the previous assertion that patients who attend specialist treatment are, on average, more disabled than their counterparts in the community.

The community sample with panic disorder or social phobia was split into those individuals who had not reported a mental health consultation in the previous 12 months, those who had seen solely a primary care physician for a mental health consultation, and those who had seen a psychiatrist or psychologist, arguably a specialist level of mental health care (Table 18.5). There appeared to be no significant relationship between level of disability and 'level of care' in the community sample ($\chi^2 = 10.03$, $df = 6$, $p = 0.12$). Of note, however, is the large proportion of individuals with high levels of disability who had not received any treatment for their anxiety disorder.

When the treatments reported by these patients are considered, there is cause for further concern. Of the 25 individuals who saw their general practitioner, 18 received medication and nine received counseling. Of the 21 individuals who saw a psychiatrist or psychologist, 16 received medication, 15 received counseling, eight received long-term psychotherapy, while only three received cognitive-behavioral therapy. Therefore, very few patients reported receiving a treatment that is known to produce clinically significant treatment effects that are maintained over time. The majority of patients had been prescribed medication and yet were still highly disabled, a finding inconsistent with the notion of an effective treatment.

Conclusions

Not everyone requires specialist treatment. Data presented in this chapter show that the outcome for some people who leave specialist care is good, and that people in the community with an anxiety disorder are, on average, less disabled than their counterparts who attend specialist treatment programs. It may be possible to identify individuals with a high level of need for treatment by assessing their disability; comorbid disorder, particularly major depression, and marked neuroticism appear to be associated with higher levels of disability. Effective treatments are available, but they are not being delivered effectively in the community. Many of those who drop out of treatment programs at a specialist anxiety disorders clinic and seek treatment elsewhere have a poor long-term outcome, particularly when compared to similar patients who complete their treatment. Data from a community sample show that a high proportion of patients with panic disorder or social phobia who have significant disability do not receive any mental health care. And when these individuals do receive mental health care, whether primary or specialist, the treatment is not optimal. Even drug treatment, albeit easy to deliver and associated with minimal side-effects, does not produce the treatment effects associated with cognitive-behavioral therapy. In the earlier reported follow-up of patients who either left or refused treatment, the majority of medications prescribed over the follow-up were benzodiazepines. There is evidence that discontinuation of such medication is associated with relapse of symptoms for 70–90% of patients (e.g., Fyer et al., 1987) and, while lowering anxiety symptoms in the short term, may subsequently decrease a patient's tolerance to anxiety and discomfort (Fava et al., 1994). There remains a high level of unmet need in individuals with panic disorder and social phobia. The challenges ahead include being better able to identify those patients who need specialist treatment and to ensure that effective treatment is available to them. It will also be important to determine whether other levels of care, such as primary health care services or models of self-help, will provide adequate care for individuals with lower levels of disability. Most importantly, all health services must deliver treatments that produce clinically significant change in both symptoms and the disability associated with a disorder.

References

Andrews, G., Crino, R., Hunt, C., Lampe, L. & Page, A. (1994). *The Treatment of Anxiety Disorders. Clinician's Guide and Patient Manuals.* New York: Cambridge University Press.

Andrews, G., Sanderson, K. & Beard, J. (1998). Burden of disease: methods of calculating the disability for mental disorder. *British Journal of Psychiatry*, **173**,

123–31.

Bandelow, B., Sievert, K., Rothemeyer, M., Hajak, G. & Ruther, E. (1995). What treatments do patients with panic disorder and agoraphobia get? *European Archives of Psychiatry and Clinical Neurosciences*, 245, 165–71.

Beck, A.T., Sokol, L., Clark, D.A., Berchick, R. & Wright, F. (1992). A crossover study of focused cognitive therapy for panic disorder. *American Journal of Psychiatry*, 149, 778–83.

Chambless, D.L. & Gillis, M.M. (1993). Cognitive therapy of anxiety disorders. *Journal of Consulting and Clinical Psychology*, 61, 248–60.

Chambless, D.L., Foa, E.B., Groves, G.A. & Goldstein, A.J. (1982). Exposure and communications training in the treatment of agoraphobia. *Behaviour Research and Therapy*, 20, 219–31.

Clark, D.M., Salkovskis, P.M., Hackman, A., Middleton, H., Anastasiades, P. & Gelder, M. (1994). A comparison of cognitive therapy, applied relaxation and imipramine in the treatment of panic disorder. *British Journal of Psychiatry*, 164, 759–69.

Craig, A., Franklin, J. & Andrews, G. (1984). A scale to measure locus of control of behaviour. *British Journal of Medical Psychology*, 57, 173–80.

Craske, M.G., Brown, T.A. & Barlow, D.H. (1991). Behavioral treatment of panic disorder: a two-year follow-up. *Behavior Therapy*, 22, 289–304.

Craske, M.G., Maidenberg, E. & Bystritsky, A. (1995). Brief cognitive-behavioral versus nondirective therapy for panic disorder. *Journal of Behavior Therapy and Experimental Psychiatry*, 26, 113–20.

Derogatis, L.R. (1977). *SCL-90 Revised Version Manual-1*. Baltimore: Johns Hopkins School of Medicine.

Eysenck, H.J. & Eysenck, S.B.G. (1975). *Manual of the Eysenck Personality Questionnaire. (Junior and Adult)*. Kent, UK: Hodder & Stoughton.

Fava, G.A., Grandi, S., Belluardo, P., Savron, G., Raffi, A.R., Conti, S. & Saviotti, F.M. (1994). Benzodiazepines and anxiety sensitivity in panic disorder. *Progress in Neuro-Psychopharmacology & Biological Psychiatry*, 18, 1163–8.

Feske, U. & Chambless, D.L. (1995). Cognitive behavioral versus exposure only treatment for social phobia: a meta-analysis. *Behavior Therapy*, 26, 695–720.

Fyer, A.J., Liebowitz, M.R., Gorman, J.M., Campeas, R., Levin, A., Davies, S.O., Goetz, D. & Klein, D.F. (1987). Discontinuation of alprazolam treatment in panic patients. *American Journal of Psychiatry*, 144, 303–8.

Gould, R.A., Otto, M.W. & Pollack, M.H. (1995). A meta-analysis of treatment outcome for panic disorder. *Clinical Psychology Review*, 15, 819–44.

Heimberg, R.G., Dodge, C.S., Hope, D.A., Kennedy, C.R. & Zollo, L.J. (1990). Cognitive behavioral treatment for social phobia: comparison with a placebo control. *Cognitive Therapy and Research*, 14, 1–23.

Heimberg, R.G., Salzman, D.G., Holt, C.S. & Blendell, K.A. (1993). Cognitive-behavioral group treatment for social phobia: effectiveness at five-year follow-up. *Cognitive Therapy and Research*, 17, 325–39.

Hollifield, M., Katon, W., Skipper, B., Chapman, T., Ballenger, J.C., Mannuzza, S. & Fyer, A.J. (1997). Panic disorder and quality of life: variables predictive of functional impairment. *American Journal of Psychiatry*, 154, 766–72.

Hunt, C. & Andrews, G. (1998). Long-term outcome of panic disorder and social phobia. *Journal of Anxiety Disorders*, 12, 395–406.

Keller, M.B. (1992). The naturalistic course of anxiety and depressive disorders. *Clinical Neuropharmacology*, 15 [Suppl. 1], 171A–173A.

Klosko, J.S., Barlow, D.H., Tassinari, R. & Cerny, J.A. (1990). A comparison of alprazolam and behavior therapy in treatment of panic disorder. *Journal of Consulting and Clinical Psychology*, 58, 77–84.

Marks, I.M., Swinson, R.P., Basoglu, M., Kuch, K., Noshirvani, H., O'Sullivan, G., Lelliott, P.T., Kirby, M., McNamee, G., Sengun, S. & Wickwire, K. (1993). Alprazolam and exposure alone and combined in panic disorder with agoraphobia. A controlled study in London and Toronto. *British Journal of Psychiatry*, 162, 776–87.

O'Brien, R.G. & Kister Kaiser, M. (1985). MANOVA method for analyzing repeated measures designs: an extensive primer. *Psychological Bulletin*, 97, 316–33.

Pollack, M.H., Otto, M.W., Rosenbaum, J.F., Sachs, G.S., O'Neil, C., Asher, R. & Meltzer-brody, S. (1990). Longitudinal course of panic disorder: Findings from the Massachusetts General Hospital Naturalistic Study. *Journal of Clinical Psychiatry*, 51 [12 Suppl. A], 12–16.

Scholing, A. & Emmelkamp, P.M.G. (1996a). Treatment of fear of blushing, sweating, or trembling. Results at long-term follow-up. *Behavior Modification*, 20, 338–56.

Scholing, A. & Emmelkamp, P.M.G. (1996b). Treatment of generalized social phobia: results at long-term follow-up. *Behaviour Research and Therapy*, 34, 447–52.

Tabachnick, B.G. & Fidell, L.S. (1989). *Using Multivariate Statistics* (2nd edition) New York: Harper & Row.

Taylor, S. (1996). Meta-analysis of cognitive-behavioral treatments for social phobia. *Journal of Behavior Therapy and Experimental Psychiatry*, 27, 1–9.

Ware, J.E., Kosinski, M. & Keller, S.D. (1994). *SF-36 Physical and Mental Health Summary Scales: A User's Manual*. Boston, MA: New England Medical Center.

Ware, J.E., Kosinski, M. & Keller, S.D. (1996). A 12-item short-form health survey: construction of scales and preliminary tests of reliability and validity. *Medical Care*, 34, 220–33.

Wittchen, H.-U. (1988). Natural course and spontaneous remissions of untreated anxiety disorders: results of the Munich follow-up study (MFS). In I. Hand & H.-U. Wittchen (eds.), *Panic and Phobias 2. Treatments and Variables Affecting Course and Outcome*, pp. 3–17. Berlin: Springer-Verlag.

19

Alcohol-use disorders: who should be treated and how?

Wayne Hall and Maree Teesson

Summary

Alcohol-use disorders are among the more prevalent mental disorders diagnosed in community surveys, yet only a small proportion of people with alcohol-use disorders seek or receive treatment from mental health or addiction treatment services. Although it is tempting to assume that these disorders are undertreated, treatment may not always be appropriate, since approximately half of the disorders detected in population surveys will remit without formal treatment. If not everyone with an alcohol-use disorder needs treatment, how should we deploy limited treatment resources to produce the greatest reduction in alcohol-related harm?

Public education about the risks of alcohol use may prevent and ameliorate the significant public health consequences of the prevalent, milder alcohol-use disorders. Education about self-help strategies for quitting or cutting down may obviate the need for professional assistance. Those whose problems resist self-help need more effective forms of treatment, more efficiently delivered than is often the case at present. *Treatment services appear to routinely provide the most expensive, intensive and least effective forms of intervention to persons who present with alcohol-use disorders.* Better triage would ensure a more rational use of scarce treatment resources.

Given the high rates of comorbidity between alcohol-use, anxiety, and affective disorders, the treatment of people with comorbid mental and alcohol-use disorders must be improved. Specialist mental health services need to recognize and treat comorbid alcohol-use disorders among their patients. Specialist alcohol treatment services need to give priority to better identification and management of anxiety and affective disorders among their patients since these are the mental disorders that are most prevalent and the most amenable to treatment.

Introduction

Alcohol-use disorders are among the most prevalent mental disorders in the general community. Managing scarce treatment resources for alcohol-use disorders requires a balance between the provision of expensive clinical interventions for alcohol-dependent people who seek treatment on the one hand, and expenditure on public health strategies that aim to reduce alcohol consumption, alcohol-related problems, and the risks of developing other physical and mental disorders on the other. The management of alcohol-use disorders should be informed by an understanding of the epidemiology of alcohol-use disorders in the population.

The epidemiology of alcohol-use disorders

Alcohol-use disorders (which include abuse and dependence) typically involve impaired control of alcohol use. Obtaining, using, and recovering from alcohol consumes a disproportionate amount of the user's time, and the user continues to drink alcohol despite associated problems. Alcohol abusers typically develop tolerance to the effects of alcohol, requiring larger doses to achieve the desired psychological effect, and abrupt cessation of use often produces a withdrawal syndrome. Many alcohol abusers experience other psychological and physical health problems, and their alcohol use often adversely affects the lives of their family members, friends and work mates.

Many health professionals think that alcohol-use disorders are relatively rare and have a poor outcome. These pessimistic views about treatment outcome are shared by many people in the population who have alcohol problems (Grant, 1997). Recent American research using standardized interviews to estimate the proportion of people with alcohol-use disorders in a random sample of the community challenged the optimistic assumption that alcohol-use disorders are rare, and the pessimistic assumption that their outcome is always poor (Helzer & Canino, 1992).

The Epidemiologic Catchment Area Study

The Epidemiologic Catchment Area (ECA) study involved personal interviews with 20,000 Americans in five states (Regier et al., 1990, 1993; Robins & Regier, 1991). A standardized interview for detecting mental disorders was used to assess the prevalence of DSM-III psychiatric diagnoses, including alcohol abuse and dependence. The results indicate that alcohol-use disorders were the second most common mental disorder among the major diagnoses that were assessed (Helzer, Burnam & McEvoy, 1991). A total of just under 14% of the population suffered from alcohol-use disorders at some time in their lives (with 8% meeting criteria for alcohol dependence), comparable to the 14% who had phobias at some time in their lives (Robins & Regier, 1991).

The prevalence of alcohol-use disorders was strongly related to gender: 24% of men and 5% of women had suffered from such disorders at some time in their lives, while 12% of men and 2% of women had experienced these disorders in the year before they were interviewed. Heavy drinking was a risk factor: the lifetime experience of those with alcohol-use disorders increased from 15% among all drinkers to 49% of those with a history of drinking more than seven drinks in a session at least once a week.

In the ECA study individuals with alcohol-use disorders were at high risk of suffering from other mental disorders. Nearly half (47%) had a second psychiatric diagnosis (compared with a third of people who were diagnosed as having a psychiatric illness other than alcohol-use disorder). The most common diagnoses were: drug abuse and dependence, antisocial personality disorder, mania, schizophrenia, panic disorders, and obsessive-compulsive disorder (Helzer et al., 1991).

Alcohol-use disorders in the ECA were disorders of 'youthful onset', with 80% of those who had ever experienced a symptom having done so before age 30. They had a high rate of remission: half of those who had ever experienced a symptom had not experienced one for at least a year. The average length of symptoms of those with alcohol-use disorders was less than five years, indicating that many who drink heavily and experience symptoms of dependence can stop drinking for periods of a year or more (Helzer et al., 1991).

Most individuals with alcohol-use disorders who stopped or moderated their drinking did so without professional assistance. Only 12% had ever told a doctor about their drinking problem (27% of those who were dependent, 8% of those who had abused alcohol, and only 3% of heavy drinkers who had experienced at least one problem). These findings indicate that alcohol-use disorders in the community have a more benign outcome than the pessimistic picture we obtain from clinical samples.

The National Comorbidity Survey

The National Comorbidity Survey (NCS) is a population survey that was undertaken between 1990 and 1992 to examine the extent of comorbidity between substance-use and nonsubstance-use disorders in the USA (Kessler et al., 1994). The survey used a modified version of the Composite International Diagnostic Interview (CIDI) schedule to make the same diagnoses as in the ECA.

The prevalence of alcohol-use disorders was higher in the NCS than the ECA. The NCS differed from the ECA in assessing dependence symptoms in any person who had ever used alcohol 12 or more times in a year (Anthony, Warner & Kessler, 1994). The proportion of the population that met lifetime criteria for alcohol dependence was 24%. The proportion of those who had ever used alcohol who met criteria for lifetime dependence was 15%. Men were more likely than women to become dependent on alcohol (Anthony et al., 1994).

As in the ECA, the treated prevalence of mental disorders in the NCS was very low. Only 12% of people with a mental disorder in the past 12 months had seen a mental health professional within that year. The likelihood of having received treatment was highest among people with three or more disorders (23% versus 12%) (Kessler et al., 1994). Rates of comorbid disorders were high among those with alcohol-use disorders: 78% of men and 86% of women with an alcohol-use disorder had another mental disorder (Kessler et al., 1997). The highest odds of comorbidity were with other forms of drug disorder, affective disorders, and anxiety disorders (Kessler et al., 1997). People with an alcohol disorder and another comorbid mental disorder were more likely to have received treatment than those without (Kessler et al., 1996).

The validity of psychiatric diagnoses in community surveys

All diagnoses in the ECA and the NCS were based upon self-reported information collected in a structured interviewed by a lay interviewer. The approach taken in validating the ECA diagnoses was to compare the diagnoses generated with the Diagnostic Interview Schedule (DIS) with those of psychiatrists who reinterviewed respondents six weeks later using DIS, a diagnostic checklist and follow-up questions (Helzer, Robins, McEvoy & Spitznagel, 1985). There was reasonable but imperfect agreement between the lay and psychiatrist diagnoses for most mental disorders, with alcohol- and substance-use diagnoses showing the best agreement. As expected, the cases about which lay interviewers and psychiatrists were most likely to disagree were those with symptoms at the threshold of the diagnostic definition, a sizeable group in community surveys. A later study produced somewhat poorer evidence for validity (Anthony et al., 1985).

Robins (1985) argued that the validity of the ECA findings could be inferred from other evidence. This included the internal consistency of the ECA findings across study sites; the consistency of the ECA findings with those of other surveys using the DIS in other countries; and the broad agreement between the ECA findings and the results of epidemiological studies based on clinical case records and validated self-report. Validity has been enhanced by the broad agreement between the findings of the ECA and the NCS, which used improved diagnostic interview schedules and various other methodological refinements (Kessler et al., 1994).

In designing the NCS study, Kessler and his colleagues had the advantage of benefiting from the considerable work that has gone into the development and validation of the CIDI. There is consequently good evidence for the reliability and validity of the modified CIDI used in the NCS (Kessler, 1995a).

Thus, while community epidemiological surveys may not provide perfect estimates of the prevalence of mental disorders in the community, they provide a reasonably valid portrait of the pattern of disorders in the community. This represents an enormous improvement on previous knowledge of the epidemiology of mental and substance-use disorders derived from clinical populations.

Who should be treated and how?

The low rates of treatment among people with alcohol-use disorders in population studies seem to suggest that we should be more active in finding and treating people with such disorders in the community. However, this may not necessarily be the case. Since a substantial proportion of these disorders are likely to remit without professional help, it would be inefficient to use scarce clinical resources to deal with time-limited and minimally disabling disorders. Furthermore, a substantial proportion of people with mild alcohol-use disorders are not interested in receiving treatment (Grant, 1997). The attempt to identify and treat all those with alcohol-use disorders in the community may also medicalize behavior that is better modified in other ways.

Public health alcohol policies

A major development in the conceptualization of alcohol-use disorders and alcohol-related health problems has been the development of a public health perspective of alcohol use. This avoids focusing exclusively on the 'alcoholic', by considering the spectrum of health problems caused by alcohol, e.g., road traffic accidents, lost productivity, violence, and diseases such as cancer, liver cirrhosis, brain damage, and heart disease (Edwards et al., 1994). The World Bank Burden of Disease Study (Murray & Lopez, 1997) recently reinforced the need for a public health perspective by identifying alcohol as a risk factor for disability caused by disease and injury. In designing an essential national package of health services based on the World Bank Burden of Disease Study, Bobadilla, Cowley, Musgrove & Saxenian (1994) included interventions to reduce the risk factor of alcohol use.

A public health approach adopts a broader explanation of the causes of alcohol-related health problems. While more traditional approaches have focused on the characteristics that predispose some drinkers to develop alcohol-use disorders, the public health approach emphasizes the characteristics of the physical and social environment which encourage hazardous drinking, such as the advertising and promotion of alcohol, and the ready availability of cheap alcohol (Edwards et al., 1994; Walsh & Hingson, 1987).

An important consequence of the public health perspective for policy is that the prevalence of alcohol-related problems in the community can be reduced by cutting down the population's alcohol consumption. Among the measures proposed are: laws and regulations which aim to reduce the availability of alcohol (e.g., licensing regulations that restrict trading hours for liquor outlets, and the enforcement of laws on underage drinking); measures that increase the price of alcohol to reduce consumption (e.g., increased taxes levied on the alcohol content of beverages); and regulations to control the promotion of alcohol (Edwards et al., 1994; Walsh & Hingson, 1987).

Public education about alcohol

The lack of popular and political support for policies that increase the price of alcohol or reduce its availability (Flaherty, Homel & Hall, 1991) has encouraged a search for other approaches to reduce the public health impact of alcohol use. Foremost among these has been the public education of drinkers about the risks of alcohol use. In Australia, guidelines about the maximum number of standard drinks that can be legally consumed before driving, in combination with random breath testing, has reduced overall road fatalities and the proportion of fatalities in which the driver had a blood alcohol level above the prescribed level (0.05%) (Homel, 1989). These campaigns enjoy widespread public support and have probably also reduced alcohol consumption by providing a reason for drinkers to moderate their consumption (Homel, 1989).

In many English-speaking countries health authorities have issued guidelines for 'safe' levels of alcohol use, typically in the form of the number of standard drinks that can be consumed per day and per week with minimum risk to health (e.g., Australian National Health and Medical Research Council, 1992). These guidelines have rarely been accompanied by an education campaign to explain their rationale or to tell the public about how to measure standard drinks. The task of complying with these guidelines has also been made more difficult in Australia by the alcohol industry's resistance to indicate the number of standard drinks on the label of alcohol containers. More recently, public understanding of 'safe' levels of consumption has been complicated by widely publicized evidence that moderate alcohol consumption benefits cardiovascular health (Hall, 1996). The primary goal of these safe drinking limits has most often been to reduce the health complications of heavy drinking, such as liver cirrhosis. More attention needs to be paid to explaining the risks of developing alcohol dependence from heavy drinking, binge drinking, and drinking to relieve withdrawal symptoms and hangovers.

Screening and brief intervention for hazardous drinkers

People who present for medical treatment can be screened for hazardous alcohol use and alcohol-related problems. Those identified as drinking at hazardous levels can be advised to reduce or stop consumption, and given simple ways to achieve these goals (Heather & Tebbut, 1989). Research has shown that screening and brief advice for excessive alcohol consumption in general practice and hospital settings reduces consumption and the problems caused by alcohol (e.g., Chick, Lloyd & Crombie, 1985; Elvy, Wells & Baird, 1988; Kristenson, Ohlin, Hulter-Nosslin, Trell & Hood, 1983; Wallace, Cutler & Haines, 1988). Given the economic costs of conventional treatment for alcohol-related problems (Holder & Blose, 1986; Holder & Schachman, 1987), there is a good economic argument for brief intervention. It usually involves an investment of one to three hours in screening and brief advice, which costs a small fraction of the intensive inpatient treatment required for alcohol dependence. Brief methods of intervention can also reach a far greater number of people whose drinking is hazardous or harmful than could ever be achieved by specialist alcohol treatment services.

The role of specialist addiction treatment

Since self-help and brief interventions will not always suffice, there will always be a role for specialist treatment for alcohol-use disorders. However, evidence from controlled evaluations suggests that the form of treatment offered should differ from that routinely provided until recently, namely inpatient or residential treatment (Heather & Tebbutt, 1989; Mattick & Jarvis, 1993). Controlled evaluations of inpatient treatment for the minority of people with alcohol-use disorders who seek treatment demonstrate that about a third of such patients remain abstinent over a year, a third substantially reduce their drinking, while the drinking in the remaining third remains largely unchanged (Heather & Tebbutt, 1989). There is good evidence that such treatment has a net economic benefit. Studies of insured people (Holder & Blose, 1986; Holder & Schachman, 1987) show that health care expenditure is substantially less in the three years after than in the three years before treatment. Furthermore, a randomized controlled trial (Walsh et al., 1991) has shown that intensive inpatient treatment for alcohol-dependent people has net economic benefits.

Nonetheless, the evidence from reviews of the research literature (e.g., Finney, Hahn & Moos, 1996; Heather & Tebbut, 1989; Mattick & Jarvis, 1993), from large-scale follow-up studies of treatment (e.g., Armor, Polich & Stambul, 1978), and from well-controlled studies comparing brief advice with more intensive treatment (e.g., Orford & Edwards, 1977) indicates that there is, at most, a small difference in outcome between inpatient treatment and simple assessment and advice to stop drinking. This indicates that residential or inpatient treatment is not routinely required for all people with moderate to severe alcohol-use disorders.

It has been suggested that those with the most severe disorders are the most likely to benefit from inpatient treatment. This 'matching hypothesis' implies that patients who are appropriately matched to treatment will do better than those who are not. This was viewed as the key to improved effectiveness of treatment for alcohol-use disorders. Project MATCH, a large, statistically powerful treatment trial, was designed to test the matching hypothesis (Project Match Research Group, 1997). Contrary to expectation, the study failed to find evidence of robust matching effects. Aside from the severity of the psychiatric illness, where small interaction effects were found, the effectiveness of treatment did not vary as a function of the patients' characteristics (Project Match Research Group, 1997).

The role of inpatient hospitalization for severely affected alcoholics remains controversial (Finney et al., 1996). Respite care with charitable and voluntary agencies, and welfare services are important for the indigent and homeless. Whether we should continue to provide residential treatment programs based on the Alcoholics Anonymous 12-step approach in hospitals is more contentious. There is no evidence for its effectiveness, but a case for some provision has been made on humanitarian grounds (Mattick & Jarvis, 1993). Enrolment in Alcoholics Anonymous groups is an important and inexpensive resource for individuals wishing to avoid relapse, and especially for the homeless and socially isolated whose drinking has cost them their family and friends (Mattick & Jarvis, 1993).

Alcohol detoxification

Detoxification is an important public health response to alcohol-related problems. It benefits the health of the drinker and the community by postponing the emergency presentation of more severe health problems, and it provides an opportunity for intervention and referral to other treatment services. It can often be accomplished under supervision in the home (e.g., Hayashida et al., 1989; Stockwell et al., 1991), although some severely dependent people and homeless alcohol-dependent people require inpatient treatment (Hall & Zador, 1997).

Dealing with comorbid mental disorders

Alcohol-use disorders complicated by other comorbid mental disorders have been recognized as having a poorer prognosis and being more difficult to treat (Drake, Bartels, Teague, Noordsby & Clark, 1993; McLelland, Luborsky, Woody, O'Brien & Druley, 1983) than those without comorbid disorders. Comorbid disorders are more likely to be chronic and disabling, and result in greater service utilization (Kessler, 1995b). Therefore, they cause considerable misery and suffering among those afflicted by them, and considerable social costs in terms of marital breakdown, social isolation, poor educational attainment, unemployment and chronic financial difficulties (Kessler,

1995*b*). The community surveys also indicate that cases with comorbid disorders are over-represented in clinical populations (Galbaud du Fort, Newman & Bland, 1993; Kessler, 1995*b*).

Accordingly, we need to improve our treatment of comorbid mental and substance-use disorders. Specialist mental health services need to better recognize and treat comorbid substance-use disorders among their clients. This is especially the case with anxiety and affective disorders, since a substantial minority of people with these disorders who seek treatment from the mental health services will have alcohol and other drug-use disorders (Hall & Farrell, 1997). Specialist drug and alcohol services also need to improve their recognition of the disorders that are most amenable to treatment, namely the anxiety and affective disorders. There are brief, valid and reliable screening tests that can detect anxiety and depressive disorders among alcohol- and drug-dependent people, yet they are rarely used (Mattick, Oliphant, Bell, & Hall, 1996).

Conclusions

Alcohol-use disorders are among the most prevalent disorders diagnosed in community surveys of mental disorders but very few people with these disorders seek or receive treatment. This does not necessarily indicate that these disorders are grossly undertreated, since many of the disorders identified in population surveys will remit without professional help. Public education about the risks of alcohol use may be the best way of preventing and ameliorating the public health impact of the prevalent, milder forms of alcohol disorders. Good advice on self-help strategies for quitting or cutting down may obviate the need for professional assistance. For those cases whose problems resist self-help, existing treatment systems need to provide more effective forms of treatment, more efficiently. Better triage would ensure a more rational use of scarce treatment resources.

References

Anthony, J.C., Folstein, M., Romanoski, A.J., Korff, M.R., von Nestadt, G.R., Chalal, R., Merchant, A., Brown, C.H., Shapiro, S., Kramer, M. & Gruenberg, E.M. (1985). Comparison of the lay Diagnostic Interview Schedule and a standardized psychiatric diagnosis. Experience in Eastern Baltimore. *Archives of General Psychiatry*, 42, 667–75.

Anthony, J.C., Warner, L.A. & Kessler, R.C. (1994). Comparative epidemiology of dependence on tobacco, alcohol, controlled substances and inhalants: basic findings from the National Comorbidity Survey. *Clinical and Experimental Pharmacology*, 2, 244–68.

Armor, D.J., Polich, J.M. & Stambul, H.B. (1978). *Alcoholism and Treatment.* New York: John Wiley and Sons.

Australian National Health and Medical Research Council (1992). *Is There a Safe Level of Daily Consumption of Alcohol for Men and Women? Recommendations Regarding Responsible Drinking Behaviour.* Canberra: Australian Government Publishing Service.

Bobadilla, J.L., Cowley, P., Musgrove, P. & Saxenian, H. (1994). Design, content and financing of an essential national package of health services. In C.J.L. Murray & A.D. Lopez (eds.), *Global Comparative Assessments in the Health Sector: Disease Burden, Expenditures and Intervention Packages.* Geneva: World Health Organization.

Chick, J., Lloyd, G. & Crombie, E. (1985). Counselling problem drinkers in medical wards: a controlled study. *British Medical Journal,* **290,** 965–7.

Drake, R.E., Bartels, S.J., Teague, G.R., Noordsby, D.L. & Clark, R.E. (1993). Treatment of substance abuse in severely mentally ill patients. *Journal of Nervous and Mental Disease,* **181,** 606–11.

Edwards, G., Anderson, P., Babor, T.F., Casswell, S., Ferrence, R., Giesbrecht, N., Godfrey, C., Holder, H.D., Lemmens, P., Mäkelä, K., Midanik, L.T., Norström, T., Österberg, E., Romelsjö, A., Room, R., Simpura, J. & Skog, O. (1994). *Alcohol Policy and the Public Good.* Oxford: Oxford University Press.

Elvy, G.A., Wells, J.E. & Baird, K.A. (1988). Attempted referral as intervention for problem drinking in the general hospital. *British Journal of Addiction,* **83,** 83–9.

Finney, J.W., Hahn, A.C. & Moos, R.H. (1996). The effectiveness of inpatient and outpatient treatment for alcohol abuse: the need to focus on mediators and moderators of setting effects. *Addiction,* **91,** 1773–96.

Flaherty, B., Homel, P. & Hall, W. (1991). Community attitudes towards public health policies on alcohol. *Australian Journal of Public Health,* **15,** 301–6.

Galbaud du Fort, G., Newman, S.C. & Bland, R.C. (1993). Psychiatric comorbidity and treatment seeking. Sources of selection bias in the study of clinical populations. *Journal of Nervous and Mental Disease,* **181,** 467–74.

Grant, B.F. (1997). Barriers to alcoholism treatment: reasons for not seeking treatment in a general population sample. *Journal of Studies in Alcohol,* **58,** 365–71.

Hall, W. (1996). Changes in the public perceptions of the health benefits of alcohol use, 1989 to1994. *Australian Journal of Public Health,* **20,** 93–5.

Hall, W. & Farrell, M. (1997). Comorbidity between substance use disorders and other mental disorders. *British Journal of Psychiatry,* **171,** 4–5.

Hall, W. & Zador, D. (1997). The alcohol withdrawal syndrome. *Lancet,* **349,** 1857–60.

Hayashida, M., Alterman, A.I., McLellan, A.T., O'Brien, C.P., Purtill, J.J., Volpicelli, J.R., Raphaelson, A.H. & Hall, C.P. (1989). Comparative effectiveness of inpatient and outpatient detoxification of patients with mild-to-moderate alcohol withdrawal syndrome. *New England Journal of Medicine,* **320,** 358–65.

Heather, N. & Tebbut, J. (eds.) (1989). *An Overview of the Effectiveness of Treatment for Drug and Alcohol Problems.* National Campaign Against Drug Abuse Monograph Series Number 11. Australian Government Publishing Service.

Helzer, J.E. & Canino, G.J. (1992). *Alcoholism in North America, Europe and Asia.* New York: Oxford University Press.

Helzer, J.E., Burnam, A. & McEvoy, L.T. (1991). Alcohol abuse and dependence. In L.N. Robins & D.A. Regier (eds.), *Psychiatric Disorders in America: The Epidemiologic Catchment Area Study*. New York: The Free Press.

Helzer, J.E., Robins, L.N., McEvoy, L.T. & Spitznagel, E. (1985). A comparison of clinical and diagnostic interview schedule diagnoses. *Archives of General Psychiatry*, **42**, 657–66.

Holder, H.D. & Blose, J.O. (1986). Alcoholism treatment and total health care utilization and costs: a four-year longitudinal analysis of federal employees. *Journal of the American Medical Association*, **256**, 1456–60.

Holder, H.D. & Schachman, R.H. (1987). Estimating health care savings associated with alcoholism treatment. *Alcoholism: Clinical and Experimental Research*, **11**, 66–73.

Homel, R. (1989). Crime on the roads: drinking and driving. In J. Vernon (ed.), *Alcohol and Crime*. Canberra: Australian Institute of Criminology.

Kessler, R.C. (1995*a*). The National Comorbidity Survey: preliminary results and future directions. *International Journal of Methods in Psychiatric Epidemiology*, **5**, 139–51.

Kessler, R.C. (1995*b*). The epidemiology of psychiatric comorbidity. In M. Tsuang, M. Tohen & G. Zahner (eds.), *Textbook of Psychiatric Epidemiology*. New York: John Wiley.

Kessler, R.C., Crum, R.M., Warner, L.A., Nelson, C.B., Schulenberg, J. & Anthony, J.C. (1997). Lifetime co-occurrence of DSM-III-R alcohol abuse and dependence with other psychiatric disorders in the National Comorbidity Survey. *Archives of General Psychiatry*, **54**, 313–21.

Kessler, R.C., McGonagh, K.A., Zhao, S., Nelson, C.B., Hughes, M., Eshleman, S. Wittchen, H.-U. & Kendler, K.S. (1994). Lifetime and 12-month prevalence of DSM-III-R psychiatric disorders in the United States. *Archives of General Psychiatry*, **51**, 8–19.

Kessler, R.C., Nelson, C.B., McGonagle, K.A., Edlund, M.J., Frank, R.G. & Leaf, P.J. (1996). The epidemiology of co-occurring addictive and mental disorders: Implications for prevention and service utilization. *American Journal of Orthopsychiatry*, **66**, 17–30.

Kristenson, H., Ohlin, H., Hulter-Nosslin, M.S., Trell, E. & Hood, B. (1983). Identification and intervention of heavy drinking in middle-aged men: results and follow-up of 24-60 months of long-term study with randomised controls. *Alcoholism*, **7**, 203–9.

Mattick, R.P. & Jarvis, T. (eds.) (1993). *An Outline for the Management of Alcohol Dependence and Abuse*. Quality Assurance Project. National Drug Strategy Monograph. Sydney: National Drug and Alcohol Research Centre.

Mattick, R.P., Oliphant, D.A., Bell, J. & Hall, W. (1996). Psychiatric morbidity in methadone maintenance patients: prevalence, effect on drug use and detection. In *Substance Use and Mental Illness: Proceedings of the Fourth Lingard Symposium*. Newcastle Hunter Institute of Mental Health.

McLelland, A.T., Luborsky, L., Woody, G.E., O'Brien, C.P. & Druley, K.A. (1983). Predicting response to alcohol and drug abuse treatments. *Archives of General Psychiatry*, **40**, 620–5.

Murray, C.J.L. & Lopez, A.D. (1997). Global mortality, disability and contribution of risk factors: global burden of disease study. *Lancet*, **349**, 1269–76.

Orford, J. & Edwards, G. (1977). *Alcoholism: A Comparison of Treatment and Advice, with a Study of the Influence of Marriage.* Oxford: Oxford University Press.

Project Match Research Group (1997). Matching alcoholism treatments to client heterogeneity: Project MATCH posttreatment drinking outcomes. *Journal of Studies on Alcohol*, **58**, 7–29.

Regier, D.A., Farmer, M.E., Rae, D.S., Locke, B.Z., Keith, S.J., Judd, L.L. & Goodwin, F.K. (1990). Comorbidity of mental disorders with alcohol and other drug abuse: results from the Epidemiologic Catchment Area (ECA) study. *Journal of the American Medical Association*, **264**, 2511–18.

Regier, D.A., Narrow, W.E., Rae, D.S., Manderscheid, R.W., Locke, B. & Goodwin, F.K. (1993). The de facto US mental and addictive disorders service system: Epidemiologic Catchment Area prospective study 1-year prevalence rates of disorders and services. *Archives of General Psychiatry*, **50**, 85–94.

Robins, L.N. (1985). Epidemiology: reflections on testing the validity of psychiatric interviews. *Archives of General Psychiatry*, **42**, 918–24.

Robins, L.N. & Regier, D.A. (eds.) (1991). *Psychiatric Disorders in America: The Epidemiologic Catchment Area Study.* New York: The Free Press.

Stockwell, T., Bolt, E., Milner, I., Russel, G., Bolderston, H. & Pugh, P. (1991). Home detoxification for problem drinkers: its safety and efficacy in comparison with inpatient care. *Alcohol and Alcoholism*, **26**, 645–50.

Wallace, P., Cutler, S. & Haines, A. (1988). Randomised controlled trial of general practitioner intervention in patients with excessive alcohol consumption. *British Medical Journal*, **297**, 663–8.

Walsh, D.C. & Hingson, R.W. (1987). Epidemiology and alcohol policy. In S. Levine & A.M. Lilienfeld (eds.), *Epidemiology and Public Policy.* New York: Tavistock.

Walsh, D.C., Hingson, R.W., Merrigan, D.M., Levenson, S., Cupples, A., Heeren, T., Coffman, G.A., Becker, C.A., Barker, T.A., Hamilton, S., McGuire, T.G. & Kelly, C.A. (1991). A randomized trial of treatment options for alcohol-abusing workers. *New England Journal of Medicine*, **325**, 775–82.

20

Putting epidemiology and public health in needs assessment: drug dependence and beyond

James C. Anthony

Summary

This chapter makes a case for intervention at early stages of drug involvement, well before a drug user meets diagnostic criteria for drug dependence. The case for early intervention rests upon a foundation of epidemiological evidence about the person-to-person spread of drug taking and the quite rapid transition into drug taking and the drug dependence process, once an opportunity to try a drug has occurred. In addition, co-occurring psychiatric and behavioral disturbances among many drug-dependent individuals complicate clinical decisions about diagnosis and therapeutics. This complexity warrants the earlier rather than later attention of skilled clinicians.

Introduction

Over the years, our agenda for international meetings on psychiatric epidemiology has ranged from the question 'what is a case?' to 'how many need treatment?' These questions appeal to basic concepts from the theory of sets. Consider one set, consisting of all inhabitants of a mental health catchment area or a church/civil parish, such as were surveyed for mental disorders in Norway more than 150 years ago (Holst, translated by Massey, 1852). The members of this set can be sorted into two mutually exclusive and exhaustive subsets: set members who qualify as active 'cases' and set members who qualify as 'noncases'. An alternative course of action is to sort the original set members into two subsets, one consisting of all people who need treatment and the other consisting of all those who do not.

Some observers will tell us that these two courses of action amount to one and the same thing. That is, cases need treatment services, whereas noncases do not. This represents a widely accepted conceptual model for needs assessment planning in the field of drug dependence. For instance, this conceptual model has guided the Center for Substance Abuse Treatment in its recent program for needs-based allocation of federal block grant funds in all 50 states and nine substate jurisdictions within the USA.

A strong argument for this conceptual model is that all societies face limits when allocating scarce mental health resources, especially the time and attention of medically trained psychiatrists. For example, at present, maintenance treatment with an opioid medicine (e.g., methadone, LAAM) is our most effective intervention for people dependent on heroin. Because these maintenance treatments can involve years of sustained opioid use, with potentially toxic consequences, there are few alternatives to diagnosis of heroin dependence and periodic monitoring by medically trained personnel. We simply would not want to start methadone or LAAM maintenance until the diagnosis of heroin dependence had been made, after confirmation of neuroadaptation, and with an assessment of opioid tolerance, so that proper dosing levels could be set. Otherwise, we might create a new iatrogenic case of dependence upon opioids where no dependence had existed before, not to mention an opioid overdosage casualty when tolerance is overestimated.

Life-threatening circumstances of this type argue in favor of placing the diagnosis of drug dependence in the hands of personnel with extensive medical training. These circumstances also favor close attention being paid to diagnostic criteria when determining who qualifies for intervention services and when assessing population-level needs for drug dependence services. We need more than just the numbers of heroin users in the population to estimate the number of heroin-dependent clients or patients who might be in need of an opioid maintenance program. Instead, we need epidemiological estimates of how many heroin users qualify as fully developed cases of heroin dependence. Alternatively, we need to rely upon an approximation method that makes use of past studies on the case/noncase ratio among heroin users. For example, in the 1990–92 United States National Comorbidity Survey, our research group estimated that there might be one case of heroin dependence among every three to five users of heroin. We found one case of cocaine dependence among every five to seven cocaine users, and one case of cannabis dependence among every nine to eleven cannabis users (Anthony, Warner & Kessler, 1994).

I intend to propose a different model for needs assessment planning in the case of drug dependence, opening the possibility that a similar model might apply to alcohol and tobacco dependence, and to certain other psychiatric conditions. My sense is that needs assessments must attend to the many individuals who suffer from mental and behavioral disturbances, but who do not meet current diagnostic criteria for case status. At least in the domain of drug dependence, I am confident that we will not have enough trained personnel if we make a serious effort to focus clinical attention solely on the subset of drug users with drug dependence who meet diagnostic criteria.

I recognize that it seems counter-intuitive and possibly illogical to say that:

(1) we must attend to the many drug users who do not meet drug dependence criteria, and (2) we will not have enough trained personnel if we focus attention on that relatively smaller subset of drug users who qualify as cases of drug dependence. The logic becomes apparent by considering *the spread of drugs from person to person*, and the apparently rapid transition from first trying a drug to become a regular drug user. Another reason for paying clinical attention to drug users involves differential diagnosis and the excess risk of co-occurring psychiatric disturbances among drug takers who do not meet diagnostic criteria.

Person-to-person spread of drugs

When describing the earliest stages of their involvement with drugs, most drug users say that it was not a 'friendly stranger' dealing drugs who first offered a chance to try them, but rather a friend or acquaintance already known to them. Based upon presently available evidence, this seems to be the case not only for controlled substances such as marijuana and cocaine (e.g., O'Donnell, Voss, Clayton, Slatin & Room, 1976), but also for tobacco and other 'legal' drugs (Biglan, 1995).

By studying what happens between the initial experience of drugs and the subsequent sharing of drugs with others, it is possible to see that much (though not all) of the person-to-person spread of drugs takes place within a year or so of starting drug use (Voss & Clayton, 1984). This apparent 'honeymoon' period between adopting a new innovation (e.g., smoking marijuana or injecting heroin) and introducing others to the experience can be seen both in quantitative time-oriented data from the study of epidemics and in observations from ethnographic studies.

During my own interviews with clinical cases who have been hospitalized for treatment of methamphetamine dependence after long-sustained 'ice-smoking', I have learned how the initial honeymoon period of sharing methamphetamine with friends and relatives changes over time. Initial 'altruistic' sharing and giving of drugs as gifts, with no money exchanging hands, is followed by concern that there might not be a big enough supply for one's own use. In fact, some ice-smokers have described how their first insight into their own dependence is the growing realization that they are no longer willing to share a hard-won drug supply with others, fearing that they might not have enough for their own use.

Hence, available evidence implies that person-to-person spread of a drug outbreak or epidemic occurs mainly during the relatively early stages of the 'honeymoon' period for each user. Drug-dependent people seem to be less likely to introduce others to drugs, perhaps because they are concerned about their own supply. A similar early 'honeymoon' period has been observed in relation to the diffusion of innovations generally (e.g., see Valente, 1995), but the truncation of this period by pharmacological tolerance and other features of neuroadaptation might well be unique to dependence on psychoactive drugs.

Rapid transitions from the initial drug opportunity to starting drug use

By asking people in epidemiological surveys how old they were when they were first offered a drug, and then how old they were when they first tried it, we can quantify the delay between these two discrete events. For example, studying data from a nationally representative sample of more than 20,000 US household residents age 12 years and older, our research group found that about 60% of males and 45% of females in this study population had already been offered cannabis. Of those who had been offered cannabis, about two-thirds went on to try it at least once. More than one-half of those who became cannabis users did so within one year of the initial opportunity (Van Etten, Neumark & Anthony, 1997). A similar picture emerges in research on hallucinogens, cocaine, and heroin: of those who become consumers, most do so within one year of the initial opportunity (Van Etten & Anthony, 1999).

To re-cap, epidemics of drug taking propagate by the combination of an early 'honeymoon' period of altruistic sharing among nondependent users, with a generally rapid transition into drug taking once a nonuser is given the opportunity to try it. In the population, the numbers of nondependent drug users tend to mount in an epidemic-like pattern, resembling person-to-person spread of infectious diseases that are most contagious early on. For every three to five new heroin users, we expect at least one to become dependent upon heroin, with the case/noncase ratios varying somewhat from drug to drug, place to place, and time to time, depending upon conditions such as local availability of drug supplies (Anthony et al., 1994).

These considerations demonstrate a weakness in needs assessment planning models that are based upon the idea that clinical attention should be focused on cases who meet diagnostic criteria and upon the more severe cases if there is a shortfall in services. At least for drug dependence, focusing on the most severely affected cases necessarily entails neglecting the pre-dependent drug users, who account for mounting numbers of new users (and eventually more new cases of drug dependence). This is the current situation in the USA and many other places in the world:

1. Clinical attention is focused on the most severely affected cases of drug dependence.
2. Preventive attention is focused on the nonusers.

3. Early intervention services do not pay enough attention to new drug users, who are most involved in the person-to-person spread of drugs.

Co-occurrence of other psychiatric disturbances among drug users

There is considerable appreciation for the evidence on co-occurrence of drug dependence with other psychiatric disturbances, especially antisocial personality disorder but also anxiety and affective syndromes (e.g., see Regier et al., 1990). A complementary body of evidence tends to support the theory that those who use drugs but are not dependent on them have a higher risk of suffering from these psychiatric disturbances. For example, even low-frequency users, i.e., not every day, of cocaine seem to be at a greater than average risk of developing panic attacks (Anthony, Tien & Petronis, 1989), and frequent cocaine users might be at a lower risk than infrequent users (Newcomb, Bentler & Fahy, 1987). In addition, cocaine users have a dramatically increased risk of attempting suicide and of developing incident obsessional thoughts or compulsive behaviors, even when they do not take cocaine daily and are not dependent on it (Anthony & Petronis, 1991; Crum & Anthony, 1993; Petronis, Samuels, Moscicki & Anthony, 1990).

Neurobiological theories about these psychiatric syndromes, pharmacological evidence, and epidemiological evidence tend to support the inference that at least some of the increased risk of psychiatric disturbances among drug users might be reduced if clinical attention were directed towards reducing or stopping drug involvement even before drug dependence has developed. Hence, primary prevention of an anxiety or affective syndrome would be possible if we paid more clinical attention to drug users who do not meet drug dependence criteria. Furthermore, the increased occurrence of these psychiatric syndromes among drug users might justify clinical attention being given to the difficult task of differential diagnosis in the presence of exposure to psychoactive drugs.

Conclusion

This chapter begins to make a case for abandoning a conceptual model that equates 'need' for clinical attention and mental health services with 'caseness' as defined by diagnostic criteria. The diagnostic criteria are just points of departure for a more public-health-oriented model of needs assessment.

By applying public health perspectives and drawing upon recently obtained epidemiological evidence, we can rediscover and strengthen the rationale for 'early intervention' directed towards individuals who do not classify as cases, according to the full diagnostic criteria. By fostering clinical attention to drug users who do not meet diagnostic criteria, we create opportunities for preventing and reducing the numbers of future drug-dependent individuals. The increased risk of other psychiatric syndromes among pre-dependent drug users reinforces the argument for earlier rather than later clinical attention being given to these drug users.

This chapter concentrates on drug dependence, but there are reasons why clinical attention should be given to early intervention in public-health-oriented mental health services generally. Of course, as with opioid maintenance therapies for heroin dependence, we must reserve the most scarce and expensive attention of medically trained specialists for when the probabilities of life-threatening circumstances and toxicity are greatest. Nonetheless, these specialists are also needed for differential diagnosis, prior to deciding the care and management of patients, whether they meet full diagnostic criteria or not. And one suspects that both preventive and early intervention services would benefit from the experience and perspectives of psychiatrists from time to time, as most service delivery is in the hands of mental health or prevention workers who do not have medical credentials.

References

Anthony, J.C. & Petronis, K.R. (1991). Epidemiologic evidence on suspected associations between cocaine use and psychiatric disturbances. *NIDA Research Monograph*, 110, 71–94.

Anthony, J.C., Tien, A.Y. & Petronis, K.R. (1989). Epidemiologic evidence on cocaine use and panic attacks. *American Journal of Epidemiology*, 129, 543–9.

Anthony, J.C., Warner, L.A. & Kessler, R.C. (1994).Comparative epidemiology of dependence on tobacco, alcohol, controlled substances, and inhalants: basic findings from the National Comorbidity Survey. *Experimental and Clinical Psychopharmacology*, 2, 244–68.

Biglan, A. (1995). *Changing cultural practices: a contextualist framework for intervention research*. Reno, NV: Context Press.

Crum, R.M. & Anthony, J.C. (1993). Cocaine use and other suspected risk factors for obsessive-compulsive disorder: a prospective study with data from the Epidemiologic Catchment Area surveys. *Drug Alcohol Dependence*, 31, 281–95.

Holst, H. (1852). On the statistics of the insane, blind, deaf and dumb, and lepers of Norway. [Translated by A.S.O. Massey.] *Royal Statistical Society of London Journal*, 15, 250–6.

Newcomb, M.D., Bentler, P.M. & Fahy, B.(1987). Cocaine use and psychopathology: associations among young adults. *International Journal of the Addictions*, 22, 1167–88.

O'Donnell, J.A., Voss, H.L., Clayton, R.R., Slatin, G.T. & Room, R.G. (1976). Young men and drugs – a nationwide survey. *NIDA Research Monograph (5): I-XIV*, 1–144.

Petronis, K.R., Samuels, J.F., Moscicki, E.K. & Anthony, J.C. (1990). An epidemiologic investigation of potential risk factors for suicide attempts. *Social Psychiatry and Psychiatric Epidemiology*, 25, 193–9.

Regier, D.A., Farmer, M.E., Rae, D.S., Locke, B.Z., Keith, S.J., Judd, L.L. & Goodwin, F.K. (1990). Comorbidity of mental disorders with alcohol and other drug abuse. Results from the Epidemiologic Catchment Area (ECA) Study. *Journal of the American Medical Association*, 264, 2511–18.

Valente, T.E. (1995). *Network Models of the Diffusion of Innovations*. Cresskill, NJ: Hampton Press.

Van Etten, M.L. & Anthony, J.C. (1999). Comparative epidemiology of initial drug opportunities and transitions to first use: marijuana, cocaine, hallucinogens, and heroin. *Drug and Alcohol Dependence*, 54, 117–25.

Van Etten, M.L., Neumark, Y.D. & Anthony, J.C. (1997). Initial opportunity to use marijuana and the transmission to first use: United States, 1979–1994. *Drug and Alcohol Dependence*, 49, 1–7.

Voss, H.L. & Clayton, R.R. (1984). 'Turning on' other persons to drugs. *International Journal of the Addictions*, 19, 633–52.

21

Why are somatoform disorders so poorly recognized and treated?

Ian Hickie, Rene G. Pols, Annette Koschera, and
Tracey Davenport

Introduction

Although somatic forms of distress are of considerable epidemiological
significance, impact adversely on health care utilization, and result in considerable economic, social, and personal burden, they occupy a rather minor
place in much clinical psychiatry research and teaching (Hickie, Scott &
Davenport, 1998). There is ongoing debate about appropriate nomenclature,
the role of genetic, psychosocial, cultural and neurobiological factors in
etiology, and the efficacy of specific pharmacological and behavioral interventions (Bass, 1990; Escobar, 1997; Hickie, Hadzi-Pavlovic & Ricci, 1997;
Hickie et al., 1998; Kleinman, 1987; Mayou, 1993; Pilowsky, 1991). Despite
these difficulties, the most striking feature of many of these disorders in
medical settings is their impact on patterns of health care utilization and
doctor–patient interactions (Clements, Sharpe, Simkin, Borrill & Hawton,
1997; Gureje, Simon, Üstün & Goldberg, 1997; Kroenke et al., 1997). As long
as doctors remain ill-informed about the significance of somatoform disorders and appropriate forms of intervention, they will continue to result in
high levels of disability. In this chapter the nature of somatization will be
explored, the epidemiology described, and research and clinical issues outlined.

Medical assessment processes

When patients present with common or unusual somatic symptoms, the
immediate response of general medical practitioners is to determine whether
such symptoms may be readily explained by a 'physical' pathology. While this
approach is understandable, it tends to be associated with a premature
narrowing of the medical practitioner's perspective. An overly medical approach, particularly towards nonspecific symptoms such as tiredness, headaches, sleep disturbance and aches and pains, tends to exclude the possibility
that psychological distress may give rise to these phenomena. The medical

practitioner is at particular risk of drawing this premature conclusion when physical symptoms form all or most of the patient's communication about their emotional distress. This interaction, with the resultant misunderstanding of the nature of the distress presented, is one factor that contributes significantly to the unmet need for psychiatric attention and treatment amongst this patient group. Continued miscommunication may set the stage for a management process which results in a chronic course and repeated inappropriate medical investigations and treatments. Additionally, the unwarranted focus on a medical explanation for the 'unexplained' symptoms results in further worry about illness for the patient and frustration in the medical practitioner, who feels responsibility for the symptoms, but cannot solve them.

Classification and epidemiology

The true prevalence of somatoform disorders in the community, and in broader medical practice, has been considerably debated (Escobar, Burnam, Karno, Forsythe & Golding, 1987a; Escobar, Manu, Lane, Matthews & Swartz, 1989a; Escobar, Rubio-Stipec, Canino & Karno, 1989b; Gureje et al., 1997; Hickie et al., 1996; Kroenke et al., 1997; Regier et al., 1988; Robins et al., 1984). If a very restrictive notion of somatization disorder is employed, as has characterized recent community-based studies in the USA (Regier et al., 1988; Robins et al., 1984), then such disorders are rare (prevalence of less than 1%). By contrast, once broader notions are used, prevalence estimates suggest that from 5% to 10% of the community (Gureje et al., 1997; Kroenke et al., 1997), and up to 25% of those consulting their general practitioner are likely to have such syndromes (Hickie et al., 1996). If one considers these disorders by looking at their effect on health care utilization and disability, then the much broader concepts are justified (Hickie et al., 1998). Currently, psychiatric epidemiology is in danger of ignoring such disorders. This is evidenced by their omission from the National Comorbidity Survey in the USA (Kessler et al., 1994) and the ongoing proposition that such disorders are better viewed simply as variants of anxiety and depressive disorders (Goldberg, 1996).

A further issue in the current classification of such disorders is whether they are best viewed as a single dimension of somatic distress (with somatoform disorders as the least severe and somatization disorders as the most extreme manifestation) or as a series of more symptom-specific domains (e.g., chronic fatigue, chronic pain, irritable bowel, chronic headache, fibromyalgia). Epidemiologically, it is simpler to record a single measure of distress; however, treatment approaches may do better to focus on reducing the specific symptom complexes. The dimensional approach is well described by Escobar et al. (1989*b*), with the development of the Somatization Symptom Index (SSI) which uses the nonspecific somatic symptoms from the Diagnostic Interview Schedule (DIS) (Escobar et al., 1989*a*). In response to the low prevalence of somatoform disorders in the Epidemiological Catchment Area (ECA) studies (0.6% average) (Regier et al., 1988; Robins et al., 1984), Escobar recalculated the prevalence using cut-off points of four unexplained somatic symptoms for men, and six for women, from eleven of the most prevalent unexplained symptoms (these are some of the original 37 somatic items in the DIS). Consequently, they reported a prevalence of 4.4% to 20% across the different ECA sites (Escobar, Swartz, Rubio-Stipec & Manu, 1991). They argued that the definition of somatoform disorder had ceased to be clinically useful and that the SSI may be a more useful indication of significant somatization.

This dimensional view of somatization also readily lends itself to cross-cultural and comorbidity studies (Escobar et al., 1991). The original symptoms used, however, emphasized many unusual pseudo-neurological, genito-urinary and gynecological experiences more typical of the rare somatization disorders encountered in consultation-liaison psychiatry. By contrast, the classic symptoms of general medical practice, notably tiredness, headaches, muscular aches and pains and gastro-intestinal disturbance, are relatively under-emphasized. Furthermore, the experience of somatic distress is not likely to be unidimensional (Kirmayer & Robbins, 1991), with certain patients (for genetic, biological or experiential reasons) preferentially experiencing somatic symptoms within certain body systems. That is, when the symptoms are more severe, the patients may simply experience more severe versions of a limited number of symptoms (e.g., chronic fatigue, chronic pain) rather than develop a wide range of the other pseudo-neurological, genito-urinary or gynecological symptoms predicted by the single dimensional model.

One syndrome or many?

Psychiatric classification systems have included the specific disorder of somatization, as well as other disorders of unknown prevalence and questionable validity. For example, DSM-IV (American Psychiatric Association, 1994), in addition to somatization disorder, lists undifferentiated somatoform disorder, conversion disorder, hypochondriasis, and body dysmorphic disorder. By contrast, ICD-10 includes the broader notion of neurasthenia (World Health Organization, 1992) to describe a prevalent and disabling disorder that has a large impact on health care utilization (Hickie et al., 1998). Other important categories from a clinical perspective, such as chronic pain disorder, have major impacts on health care utilization across a wide range of disciplines. This is also true of other specific disorders such as chronic fatigue syndrome (Fukuda et al., 1994), irritable bowel syndrome (Drossman, Richter & Talley, 1994), and fibromyalgia (Buchwald, 1996), which are largely ignored by clinical psychiatrists and placed under the care of specialist physicians and general practitioners.

An integrated model of somatoform disorders

As all sensory modalities register sensations continuously, normally we accommodate to these sensations and appropriately respond to, or ignore, these exteroceptive stimuli. Most people are much less sensitive to enteroceptive stimuli, which are autonomically mediated and do not normally register in our consciousness. We may notice these sensations when they are intense, or cause additional sensations that stimulate exteroceptive sensors. For example, a patient may report hearing the gurgling of the intestine or the noise of wind being passed.

Most often, these symptoms are noticed and interpreted as normal and no specific response follows. Even when the symptoms persist, individuals normally habituate to the stimulus and do not attach medical significance to its occurrence. Thus, to keep registering the sensory stimuli as abnormal depends on changes in the somatic stimulus, and/or its frequency, and requires the individual to consciously pay attention to it. The latter is more likely to occur if the individual associates such stimuli with illness (because of a prior experience or pre-existing beliefs), or if the sensation is linked with anxiety or an abnormal mood state. That is, cognitive and/or mood factors, by creating ongoing arousal, may interfere with the normal process of habituation. As such stimuli depend on ongoing attention for their significance, they may also be diminished by shifts of attention. For example, many people find that getting on with some work distracts them from a headache.

For somatic symptoms to be reported to a medical practitioner as abnormal there needs to be a physical stimulus, cognitive attention, arousal and a consequent failure of the normal habituation process. That is, the patient has to interpret the somatic stimuli as significant and abnormal, and attribute them to a possible underlying illness. The conclusion of abnormality and/or underlying pathology by the patient then generates further anxiety which can only be relieved (or exacerbated) by consulting an appropriate health practitioner. In the general population, a wide variety of nonspecific somatic sensations (pain, tiredness, headaches) are experienced, but only a restricted group of patients report these to medical practitioners (Crook, Redeout & Browne, 1984; Simon & VonKorff, 1991). Thus, it is often more important to consider the cognitive, affective, developmental, cultural, and neurobiologi-

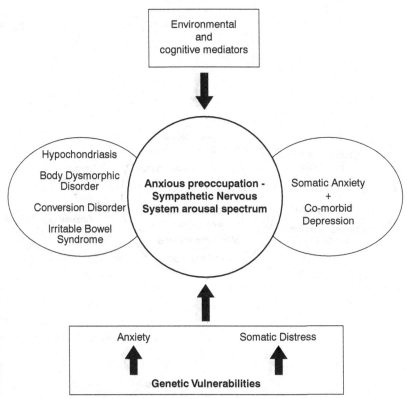

Figure 21.1 Somatic and psychological presentation of anxious preoccupation – sympathetic nervous system arousal.

cal characteristics of those patients, rather than to seek exotic explanations for the symptoms themselves.

From an etiological perspective, therefore, a wide range of factors may serve as risk factors for these disorders (see Figures 21.1 and 21.2). Neurobiological factors, which are themselves likely to be genetically determined (Bohman, Cloninger, von Knorring & Sigvardsson, 1984; Hickie, Bennett, Lloyd, Health & Martin, 1999*a*; Hickie, Kirk & Martin, 1999*b*), may well determine the level of symptoms generated, their intensity, and their specific form. Such inherited factors may consist of either a general liability to somatic distress or more discrete sets of vulnerabilities. For example, different genetic and neurobiological factors may predispose to bowel-related symptoms rather than headache and chronic fatigue. The vulnerability to somatic distress is not likely to occur simply secondarily to a general liability to the common forms of anxiety and depression (Hickie et al., 1999*a*, *b*). It is

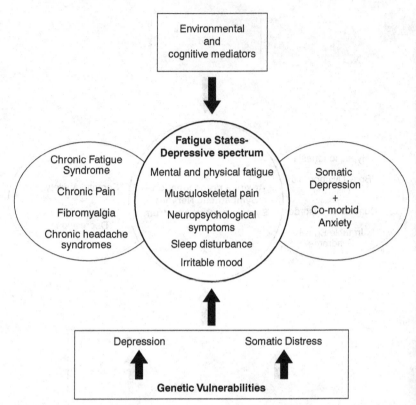

Figure 21.2 Somatic and psychological presentation of fatigue states – depressive spectrum.

likely, however, that many patients who present for medical attention do share both sets of vulnerabilities, leading to a continuous interaction between affective, cognitive and somatic factors, with escalation of the somatic and psychological forms of distress experienced by the patient over their lifetime (Figures 21.1 and 21.2).

Clinically, it may be useful to consider these patients' problems as broadly falling into two categories. First, an anxious disposition gives rise to many disorders, ranging from the common anxiety disorders to those somatoform disorders characterized by anxious preoccupation about body parts and/or function (primary hypochondriasis, body dysmorphic disorder, conversion disorder, irritable bowel syndrome; see Figure 21.1). Second, fatigue and depressive states may give rise to depressive disorders that range from those with strong somatic features to chronic fatigue, chronic pain and headache-type syndromes (Figure 21.2). Interestingly, longitudinal studies show that somatic distress persists for longer than psychological distress (Merikangas & Angst, 1994).

Somatic symptoms as a communication of emotional distress

Within primary care and general medical settings it is more common for patients to present their symptoms of distress as a mixture of anxiety, depression and vague somatic complaints than to present any pure form alone (Goldberg & Bridges, 1988; Hickie et al., 1996; Katon & Russo, 1992; Wessely, Chalder, Hirsch, Wallace & Wright, 1996). When specific somatic complaints such as fatigue are systematically evaluated, it is clear that psychological syndromes such as anxiety and depression are major risk factors (Hickie et al., 1996; Wessely et al., 1996). Depressive disorders are particularly associated with symptoms of fatigue and pain, while anxiety disorders are clearly associated with a wide range of cardiovascular and gut symptoms. In the World Health Organization's multicenter study of psychological problems in primary health care, one-third of the sample had clear-cut and probable psychological disorders. Of these psychological disorders, over half presented with mixed somatic and psychological features, 35% presented with physical symptoms alone and only 16% presented with psychological symptoms alone (Üstün & Sartorius, 1995).

It is most likely, therefore, that nonspecific somatic symptoms in patients consulting general practitioners indicate underlying distress. Often too much emphasis is given to the somatic symptoms reported by the individual, both in everyday life and when dealing with the medical profession. Unfortunately, this may convince the doctor and the patient that a physical illness is causing the symptoms rather than a primary psychological disorder such as anxiety or depression.

Chronic pain

Primary psychogenic pain disorder is relatively rare. In a survey of 158 patients, who were assessed by a multidisciplinary team in a pain management unit over a year, only three patients did not have organic pathology related to their pain. Only five patients did not have a psychiatric disorder, and the majority had a pain disorder with psychogenic features. The response to pain is embedded into the spinal reflex arc to protect bodily integrity. The avoidance response to pain often results in complex and even bizarre pain behaviors which are relatively common in pain-unit patients.

Not only does pain involve avoidance, it also demands attention. This makes the person more vigilant and sensitive to pain, and they develop further maneuvers to avoid it. This pattern of operant learning can readily increase the somatic symptoms. The person becomes more afraid of pain (secondary morbidity), and they may adopt an abnormal posture and misuse medications. The result is that their experience of pain worsens.

Somatization as an economic issue

In a South Australian study of patients with somatization, the estimated cost to the health services was at least Aus$11,000 to Aus$31,000 per annum per patient (according to data identified from hospital admission records – Battersby & Gruzin, 1996). In the way that health services are currently structured, patients with significant somatization will have a substantial number of investigations and/or hospital stays. A number of controlled studies show that a containment approach can be extremely effective in reducing hospitalization by 70% and costs by 50%, but with increased involvement of the general practitioner (Smith, Rost & Kashner, 1995). Similarly, cognitive-behavioral treatment, both individually (Warwick, Clark, Cobb & Salkovskis, 1996) and in groups, is extremely effective.

On the basis of this research, this approach is being trialled for the intervention group ($n = 310$) in the South Australian HealthPlus randomly controlled trial ($n = 620$ subjects total) of coordinated care for the broad spectrum of somatization seen in anxiety, pain, and somatoform disorders. We are interested to see whether such efficacy can be repeated in a field trial. At present, there are no accurate data on the prevalence and incidence of these symptoms, syndromes and disorders, and the cost implications cannot be accurately estimated without further surveys of the community, general practice, and hospitals.

Disability due to neurasthenia

Community-based and general practice studies in Australia make it clear that neurasthenia and other prolonged fatigue syndromes are major sources of disability (Table 21.1). Interestingly, such disability is greater than that attributed to other psychological disorders such as depression and that due to other physical disorders. Given the current interest in the disability caused by psychological conditions, these studies indicate the importance of including specific somatic syndromes, particularly the prevalent ones (such as chronic fatigue and chronic pain), in future epidemiological studies that try to measure the burden of psychological disorders in the community (Escobar et al., 1987a, b; 1989b).

Table 21.1. Comparison of disability levels for patients with neurasthenia and other psychological disorders

Community sample ($n = 1364$)	Neurasthenia[a] ($n = 53^c$)	Major depression[b] ($n = 187^c$)	Any physical disorder ($n = 696^c$)
Disability	Mean (SD)	Mean (SD)	Mean (SD)
BDQ[d] – total	9.4 (5.0)	7.2 (6.0)	6.5 (5.8)
days disabled	9.1 (10.9)	6.1 (9.7)	4.3 (8.5)
days in bed	2.0 (5.5)	1.0 (2.4)	1.1 (3.7)
SF12[e] – physical	41.6 (10.6)	45.5 (12.6)	43.3 (12.7)
mental	38.3 (11.9)	40.0 (13.0)	48.9 (10.8)

Primary care sample ($n = 471$)	Prolonged fatigue syndromes[f] (PFS only) ($n = 50$)	Psychological distress[g] (only) ($n = 44$)	PFS and psychological distress ($n = 92$)
Disability	mean (SD)	mean (SD)	mean (SD)
BDQ[d] – total	8.4 (5.3)	4.9 (4.3)	10.1 (6.0)
days disabled	4.8 (8.1)	2.5 (5.0)	6.9 (8.7)
days in bed	1.0 (3.2)	1.0 (2.1)	2.7 (5.9)

Source: Andrews, Sanderson & Beard (1998).
[a] Neurasthenia (ICD-10): duration $\geq$ 3 months.
[b] Major depression (ICD-10): duration $\geq$ 2 weeks.
[c] As co-morbidity is not accounted for, respondents may appear in more than one column in the table. Consequently, there is no statistical comparison between the groups.
[d] BDQ, Brief Disability Questionnaire (VonKorff, Üstün, & Ormel, 1996).
[e] SF-12: Short Form 12 of the Medical Outcomes Study (with lower scores indicating greater disablement – Ware, Kosinski, & Keller, 1996).
[f] Prolonged Fatigue Syndromes (PFS): fatigue cases (Duration $\geq$ 2 weeks). Total = 30.1%.
[g] Psychological distress: [General Health Questionnaire caseness from SPHERE]. Total = 28.8%.

Treatment approaches for somatoform disorders

The usual clinical approach to somatic symptoms that accompany other major disorders is to treat the other disorder first. For example, with major depression and profound tiredness or chronic pain, traditionally the emphasis is on pharmacological treatment of the depression. When there is panic disorder and significant focusing on cardiovascular symptoms, pharmacological or behavioral treatments are used to prevent panic attacks. In both these situations, however, it is common for the somatic symptoms to persist after the symptoms of depression or anxiety have been reduced or resolved, and for the patient to remain disabled.

When the specific somatic symptoms or resultant disability do persist then specific behavioral treatment should be offered. A range of specific cognitive-behavioral approaches have been developed for chronic pain (Pilowsky, Spence, Rounsefell, Forsten & Soda, 1995), chronic fatigue (Sharpe, Chalder, Palmer & Wessely, 1997), and hypochondriasis (Warwick et al., 1996). The different approaches share common elements aimed at reducing autonomic arousal, increasing physical and social activity (encouraging the person to put a time limit on the activity rather than stopping because it has made their symptoms worse), treating comorbid mood symptoms, correcting misconceived ideas about the illness, and emphasizing a reduction in disability instead of searching for elusive 'curative' treatments. More contentious, however, is which set of specific approaches to include within each package. Clearly for chronic pain disorder the role of analgesic therapies needs to be closely supervised. For fibromyalgia and chronic fatigue it is important to consider any pharmacotherapy that may improve sleep and relieve pain (e.g., low-dose tricyclic antidepressants, nefazodone, and nonsteroidal anti-inflammatory agents). Agents that may affect subjective energy directly, such as moclobemide, are worthy of consideration in chronic fatigue. For irritable bowel syndrome there are a range of agents that alter gut motility (Talley, 1995). Patients are particularly unlikely to comply with cognitive-behavioral approaches if they feel that such strategies will just result in their symptoms worsening, unless the physician also provides relevant symptom relief.

A framework for future research

The large overlap between anxiety and depressive disorders and somatic syndromes suggests that etiological research needs to clarify which risk factors are shared and which are not. There is a clear need to conduct multimodal studies evaluating the genetic, neurobiological, cognitive, social, and cultural factors. Our recent longitudinal design and twin studies of fatigue syndromes (Hickie et al., 1999a, b) highlight these issues. Such research may then determine useful intervention strategies. For example, one such common factor may be a disturbance of attention, which is seen across all these disorders. In this model, anxiety disorders could be thought of as disorders of exteroception; posttraumatic stress disorder and pain disorders as both exteroception and enteroception; and somatoform disorders as disorders of excessive attention to enteroceptive stimuli. The cognitive-behavioral approaches aim ultimately to teach the patients to reduce the attention they pay to these stimuli in order to restore normal levels of arousal.

An enterprising alternative to concentrating on symptoms is to look at use of the health care system. In this approach, patients who use the health care system to excess, regardless of their exact diagnosis, would be taught specific behavioral strategies designed to reduce their disability and health care costs. Since many factors are shared (autonomic arousal, failure to habituate to common physical symptoms, illness fears, preoccupation with seeking medical attention, decreased physical and social activity), the emphasis could well be on providing accurately targeted strategies that can be implemented across a wide range of general medical services.

Meeting the need for treatment of somatoform disorders

Given the high prevalence of somatoform disorders, the resultant disability and their impact on health care costs, there is clearly a need to develop educational and intervention strategies that address this large area of unmet need. A medical education agenda needs to:

1. Change medical undergraduate degrees so that more time and emphasis are given to identifying and treating these common and disabling forms of illness.
2. Shift the medical training objectives at the undergraduate, initial postgraduate and specialist training levels, from emphasizing the endless search for rare physical pathologies to appreciating the role of psychological factors in the presentation of common nonspecific somatic symptoms, such as tiredness, headaches, and musculoskeletal aches and pains.
3. Develop specific objectives for family practice trainees in the efficient identification and treatment of these disorders within general practice and other general medical settings.
4. Provide specific training programs for family practice trainees in the behavioral management of the common somatoform disorders (i.e., chronic fatigue, chronic pain, chronic headache, and irritable bowel syndromes).

Correspondingly, a public health and services agenda needs to:

1. Recognize the importance of such disorders independent of the common anxiety and depressive disorders.
2. Give practical support, and financial and professional incentives to current practitioners so that they can become more skilled at treating these disorders.
3. Provide specific materials (e.g., case-identification instruments (Escobar et al., 1989b), educational booklets (World Health Organization, 1997), and treatment manuals for use in the primary care sector.

4. Develop incentives for cost-containment through long-term management of such patients in the primary care sector, thus minimizing specialist referral and complex and intrusive medical investigations.
5. Evaluate innovative treatment models in primary care that emphasize reduction in disability, cost-containment and long-term continuous care.

Currently, the initiatives for service changes in this area are being driven largely by cost-containment models. Clearly, we need to build on such initiatives and modify such service developments so that specific behavioral and relevant pharmacological treatments are also provided. To date, specialist psychiatry has had little impact on these disorders outside the teaching hospital and specialist referral center environments. The challenge now lies in taking the theoretical initiatives and clinical practices developed within such settings out into the general medical and family practice environments, where they can be provided to much broader groups of patients.

References

American Psychiatric Association (1994). *Diagnostic and Statistical Manual of Mental Disorders* (4th edition). Washington, D. C.: American Psychiatric Association.
Andrews, G., Sanderson, K. & Beard, J. (1998). Burden of disease: methods of calculating disability from mental disorder. *British Journal of Psychiatry*, 173, 123–31.
Bass, C. (ed.) (1990). *Somatisation: Physical Symptoms and Psychological Illness.* Oxford: Blackwell Scientific Publications.
Battersby, M. & Gruzin, S. (1996). *SA HealthPlus Unit of the South Australian Health Commission.* Final Report to the Ambulatory Care Reform Program. Adelaide: South Australian Health Commission.
Bohman, M., Cloninger, C.R., von Knorring, A.L. & Sigvardsson, S. (1984). An adoption study of somatoform disorders. III. Cross-fostering analysis and genetic relationship to alcoholism and criminality. *Archives of General Psychiatry*, 41, 872–8.
Buchwald, D. (1996). Fibromyalgia and chronic fatigue syndrome: similarities and differences. *Rheumatic Disease Clinics of North America*, 22, 219–43.
Clements, A., Sharpe, M., Simkin, S., Borrill, J. & Hawton, K. (1997). Chronic fatigue syndrome: a qualitative investigation of patients' beliefs about the illness. *Journal of Psychosomatic Research*, 42, 615–24.
Crook, J., Rideout, E. & Browne, G. (1984). The prevalence of pain complaints in a general population. *Pain*, 18, 299–314.
Drossman, D.A., Richter, J.E. & Talley, N.J. (eds.) (1994). *The Functional Gastrointestinal Disorders.* Boston, MA: Little Brown.
Escobar, J.I. (1997). Developing practical indexes of somatization for use in primary care. *Journal of Psychosomatic Research*, 42, 323–8.

Escobar, J.I., Burnam, M.A., Karno, M., Forsythe, A. & Golding, J.M. (1987a). Somatization in the community. *Archives of General Psychiatry*, **44**, 713–18.

Escobar, J.I., Golding, J.L., Hough, R.L., Karno, M., Burnam, M.A. & Wells, K.B. (1987b). Somatization in the community: relationship to disability and use of services. *American Journal of Public Health*, **77**, 837–40.

Escobar, J.I., Manu, P., Lane, T., Matthews, D. & Swartz, M. (1989a). Medically unexplained physical symptoms, somatization disorder and abridged somatization: studies with the DIS. *Psychiatric Developments*, **7**, 235–45.

Escobar, J.I., Rubio-Stipec, M., Canino, G. & Karno, M. (1989b). Somatic Symptom Index (SSI): a new and abridged somatization construct: prevalence and epidemiological correlates in two large community samples. *Journal of Nervous and Mental Disease*, **177**, 140–6.

Escobar, J.I., Swartz, M., Rubio-Stipec, M. & Manu, P. (1991). Medically unexplained symptoms: distribution, risk factors, and comorbidity. In L.J. Kirmayer & J.M. Robbins (eds.), *Current Concepts of Somatization: Research and Clinical Perspectives*. Washington, D.C.: American Psychiatric Press.

Fukuda, K., Straus, S.E., Hickie, I., Sharpe, M.C., Dobbins, J.G., Komaroff, A. & the International Chronic Fatigue Syndrome Study Group (1994). The chronic fatigue syndrome: a comprehensive approach to its definition and study. *Annals of Internal Medicine*, **121**, 953–9.

Goldberg, D. (1996). A dimensional model for common mental disorders. *British Journal of Psychiatry*, **168** [Suppl. 30], 44–9.

Goldberg, D.P. & Bridges, K. (1988). Somatic presentations of psychiatric illness in primary care setting. *Journal of Psychosomatic Research*, **32**, 137–44.

Gureje, O., Simon, G.E., Üstün, T.B. & Goldberg, D.P. (1997). Somatization in cross-cultural perspective: a World Health Organization study in primary care. *American Journal of Psychiatry*, **154**, 989–95.

Hickie, I., Bennett, B., Lloyd, A., Heath, A. & Martin, N. (1999a). Complex genetic and environmental relationships between psychological distress, fatigue and immune functioning: a twin study. *Psychological Medicine*, **29**, 269–77.

Hickie, I., Hadzi-Pavlovic, D. & Ricci, C. (1997). Reviving the diagnosis of neurasthenia. *Psychological Medicine*, **27**, 989–94.

Hickie, I., Hooker, A., Hadzi-Pavlovic, D., Bennett, B., Wilson, A. & Lloyd, A. (1996). Fatigue in selected primary care settings: sociodemographic and psychiatric correlates. *Medical Journal of Australia*, **164**, 585–8.

Hickie, I., Kirk, K. & Martin, N. (1999b). Unique genetic and environmental determinants of prolonged fatigue: a twin study. *Psychological Medicine*, **29**, 259–68.

Hickie, I.B., Scott, E.M. & Davenport, T.A. (1998). Somatic distress: Developing more integrated concepts. *Current Opinion in Psychiatry*, **11**, 153–8.

Katon, W. & Russo, J. (1992). Chronic fatigue syndrome criteria: a critique of the requirements for multiple physical complaints. *Archives of Internal Medicine*, **152**, 1604–9.

Kessler, R.C., McGonagle, K.A., Zhao, S., Nelson, C.B., Hughes, M., Eshleman, S., Wittchen, H. & Kendler, KS. (1994). Lifetime and 12-month prevalence of DSM-III-R psychiatric disorders in the United States: Results from the National Comorbidity Survey. *Archives of General Psychiatry*, **51**, 8–19.

Kirmayer, L.J. & Robbins, J.M. (1991). Functional somatic syndromes. In L.J. Kirmayer & J.M. Robbins (eds.), *Current Concepts of Somatization: Research and Clinical Perspectives*. Washington, D.C.: American Psychiatric Press.

Kleinman, A. (1987). Anthropology and psychiatry: the role of culture in cross-cultural research on illness. *British Journal of Psychiatry*, 151, 447–54.

Kroenke, K., Spitzer, R.L., deGruy, F.V., Hahn, S.R., Linzer, M., Williams, J.B.W., Brody, D. & Davies, M. (1997). Multisomatoform disorder: an alternative to undifferentiated somatoform disorder for the somatizing patient in primary care. *Archives of General Psychiatry*, 54, 352–8.

Mayou, R. (1993). Somatization. *Psychotherapy and Psychosomatics*, 59, 69–83.

Merikangas, K. & Angst, J. (1994). Neurasthenia in a longitudinal cohort study of young adults. *Psychological Medicine*, 24, 1013–24.

Pilowsky, I. (1991). Somatic symptoms and other related disorders. *Current Opinion in Psychiatry*, 4, 220–4.

Pilowsky, I., Spence, N., Rounsefell, B., Forsten, C. & Soda, J. (1995). Out-patient cognitive-behavioural therapy with amitriptyline for chronic non-malignant pain: a comparative study with 6-month follow-up. *Pain*, 60, 49–54.

Regier, D.A., Boyd, J.H., Burke, J.D., Rae, D.S., Myers, J.K., Kramer, M., Robins, L.N., George, L.K., Karno, M. & Locke, B.Z. (1988). One-month prevalence of mental disorders in the United States: based on five epidemiologic catchment area sites. *Archives of General Psychiatry*, 45, 977–86.

Robins, L.N., Helzer, J.E., Weissman, M.M., Orvaschel, H., Gruenberg, E., Burke, J.D. Jr. & Regier, D.A. (1984). Lifetime prevalence of specific psychiatric disorders in three sites. *Archives of General Psychiatry*, 41, 949–58.

Sharpe, M., Chalder, T., Palmer, I. & Wessely, S. (1997). Chronic fatigue syndrome. a practical guide to assessment and management. *General Hospital Psychiatry*, 19, 185–99.

Simon, G.E. & VonKorff, M. (1991). Somatization and psychiatric disorder in the NIMH Epidemiologic Catchment Area study. *American Journal of Psychiatry*, 148, 1494–500.

Smith, G.R., Rost, K. & Kashner, M. (1995). A trial of the effect of a standardised psychiatric consultation on health outcomes and costs in somatizing patients. *Archives of General Psychiatry*, 52, 238–43.

Talley, N.J. (1995). Review article: functional dyspepsia – should treatment be targeted on disturbed physiology? *Alimentary Pharmacology and Therapeutics*, 9, 107–15.

Üstün, T.B. & Sartorius, N. (eds.) (1995). *Mental Illness in General Health Care: An International Study*. Chichester: John Wiley & Sons Ltd.

VonKorff, M., Üstün, T.B. & Ormel, J. (1996). Self-report disability in an international primary care study of psychological illness. *Journal of Clinical Epidemiology*, 49, 297–303.

Ware, J.E., Kosinski, M. & Keller, S.D. (1996). A 12-item short-form health survey: construction of scales and preliminary tests of reliability and validity. *Medical Care*, 34, 220–33.

Warwick, H.M.C., Clark, D.M., Cobb, A.M. & Salkovskis, P.M. (1996). A controlled trial of cognitive-behavioural treatment of hypochondriasis. *British Journal of*

Psychiatry, **169**, 189–95.

Wessely, S., Chalder, T., Hirsch, S., Wallace, P. & Wright, D. (1996). Psychological symptoms, somatic symptoms, and psychiatric disorder in chronic fatigue and chronic fatigue syndrome: a prospective study in the primary care setting. *American Journal of Psychiatry*, **153**, 1050–9.

World Health Organization (1992). *The Tenth Revision of the International Classification of Diseases and Related Health Problems* (ICD-10). Geneva: World Health Organization.

World Health Organization. (1997). *Mental Disorders Educational Package*. Geneva: World Health Organization.

Part IV

Unmet need: specific issues

Introduction

Scott Henderson

The unmet needs of specific groups

Some groups in the human population have greater unmet needs than others – and some lesser. In this penultimate section of the book, our contributors look at this issue. Sawyer and Patton (Chapter 22), then Cottler et al. (Chapter 23) consider the situation for children and young people. Hunter (Chapter 24) spells out the social disaster caused by European contact for indigenous or Aboriginal Australians after some 60,000 years presence in Australia. Then Patel (Chapter 25) reminds us of the situation for the majority of people today – those living in low-income countries. We could continue to list specific groups. Our book would then have covered the elderly, women, migrants, refugees, the poor, those in war zones, those afflicted by natural disasters, and many more who are disadvantaged and have poor health. Since the list is endless, we urge the reader to consider the deeper principles that can be discerned in the contributions by Sawyer and Patton, Cottler et al., Hunter, and by Patel. Along with the preceding chapters, these help to set the agenda for answering that awesome question, 'what is to be done?'

Sawyer and Patton see three complementary tasks: how to identify the needs of children; what treatments are available and effective; and, lastly, what can be done to *prevent* childhood mental disorders. Readers should remember that some remarkable claims are currently being made about the effect of group interventions for young people in schools (e.g., Kellam & Anthony, 1998; Kellam, Mayer, Rebok, & Hawkins, 1998). Cottler et al. lucidly recount how children's need can be measured. This is difficult to do with precision and validity, because the child, parent, and teacher may give different information about symptoms and behavior, and their conse-quences.

Hunter says, quite starkly, that the, '*Aborigines and Torres Strait Islanders are the most disadvantaged distinct population in Australia*' (our italics). Of all humankind, he would know. He worked in the tropical North of Australia for many years, visiting his vastly dispersed parish in a four-wheel drive vehicle and coming to be deservedly accepted by the black communities of Cape

York. Hunter directs us to their two imperative needs, neither of which is met: social justice and services.

Patel's chapter on how to meet needs in low-income countries is a combined challenge and appeal. He says that two kinds of psychiatric research have emerged, universalism and cultural relativism; and that these are polar opposites. Be that as it may, he goes on to say that, 'neither pole of research has made any significant impact on the understanding of mental disorders by general health workers in low-income countries because of the uneven emphasis placed on either biology or culture.' A remedy, Patel argues, is to use the model of Health Systems Research. He illustrates the successful application of this in his own contribution to a major project in Zimbabwe.

Another special issue is need caused by disablement. This is dealt with by Pull et al. (Chapter 26), who describe their careful study of a small sample of patients and mental health professionals in Luxembourg. The whole matter of measuring need has been perceptively examined by Meadows et al. (Chapter 27). They bring the reader back to the central issue of what need is, and how it can be measured in a way that planners could use to make changes.

Mental health literacy

Do most people know when they are mentally unwell? Do they know when someone close to them is unwell? And do they know what help they should get from professionals? These are not trivial questions for this book. An understanding of common mental disorders is a necessary, though not sufficient, preliminary to help-seeking. Notice that the above questions are from the individual's viewpoint, not the professional's, yet much of the thinking about psychiatric services is based on the provider's rather than the consumer's viewpoint. So Jorm and his colleagues (Chapter 28) are right to point to the reciprocal but entirely overlooked other half of Goldberg and Huxley's 'pathways to care' (Goldberg & Huxley, 1980). Their chapter is a synthesis of entirely independent studies of knowledge and beliefs about mental disorders conducted in three countries.

The notion of mental health literacy points to a tough agenda: improving the public's level of knowledge about the common mental disorders; and the goodness of fit between the treatments *they* think appropriate and the treatments we professionals currently recommend – sometimes on the basis of scientific evidence. So there is much education to be achieved in the coming century, and it may take all of it to significantly improve people's knowledge of, and attitudes to, mental disorders. If patients and their doctors have different ideas about what would help these disorders, the outcomes – a now highly valued construct – will be worse than they need be. And for planners and policy makers, Jorm et al. (Chapter 28) say that, 'Any attempt at top-down planning of the distribution of mental health services will run into difficulties if it conflicts with the public's beliefs about treatment.'

The automation of psychiatry?

In his personal overview in Part V, Copeland suggests how we can distribute our resources to wherever they are needed. His Aunt Sally is presented as a provocative idea to elicit our interest and criticism: the automation of clinical psychiatry wherever this may be practicable, using computers. Such an idea may seem far-fetched, yet it is wholly in line with global technical developments. We think it is more likely to be a prediction than a suggestion.

References

Goldberg, D.P. & Huxley, P. (1980). *Mental Illness in the Community: the Pathway to Psychiatric Care.* London: Tavistock Publications.

Kellam, S. & Anthony, J. (1998). Targeting early antecedents to prevent tobacco smoking: findings from an epidemiologically based randomized field trial. *American Journal of Public Health*, **88**, 1490–5.

Kellam, S.G., Mayer, L.S., Rebok, G.W. & Hawkins, W.E. (1998). The effects of improving achievement on aggressive behavior and of improving aggressive behavior on achievement through two prevention interventions: an investigation of etiological roles. In B. Dohrenwend (ed.), *Adversity, Stress, and Psychopathology.* Washington, D.C.: American Psychiatric Press.

22

Unmet need in mental health service delivery: children and adolescents

Michael Sawyer and George Patton

Mental disorders impose a substantial burden of illness and disability on children and adolescents. Prevalence rates of these disorders are high and the prognoses of many of the disorders are poor (Robins, 1966). There is also growing evidence of continuities between childhood and adult disorders (Ferdinand & Verhulst, 1995; Harrington, 1992; Robins, 1966). Currently, only a small proportion of the large number of children with mental disorders receive treatment, in part because of the limited number of trained clinicians available to provide help (Burns, 1996; Offord et al., 1987; Sawyer, Sarris, Baghurst, Cornish & Kalucy, 1990). As a result, in the medium term it is unlikely that treatment programs based in secondary or tertiary services will be able to provide effective help for the majority of children with mental disorders. A range of approaches is needed to identify children with unmet need and to provide effective help. This chapter focuses on three issues relevant to the unmet need for treatment of children and adolescents: (1) identification of the needs of children with mental disorders; (2) treatment of children's mental disorders; and (3) prevention of children's mental disorders. The chapter does not address a number of issues such as exploitative work practices, sexual exploitation, or the impact of wars and natural disasters on children, all of which can have a major adverse influence on children's mental health and are of increasing concern, particularly for children living in third world countries (Desjarlais, Eisenberg, Good & Kleinman, 1995).

Key features of childhood mental disorders

Responses to the unmet needs of children and adolescents with mental disorders must take into account a number of key features of childhood disorders if they are to successfully address this issue (for brevity, the term children will be employed in this chapter to refer to children and adolescents). First, younger children rarely make their own appointments to attend mental health services. Instead, they depend on parents or teachers for referral to these services. As a result, parents' and teachers' knowledge of mental health services and their attitudes towards these services can have a significant impact on patterns of mental health service utilization. There is also extensive evidence of poor agreement between parents, teachers and children about the existence of emotional and behavioral disorders (Achenbach, McConaughy & Howell, 1987). This may particularly disadvantage children with emotional disorders. While emotional disorders can cause considerable distress, their presence may not be readily evident to an observer. As a result, parents or teachers may fail to recognize and provide help to children experiencing significant emotional problems. Emotional disorders are common amongst adolescents and it is possible that a failure to recognize problems amongst this age group contributes to the under-representation of adolescents in mental health services (Garland & Besinger, 1996). It may also contribute to their high rate of suicide.

Second, children's problems reflect unique interactions between intra-individual difficulties and environmental conditions (Saxe, Cross & Silverman, 1988). Children are closely entwined in family and school systems and are highly dependent on their environment in both these settings. Interventions designed to help children with mental disorders must take into account the profound influence of these environments. This requires the close involvement of schools and families in treatment directed towards children living at home. In Western countries, the vast majority of children attend school for long periods of their lives. As a result, school staff can play an important role in the provision of mental health services for children. For example, results from the study by Burns et al. (1995) highlight the extent to which children with mental disorders receive help from education services in North America. In their study, Burns et al. reported that the education system plays a key role in the provision of services with 70% to 80% of children who received services for mental disorders being seen by staff working in the education sector. In contrast, only 11% to 13% of children received help through the health sector.

Third, in many countries primary care physicians and pediatricians, but not mental health specialists, are the professionals who most frequently provide health care to children (Offord et al., 1987; Sawyer et al., 1990). As a result, these professional groups have the potential to play an important role in facilitating referral of children to mental health services. However, recent evidence suggests that factors other than the severity of children's mental disorders – for example mental disorders in mothers or family stress – may influence whether children are referred to mental health services by these practitioners (Garralda & Bailey, 1988). Child and adolescent mental health services must consider the impact of these factors on referral patterns when planning treatment programs for children.

Fourth, the treatment 'needs' of children change markedly as they develop. As a result, treatment programs focusing on children of different ages must account for the unique needs of children at particular developmental stages. For example, the effective treatment of younger children invariably requires the involvement of parents or guardians, while treatment programs for adolescents must respect and encourage the autonomy of this older age group. This requires careful attention to the nature of the setting in which services for children of different ages are provided. For example, settings which are orientated primarily to the treatment of younger children may be unacceptable to adolescents.

Fifth, in epidemiological studies the prevalence of mental disorders is typically assessed using a categorical approach in which children are classified into one of two groups according to whether they are assessed as having a disorder. However, this approach does not accurately describe the full extent of childhood mental health problems because many childhood problems lie on a continuum and cannot readily be described as unique disease entities (Achenbach, 1985). Furthermore, as highlighted by Stallard (1993), the use of symptom checklists to categorize children may lead to a failure to identify children who have very severe problems limited to one area. Although these children may score in the highest range on a small number of items, overall they will not score highly on screening questionnaires and thus may not be identified as having a disorder.

Finally, concern has been expressed about the lack of resources available to provide clinical services for children, and also to support research investigating the etiology and treatment of childhood mental disorders (Institute of Medicine, 1989). In many areas, such as pediatric psychopharmacology, the research base is much weaker for children than it is for adults. This limits understanding, both about the etiology of childhood mental disorders and the approaches that can be employed to provide help. At a time when governments and funding agencies are putting a higher priority on the use of *evidence-based medicine*, there is a risk that the relatively sparse research base of child and adolescent mental health may lead to a reduction in the availability of mental health services for children.

Identification of needs

In the past, need was often seen as 'an unambiguous and objective attribute of clients, subject to measurement and essentially static' (Clayton, 1983, p. 223). More recently, the term 'need' has been used in a range of different ways. For example, Brewin (1992) noted that the term is used to refer both to health problems and to the deficiency of interventions to help these problems. Boyle & Offord (1988) pointed out that 'need' is often based on 'the demand for services, the articulateness of professionals who are able to argue the case for the existence of need within their jurisdictions, and political concerns of legislators' (p. 385). This lack of an agreed definition of need is a common cause of confusion when describing the unmet needs of children with mental disorders.

The approach to need described by Bradshaw (1972) provides a useful framework within which the unmet needs of children with mental disorders can be considered. Bradshaw suggests that the concept of need includes: *normative need, felt need, expressed need,* and *comparative need.* These four categories of need will be used in this chapter as a framework to highlight various aspects of the needs of children with mental disorders.

Normative need refers to what experts define as need in a given situation. Epidemiological research that uses the concept of normative need has played a key role in identifying the prevalence of childhood mental disorders in the community (Verhulst & Koot, 1995). Using symptom scales or structured interviews to measure the prevalence of childhood mental disorders in this way provides information about the number of children who meet 'expert-defined' criteria for a disorder. Although estimates of the prevalence of child and adolescent mental disorders varies between studies, partly because of the use of different methodologies and definitions of disorder, it is clear that childhood disorders are highly prevalent (Costello et al., 1996; Offord et al., 1987; Verhulst & Koot, 1995). It also appears that the prevalence of some problems, such as adolescent depression and suicide, is increasing (Rutter & Smith, 1995).

When normative need is the focus of epidemiological studies, 'unmet need' is defined as not receiving services despite the existence of an emotional or behavioral disorder (Burns, 1996). Studies that employ this concept of need consistently report that only a minority of children and adolescents with mental disorders attend mental health services. For example, Offord et al. (1987) reported a six-month prevalence rate of 18.1% for one or more of the disorders assessed in the Ontario Child Health Study. Although children with these disorders were four times more likely to have received help from mental health or social services in the preceding six months, five of six children with disorders had not received help from either of these services. A more serious pattern was identified in the study by Burns et al. (1995), who reported that during the three months prior to their assessment only 20% of children with a diagnosis and impairment had attended a mental health service, although a somewhat higher percentage had received help from other health services over this time. It should be noted that caution is necessary when comparing results from studies describing service utilization in different countries because similar services may have different roles in the provision of health care for children in different countries. For example, pediatricians and family practitioners have quite different roles in the provision of health care for children in Australia and North America.

Many children identified in epidemiological studies as having disorders will recover from their disorder without treatment, even children with disorders considered to have the worst prognosis. For example, a follow-up assessment of the children who participated in the Ontario Child Health Study found that only 45% of the 4- to 12-year-old children who were identified as having a conduct disorder at the first assessment continued to have the disorder four years later (Offord & Bennett, 1994). Admittedly the risk for continuing problems is high, but it cannot be assumed that all children with a disorder at one point in time who are not treated will continue to have the disorder. As a result, preventive programs that simply screen large populations of children for a disorder and then plan to treat all identified children may be an inefficient use of resources. As will be discussed later, it is also important not to assume that all children who attend mental health services are having their needs met. It is possible that ineffective or inappropriate interventions are provided which have little effect on children's problems.

Felt need refers to the views of potential consumers about whether they need a service. In the Ontario Child Health Study, Boyle & Offord (1988) sought information from parents about their 'felt need' for help for their children, by asking three related questions focusing on the extent to which parents perceived their children had problems and needed help. The last of these three questions was, 'Do you think that [name] needs or needed any professional help with these problems?' A positive response to this question defined a child as having 'felt need'. Across several geographical regions of Ontario, the percentage of parents who felt that their children needed professional help was consistently lower than the percentage of children identified as having a mental disorder. This suggests that not all parents of children classified as having mental disorders in epidemiological studies feel that their child needs professional treatment. While it is intuitively attractive, Clayton (1983) has criticized this approach to needs assessment because of the risk that, without an indication of the financial cost that respondents are prepared to pay for the service, the concept of felt need may simply reflect a form of 'wishful thinking' (p. 220).

Within the framework described by Bradshaw, *expressed need* focuses on whether a felt need is turned into action, such as by actually seeking help from a mental health service. This approach to need is commonly employed by staff in mental health services who highlight their long waiting lists when advocating additional funds for their service. Limitations to the approach are its focus on the relatively small proportion of children with mental disorders referred to services, and the difficulty in comparing levels of expressed need across regions which contain varying numbers of health services. For example, it is clearly more difficult for children and parents to demonstrate expressed need in regions where no child and adolescent mental health services are available, than in regions which are well provided with these services.

The final category identified by Bradshaw is *comparative need*. This approach to need utilizes the characteristics of people in receipt of a service to create a 'gold standard'. If people with similar characteristics to those attending services are identified in the community but are not receiving services, they are defined as being 'in need'. This is similar to the approach employed to identify cut-off scores on the child behavior checklist, which has been widely used to identify the prevalence of childhood mental disorders in the community (Achenbach, 1991). Children scoring in the range typically reported for children attending mental health services are considered to be 'cases'. A limitation of this approach to assessing need is the possibility that factors other than the severity of children's problems influence their use of mental health services.

Reports from parents, teachers and children are used to assess childhood mental disorders. As the level of agreement about the existence of childhood mental disorders amongst these informants is often poor (Achenbach et al., 1987), it is unlikely that these informants will agree about the need for treatment amongst children in the community. For example, children are often referred to mental health services by teachers because of school-related problems but attend services with parents who may be unconcerned about their children's behavior at home and lack information about problems at school. When this occurs, it can be difficult for mental health professionals to satisfy the needs of children, parents and teachers. Also it cannot be assumed that the views of the parents, teachers and children do not change over time. For example, changes in knowledge or attitudes about child mental health services may encourage parents or teachers to identify more children as being in need of treatment, leading to increased felt and expressed need. Finally, there is evidence that different professional groups responsible for children may have different views about the needs and desired treatment outcomes for children with mental disorders (Rugs & Kutash, 1994; Sawyer, Meldrum, Tonge & Clark, 1992). For example, in the study by Sawyer et al. (1992), it appeared that youth workers and teachers had different expectations from mental health staff about the type of help that should be provided by mental health services. These issues can make it difficult to reach agreement across different professional groups about the needs of children with mental disorders.

Treatment of disorders

Any discussion of unmet need for treatment must consider the extent to which effective treatment interventions are available. Recently, a number of factors have increased interest in the effectiveness of treatment interventions, including concern about the unmet need for treatment, the increasing cost of treatment and increasing demands for greater accountability of mental health services (Lyons, Howard, O'Mahoney & Lish, 1997). The availability of new computer technology has also enabled service planners to make more effective use of the information describing patients and treatment programs that is now routinely collected by mental health services (Lyons et al., 1997). In general, although the potential impact of treatment interventions in child and adolescent mental health is limited by low rates of presentation to services (Burns, 1991), treatment trials have provided some of the best evidence that interventions have the potential to reduce the rates of common childhood disorders (Kendall & Panichelli-Mindel, 1995).

Clinical interventions based in treatment settings can be grouped into three categories: (1) indicated interventions, (2) treatment of discrete episodes, and (3) maintenance of remission and prevention of relapse. Indicated interventions employ treatments of proven clinical effectiveness for the management of sub-syndromal disturbance. To achieve success, indicated interventions require the provision of sufficient clinical resources to properly deliver the intervention, and a strong risk relationship between the sub-syndromal disturbance and the clinical disorder that is the target of the intervention. Ultimately, however, the public health impact of indicated interventions is determined by the proportion of children with sub-syndromal disorders who can be identified in the community either by primary care services or population screening with questionnaires.

Indicated interventions have been developed for the management of sub-syndromal psychotic disorder, sub-syndromal depression and conduct disorder (Offord & Bennett, 1994; Yung et al., 1996). Examples of indicated interventions for depressive symptoms include 'Coping with Stress' and the Penn Prevention Program, both of which are based on the principles of cognitive-behavioral therapy (Clarke, Hawkins, Murphy & Sheeber, 1993; Jaycox, Reivich, Gillham & Seligman, 1994). However, while initial reports suggest that significant improvements in depressive symptoms are possible using these programs, more definitive evidence of their effectiveness requires studies that address the problems of low participation, differential attrition and lack of blind assessment evident in these preliminary studies. Clearer evidence is available for the efficacy of clinical interventions for established disorders. For adolescent depression, for example, three treatment approaches have been explored: cognitive-behavioral therapy, interpersonal therapy, and antidepressant medication. At least in the short-term, there is good evidence that cognitive-behavioral therapy effectively reduces the symptoms of depression experienced by adolescents (Lewinsohn, Clarke, Hops & Andrews, 1990; Wood, Harrington & Moore, 1996). There is also evidence that serotonin reuptake inhibitors may effectively reduce the rates of disorder in the short-term (Emslie et al., 1995; Kutcher, 1997).

In his review of interventions for childhood mental disorders, Fonagy (1997*b*) points out that the era of generic therapies is over and professionals responsible for the treatment of children with mental disorders must be familiar with the most effective intervention available to treat each childhood disorder. As noted earlier, it cannot be assumed that because children are attending a health service, their needs are always being met. Children may continue to experience unmet needs because they are being managed at an inappropriate service level; for example, in a primary health care service rather than a more specialized service or because no effective treatment exists for their condition. However, children may also experience unmet needs despite attending a specialized service because the treatment they receive is not the most effective intervention available to treat their disorder.

Hoagwood, Jensen, Petti & Burns (1996) highlight two further issues that are important in any consideration of the treatment needs of children with mental disorders. First, they note the paucity of outcome studies that have examined treatment effectiveness in naturalistic settings. For example, they report that while over 400 studies have examined the effectiveness of psychotherapy, fewer than a dozen studies have investigated the effectiveness of this treatment approach outside research settings. This is a significant omission because it cannot be assumed that the efficacy of individual psychological therapies identified in formal outcome studies accurately reflects the results achieved in clinic settings. Fonagy (1997b) also points out the relative lack of research trials investigating the effectiveness of the traditional mix of psychosocial treatment approaches used in mental health clinics.

The second issue is the need to conceptualize outcomes more broadly than just the reduction of symptoms of mental disorders. Hoagwood et al. (1996) suggest that approaches to outcomes should include: (1) functioning, i.e., the ability of children to adapt to the varying demands of home, school, peers and neighborhood, (2) consumer perspectives, i.e., the subjective experience of the consumer, including constructs such as quality of life and satisfaction, (3) environments, i.e., potentially modifiable features of children's school and family environments, and (4) systems, i.e., the relationships between the service organizations responsible for children's care. These are important issues because there is limited evidence for the ability of treatment programs to reduce relapse and the complications of childhood-onset disorder. For example, although there have been suggestions that cognitive-behavioral approaches may prevent relapse in adolescent-onset depression, as yet there is no strong evidence for the effectiveness of these approaches (Kroll, Harrington, Gowers, Frazer & Jayson, 1996). Similarly, there is little evidence that treatment interventions reduce suicidal behavior or the social and educational impairments associated with depression amongst adolescents.

Although much has been written about the importance of coordination and providing a continuum of care, the recent study by Bickman et al. (1995) highlights the limitations of coordination and emphasizes the importance of using interventions with proven effectiveness in mental health services. In their study, Bickman et al. compared the effectiveness of coordinated care with conventional treatment in a nonrandom, controlled trial. Extra resources were provided to allow better coordination of services and greater accessibility to clients in the experimental service. Patient satisfaction in this service rose significantly but, despite increased coordination between the various components of the service, treatment outcomes did not differ between the experimental and control services.

Recently Jensen, Hoagwood & Petti (1996) identified three areas where further research is required to help improve treatment outcomes. These are: (1) studies investigating the differential long-term effects of various treatment alternatives, (2) studies that package multifaceted treatments and apply them in natural settings where they can be incorporated into routine practices, and (3) studies that examine and incorporate consumer perspective's with other outcome assessments. Studies that address these issues have the potential to play an important role in reducing the unmet needs for treatment of children and adolescents with mental disorders.

Prevention of disorders

One response to the increasing evidence of a high prevalence of childhood mental disorders has been the development of treatment services that are more accessible and responsive to client needs. Another response has been the development of preventive interventions. This is an attractive option given the high prevalence of childhood disorders, the uncertain effectiveness of treatment in the medium to long term and the knowledge that only a small proportion of children with mental disorders attend services. A greater awareness of the link between childhood risk factors and mental disorders in adulthood has also encouraged attempts to develop more effective strategies to intervene on behalf of children exposed to key risk factors such as sexual abuse and adverse childhood parenting styles (Mullen, Martin, Anderson, Romans & Herbison, 1993; Parker, 1993).

Preventive interventions in childhood can be divided into two broad groupings: universal and selective (Table 22.1). Universal interventions focus on modifying risk for whole populations and can be further divided into interventions that center on populations and on individuals. Both types of interventions have three requirements for effectiveness. First, risk factors must be identified which have a strong causal relationship with the mental disorders that are the focus of the intervention. Second, these risk factors must be modifiable. Third, there must be the capacity to deliver the intervention to all members of the target population. Population-focused interventions with proven efficacy include, 'Mastery of Learning' and the 'Good Behaviour Game' both of which have been used to modify social interactions

Table 22.1. Evidence base for preventive interventions that target some risk factors for child and adolescent mental disorders

Risk factor	Universal	Selective
Individual factors		
Depressive symptoms	+	−
Antisocial behavior	++	++
Parental loss	−	++
Life events	−	−
Family risk factors		
Family psychopathology	−	+
Family cohesion	++	++
Family conflict	++	++
Education risk factors		
Academic failure	++	++
School disengagement	++	++

Note: ++, evidence of efficacy from experimental or pseudo-experimental studies; +, intervention devised but not yet assessed for efficacy; −, no report of intervention program.

within primary school classes (Kellam et al., 1991). Examples of population-focused interventions are 'Whole-of-School' interventions, which have been employed to reduce bullying in schools (Olweus, 1993). Examples of effective individually focused interventions include those based on life skills designed to prevent substance abuse (Botvin, Baker, Dusenbury, Botvin & Diaz, 1995).

Selective interventions focus on population subgroups that have a particularly high risk for mental disorders. These interventions can be broadly divided into those centered on vulnerability and on events. Once again, to be effective the interventions must focus on risks that have a strong causal relationship with the disorder to be prevented; and the risks must have the potential to be modified as a result of an intervention. There must also be the capacity to maintain the intervention for long enough to significantly reduce the risk factors. Vulnerability-focused interventions with proven efficacy include those focusing on academic failure (Hawkins, Doueck & Lishner, 1988) and on groups disadvantaged by their ethnic and social background (Comer, 1985). Examples of effective event-centered interventions include those focusing on parental death (Sandler, West, Baca & Pillow, 1992) and juvenile offending (Klein, Alexander & Parsons, 1997).

Three characteristics of preventive interventions determine their potential usefulness in responding to unmet needs: efficacy, cost-effectiveness, and evidence of effectiveness in broader implementation. The current knowledge base in each of these areas is limited. Evidence of the efficacy of preventive interventions has largely been derived from trials using an experimental or pseudo-experimental design. However, most of these trials focus on the short-term reduction of risk factors or symptoms. Few trials have examined the ability of interventions to reduce risks or symptoms in the longer term; therefore, the impact of childhood interventions on mental disorder in adulthood is unknown. Similarly, there is little information about the cost-effectiveness of preventive interventions in childhood. There have also been few attempts to examine the broader range of effects on symptoms, behavior and social functioning which might be anticipated when interventions focus on risk factors that have a causal relationship with multiple disorders. Finally, it is important to note that even if they are shown to be effective in research trials, new prevention programs will have little impact on reducing the prevalence of childhood mental disorders unless they can be easily incorporated into the settings where young people and their parents are found. There is a great need for more information about factors that can facilitate the translation of research-based preventive interventions into routine practice in health and education services.

Conclusions

Responding to the unmet needs of children and adolescents with mental disorders presents a number of challenges. First, there is a need to achieve a better understanding of the help desired by the parents and children with mental disorders. It is known that most children with mental disorders do not receive help from mental health services. As well, however, a large proportion of children and families who attend mental health services *discontinues contact after a couple of appointments*. What is this telling us about how well the services are meeting the needs of children and parents? There is a need for greater dialogue between mental health professionals and potential consumers of mental health services, such as parents and children. Children and parents need to be more aware of the treatment alternatives and the potential outcomes of treatment available from the mental health services. Mental health professionals need to know more about the type of help desired by children with mental disorders and their parents (Rugs & Kutash, 1994).

Second, a better understanding is needed about the factors which place children at risk of continuing problems. Knowledge about factors that are amenable to change as a result of interventions will make it possible to better identify children who have the least likelihood of early recovery and hence the greatest need for help. This will make it possible to better target scarce resources to help children in greatest need. Third, mental health services have to achieve an appropriate balance between prevention and treatment programs. While there is currently limited knowledge about how to accurately judge the resources which should be committed to each of these approaches, it is important for the credibility of child and adolescent mental health that interventions focusing on individuals and on populations are provided.

Achieving these aims requires well-trained researchers in child mental health services, yet in many countries there are few mental health professionals with research skills, and progress in developing training programs is slow (Institute of Medicine, 1989). There is also a great need to translate research into routine practice more effectively. There is evidence that some clinicians do not value research and spend little time reading journals (Fonagy, 1997a). This was reflected in a recent study of the attitudes of health, welfare and education staff towards research. Some staff expressed little support for research trials and research was often described as irrelevant and of little practical help (Sawyer et al., 1992). However, many of the same staff indicated a great willingness to develop and assess new approaches to help children with mental disorders. There is also evidence that decision-makers in health services do not see health services research as particularly relevant to their needs (Woodward, Feldman & Snider, 1997). To overcome these problems the different skills available in academic settings, mental health services and other community treatment settings must be better integrated.

In summary, a range of effective preventive and treatment interventions are required to respond adequately to the unmet needs of children and adolescents with mental disorders. Evaluation of treatment and prevention approaches must give greater consideration to their effect on the longer term outcomes of children and to their impact on the ability of children to function adequately in their home and school environments, with peers, and in the wider community. Evaluation must also consider the economic benefits of successful interventions and the economic costs of failure. An increasing political will must be achieved to address the major public health problem posed by childhood and adolescent mental disorders. This requires a strong alliance between the consumers and professionals responsible for providing help to children and adolescents with mental disorders. The extent to which these alliances can be forged and their ability to achieve greater political influence will do much to shape the mental health of children and adolescents in the twenty-first century.

References

Achenbach, T.M. (1985). *Assessment and Taxonomy of Child and Adolescent Psychopathology*, Volume 3. California: Sage Publications Ltd.

Achenbach, T.M. (1991). *Manual for the Child Behavior Checklist/4-18 and 1991 Profile*. Burlington, VT: University of Vermont Department of Psychiatry.

Achenbach, T.M., McConaughy, S.H. & Howell, C.T. (1987). Child/adolescent behavioral and emotional problems: implications of cross-informant correlations for situational specificity. *Psychological Bulletin*, 101, 213–32.

Bickman, L., Guthrie, P.R., Foster, E.M., Lambert, E.W., Summerfelt, W.T., Breda, C.S. & Heflinger, C.A. (1995). *Evaluating Managed Mental Health Services: The Fort Bragg Experiment.* New York: Plenum Press.

Botvin, G.J., Baker, E., Dusenbury, L., Botvin, E.M. & Diaz, T. (1995). Long-term follow-up results of a randomized drug abuse prevention trial in a white middle-class population. *Journal of the American Medical Association*, 273, 1106–12.

Boyle, M.H. & Offord, D.R. (1988). Prevalence of childhood disorder, perceived need for help, family dysfunction and resource allocation for child welfare and children's mental health services in Ontario. *Canadian Journal of Behavioral Science*, 20, 374–88.

Bradshaw, J. (1972). The concept of social need. *New Society*, 19, 640–2.

Brewin, C.R. (1992). Measuring individual needs for care and services. In G. Thornicroft, C. R. Brewin, & J. Wing (eds.), *Measuring Mental Health Needs*, pp. 220–36. London: The Royal College of Psychiatrists.

Burns, B.J. (1991). Mental health service use by adolescents in the 1970s and 1980s. *Journal of the American Academy of Child and Adolescent Psychiatry*, 30, 144–50.

Burns, B.J. (1996). What drives outcomes for emotional and behavioral disorders in children and adolescents? *New Directions for Mental Health Services*, 71, 89–102.

Burns, B.J., Costello, E.J., Angold, A., Tweed, D., Stangl, D., Farmer, E. & Erkanli, A. (1995). Children's mental health service use across service sectors. *Health Affairs*, 14, 147–59.

Clarke, G.N., Hawkins, W., Murphy, M. & Sheeber, L.B. (1993). Cognitive behavioural treatment of depressive symptomatology in adolescents. *Journal of Adolescent Research*, 8, 183–204.

Clayton, S. (1983). Social need revisited. *Journal of Social Policy*, 12, 215–34.

Comer, J.P. (1985). The Yale-New Haven Primary Prevention Project: a follow-up study. *Journal of the American Academy of Child Psychiatry*, 24, 154–60.

Costello, E.J., Angold, A., Burns, B.J., Erkanli, A., Stangl, D.K. & Tweed, D.L. (1996). The great Smoky Mountains study of youth: functional impairment and serious emotional disturbance. *Archives of General Psychiatry*, 53, 1137–43.

Desjarlais, R., Eisenberg, L., Good, B. & Kleinman, A. (1995). *World Mental Health. Problems and Priorities in Low-Income Countries.* New York: Oxford University Press.

Emslie, G., Rush, A.J., Weinberg, W.A., Kowatch, R.A., Carmody, T. & Rintelmann, J. (1995). Fluoxetine in child and adolescent depression: acute and maintenance treatment. *Depression and Anxiety*, 7, 32–9.

Ferdinand, R.F. & Verhulst, F.C. (1995). Psychopathology from adolescence into young adulthood: an 8-year follow-up study. *American Journal of Psychiatry*, 152, 1586–94.

Fonagy, P. (1997a). Evaluating the effectiveness of interventions in child psychiatry: the state of the art – part 1. *Canadian Child Psychiatry Review*, 6, 31–47.

Fonagy, P. (1997b). Evaluating the effectiveness of interventions in child psychiatry: the state of the art – part 2. *Canadian Child Psychiatry Review*, 6, 64–80.

Garland, A.F. & Besinger, B.A. (1996). Adolescents' perceptions of outpatient mental health services. *Journal of Child and Family Studies*, 5, 355–75.

Garralda, M.E. & Bailey, D. (1988). Child and family factors associated with referral to child psychiatrists. *British Journal of Psychiatry*, 153, 81–9.

Harrington, R. (1992). The natural history and treatment of child and adolescent affective disorders. *Journal of Child Psychology and Psychiatry and Allied Disciplines*, 33, 1287–302.

Hawkins, J.D., Doueck, H.J. & Lishner, D.M. (1988). Changing teaching practices in mainstream classrooms to improve bonding and behavior of low achievers. *American Journal of Educational Research*, 25, 31–50.

Hoagwood, K., Jensen, P.S., Petti, T. & Burns, B.J. (1996). Outcomes of mental health care for children and adolescents: I. A comprehensive conceptual model. *Journal of the American Academy of Child and Adolescent Psychiatry*, 35, 1055–63.

Institute of Medicine (1989). *Research on Children and Adolescents with Mental, Behavioral, and Developmental Disorders: Mobilizing a National Initiative*. Washington D.C.: National Academy Press.

Jaycox, L.H., Reivich, K.J., Gillham, J. & Seligman, M.E. (1994). Prevention of depressive symptoms in school children. *Behaviour Research & Therapy*, 32, 801–16.

Jensen, P., Hoagwood, K. & Petti, T. (1996). Outcomes of mental health care for children and adolescents: II. Literature review and application of a comprehensive model. *Journal of American Child and Adolescent Psychiatry*, 35, 1064–77.

Kellam, S.G., Werthamer-Larsson, L., Dolan, L.J., Brown, C.H., Mayer, L.S., Rebok, G.W., Anthony, J.C., Laudolff, J. & Edelsohn, G. (1991). Developmental epidemiologically based preventive trials: baseline modeling of early target behaviors and depressive symptoms. *American Journal of Community Psychology*, 19, 563–84.

Kendall, P.C. & Panichelli-Mindel, S.M. (1995). Cognitive-behavioural treatments. *Journal of Abnormal Child Psychology*, 23, 107–23.

Klein, N.C., Alexander, J.F. & Parsons, B.V. (1997). Impact of family systems intervention on recidivism and sibling delinquency. *Journal of Consulting Clinical Psychology*, 45, 469–74.

Kroll, L., Harrington, R.C., Gowers, S., Frazer, J. & Jayson, D. (1996). Continuation of cognitive-behavioural treatment in adolescent patients who have remitted from major depression. *Journal of the American Academy of Child and Adolescent Psychiatry*, 35, 1156–61.

Kutcher, S. (1997). The pharmacotherapy of adolescent depression. *Journal of Child Psychology and Psychiatry and Allied Disciplines*, 38, 755–67.

Lewinsohn, P.W., Clarke, G.N., Hops, H. & Andrews, J. (1990). Cognitive-behavioural treatment for depressed adolescents. *Behaviour Therapy*, 21, 385–401.

Lyons, J.S., Howard, K.I., O'Mahoney, M.T. & Lish, J.D. (1997). *The Measurement and Management of Clinical Outcomes in Mental Health*. New York: John Wiley.

Mullen, P.E., Martin, J.L., Anderson, J.C., Romans, S.E. & Herbison, G.P. (1993). Childhood sexual abuse and mental health in adult life. *British Journal of Psychiatry*, 163, 721–32.

Offord, D.R. & Bennett, K.J. (1994). Conduct disorder: long-term outcomes and intervention effectiveness. *Journal of the American Academy of Child and Adolescent*

Psychiatry, **33**, 1069–78.

Offord, D.R., Boyle, M.H., Szatmari, P., Rae-Grant, N.I., Links, P.S., Cadman, D.T., Byles, J.A., Crawford, J.W., Blum, H.M., Byrne, C., Thomas, H. & Woodward, C.A. (1987). Ontario child health study. II. Six-month prevalence of disorder and rates of service utilization. *Archives of General Psychiatry*, **44**, 832–6.

Olweus, D. (1993). *Bullying at School*. Oxford: Blackwell Publishers.

Parker, G. (1993). Parental rearing style: examining for links with personality vulnerability factors for depression. *Social Psychiatry and Psychiatric Epidemiology*, **28**, 97–100.

Robins, L.N. (1966). *Deviant Children Grown Up*. Baltimore: Williams & Wilkins.

Rugs, D. & Kutash, K. (1994). Evaluating children's mental health service systems: an analysis of critical behaviors and events. *Journal of Child and Family Studies*, **3**, 249–62.

Rutter, M. & Smith, D.J. (eds.) (1995). *Psychosocial Disorders in Young People: Time Trends and Their Causes*. Chichester, UK: John Wiley.

Sandler, O.N., West, S.G., Baca, L. & Pillow, D.R. (1992). Linking empirically based theory and evaluation: The Family Bereavement Program. *American Journal of Community Psychology*, **20**, 491–523.

Sawyer, M., Meldrum, D., Tonge, B. & Clark, J. (1992). *Mental Health and Young People*. Tasmania: National Clearing House for Youth Studies.

Sawyer, M.G., Sarris, A., Baghurst, P.A., Cornish, C.A. & Kalucy, R.S. (1990). The prevalence of emotional and behavioural disorders and patterns of service utilisation in children and adolescents. *Australian and New Zealand Journal of Psychiatry*, **24**, 323–30.

Saxe, L., Cross, T. & Silverman, N. (1988). Children's mental health: the gap between what we know and what we do. *American Psychologist*, **43**, 800–7.

Stallard, P. (1993). The behaviour of 3-year-old children: prevalence and parental perception of problem behaviour: a research note. *Journal of Child Psychology and Psychiatry*, **34**, 413–21.

Verhulst, F.C. & Koot, H.M. (eds.) (1995). *The Epidemiology of Child and Adolescent Psychopathology*. New York: Oxford University Press.

Wood, A.J., Harrington, R.C. & Moore, A. (1996). Controlled trial of a brief cognitive-behavioural intervention in adolescent patients with depressive disorders. *Journal of Child Psychology and Psychiatry and Allied Disciplines*, **37**, 737–46.

Woodward, C.A., Feldman, W. & Snider, A. (1997). Health-services researchers and decision-makers: are there really two solitudes? *Annals of The Royal College of Physicians and Surgeons of Canada*, **30**, 417–23.

Yung, A., McGorry, P., McFarlane, C., Jackson, H., Patton, G. & Rakkar, A. (1996). Monitoring and care of young people at incipient risk of psychosis. *Schizophrenia Bulletin*, **22**, 283–304.

23

Assessing psychopathology among children aged four to eight

Linda Cottler, Wendy Reich, Kathy Rourke, Renee M. Cunningham-Williams, and Wilson M. Compton

Introduction

Although changes in mental health care financing are occurring globally, little data are available on the effect this may have on access to treatment, treatment outcome, and services themselves. What is known is based on adult data; thus, the impact of health care reform on children and adolescents is largely unknown. To improve service availability and treatment of mental disorders for children and adolescents, we need to know more about the cost of treating childhood disorders, and the barriers to accessing that care. This begins with knowledge of the number of children and adolescents who 'need' services, and the proportion of those 'in need' who receive mental health services.

Assessing need

Need is defined in several ways: from receiving mental health care, to functional impairment, to meeting criteria according to standardized DSM or ICD criteria (Costello, Burns, Angold & Leaf, 1993). Estimating need based on service use requires: (1) a system of care that documents in a standardized way the symptoms that are experienced by children and adolescents; (2) valid data collection; and (3) a clear understanding of all service arenas used by children and adolescents. Knowing how to identify the repertoire of service agencies and providers in all regions of a country is one of the major difficulties of defining need as 'use of services'. In the USA, services related specifically to children typically include those received through the social welfare office, and visits to a juvenile justice program, a counselor at school, a psychologist, primary care provider or a psychiatrist. Data show that approximately 1% of children receive mental health services in mental health settings (Burns & Friedman, 1990) and approximately 6%

receive services related to mental health within the primary care and school systems (Costello, 1989; Horwitz, Leaf, Leventhal, Forsyth & Speechley, 1992).

When need is defined by having met diagnostic criteria, it is important to consider the criteria, the social development of the child, the informants providing the information, the scoring algorithms for defining the disorder – whether a diagnosis is defined by lifetime or recent status – and the assessment itself. Available data indicate that 20% of children (usually children 9 to 17 years old) meet criteria for at least one DSM disorder (Costello, 1989). This is a much higher rate of need than that defined by use of services as stated above, and this definition accentuates the issue of determining what constitutes need among children and adolescents. Recently, there has been discussion about the appropriateness of DSM and ICD criteria for children in the youngest cohort, which has led to an alternative approach – the Diagnostic Classification of Mental Health and Developmental Disorders of Infancy and Early Childhood (National Center for Clinical Infant Programs, 1994). The developers argue that using this provisional multiaxial system, which may or may not overlap with the DSM and ICD systems, reduces misclassification bias attributed to the traditional diagnostic nosology.

Need for service is also defined as impairment in adaptive behavior, social functioning, or family, school and work environments, regardless of service use and symptom counts. In young children, impairment in basic social interactions and the slowed development of self-care behaviors are thought to predict psychopathology and consequent mental health service use. Work is underway to determine the relationship between service use and impairment in these areas. Studies that seek to measure the youth needs for service use by measuring impairment must include emotional, behavioral, and substance-use problems and should cover the child's functional impairment, social developmental, cognitive ability, and academic achievement.

Multiple informants: parents and teachers

Since psychiatric disorders cannot be diagnosed with biological markers, all of the above classifications require information to be obtained from collateral and self-reports. As early as the 1950s, Lapouse & Monk (1958) demonstrated discrepancies in information given by different informants about the mental health of children. A debate then began as to who is the 'best' informant for a child. Most studies rely on data from the teacher and the parent and use an analytical strategy that combines data for classifying disorders in children. Four strategies have recently been proposed for classifying disorders in children, and include using: separate parent- and teacher-endorsed diagnoses; a combination of diagnoses endorsed by either informant; combinations of items from the teacher or parent; combinations where both inform-ants agree (Offord et al., 1996).

The child as informant

Citing poor agreement between parents and teachers (Gagnon, Vitaro & Tremblay, 1992; Verhulst & Akkerhuis, 1989), some investigators have been reluctant to add a third informant to the algorithm – the child. They argue that children cannot reliably report on their own behavior. For example, when children are interviewed about a behavior interpreted as 'oppositional' by the mother, the symptom is more clearly defined as a depressive symptom by the child (Reich, Herjanic, Welner & Gandhy, 1982). Poor agreement between parents and children (Andrews, Garrison, Jackson, Addy & McKeown, 1993; Angold, Weissman & John, 1987; Bird, Gould & Staghezza, 1992; Edelbrock, Costello, Dulcan, Conover & Kalas, 1986) remains one of the classification issues that plagues child psychiatric epidemiology at pres-ent. Specifically, a parent may be more likely to identify externalizing dis-order symptoms, while a child may report the same behavior as an internaliz-ing depression symptom. Parents and children should be expected to disagree on the information reported, since they have fundamentally different knowl-edge bases. As Reich & Earls (1987) point out, agreement between informants should not be the goal, as there are some behaviors a parent or teacher may know about a child, and there are behaviors that only a child can report. Thus, rather than striving for perfect agreement between informants, the goal should be to achieve a meaningful way to integrate data from all sources.

Children under the age of nine

In addition to investigators disagreeing on what disagreements herald, and on whether children should be interviewed, there are disputes over how young children should be used as informants. Can young children report on their own life events? Can they report psychiatric symptoms? There is a prevailing concern in the field of child psychiatry that children under 9 years old cannot provide reliable and accurate self-reports of their own behavior, and should not be asked to report on it. Although findings that show poor reliability are used to defend this claim, the same findings may be used to argue on behalf of young child informants. For example, Edelbrock et al. (1986) found that 6- to 9-year-old children were less reliable than 10- to 14-year-old children in reporting clusters of symptoms with the structured Diagnostic Interview Schedule for Children (DISC). Schwab-Stone, Fallon, Briggs & Crowther (1994) similarly found that age influences the reliability of

obtained from self-reports diagnoses and symptoms in school-age children –
that younger children were less reliable than older children. Reasons for
unreliability may be the use of developmentally mature abstract constructs
such as the age of onset or duration of symptoms.

The child versions of semistructured interviews such as the Child Assessment Scale (CAS), the Diagnostic Interview for Children and Adolescents
(DICA), the Child and Adolescent Psychiatric Assessment (CAPA) and the
Schedule for Affective Disorders and Schizophrenia for School-age Children
(K-SADS) tend to have higher reliability with the younger children, perhaps
because the interviewer can use additional probes when the child does not
seem to understand the intent of the question.

Misclassification of service use and need

As just described, there are barriers to the accurate classification of self-
reports of behavioral symptoms; however, to understand the extent of unmet
need for mental health services among children, accurate data must also be
available on service use. Since young children living at home can only enter
treatment with the permission of their parents, misclassification of service
use can be attributed primarily to investigators' excluding the complete
repertoire of service providers from the assessment. Services used by children,
in addition to psychiatrists and psychologists, include speech and language
services, services for learning problems, visits to social workers, support
services related to parental psychopathology and special education services.

As shown in Figure 23.1, in Pollyanna's world (the ideal world) only
children who need services receive them, and children who do not receive
services do not need them. Thus, in the ideal world, one without classification
bias, children do not receive services unless they need them. Conversely, in
the real world, there is an increased probability of misclassification bias
(Figure 23.2). Children who use mental health services and are classified as
having a need may be correctly classified in the 'met need' group, or they may
be misclassified and receive unnecessary services if reports of need are
exaggerated by informants. Bias also occurs when children who use mental
health services have no reported need. This classification bias would be more
prevalent in adolescents who seek counseling for problems their parents and
teachers are unaware of; for example, help with substance-abuse problems, or
from self-help hotlines. Bias would also occur if children received services
that parents thought they needed when in fact the children denied the
symptoms. Additionally, reporting errors about symptoms with the resultant
lack of services would result in an inappropriate lack of services. Lastly, true
unmet need could result from the correct reporting of symptoms that are not
matched with services. This unmet need might be due to a number of barriers

Assessed Need

		yes	no
Service Use	yes	Everything is groovy	Doesn't exist
	no	You don't really need treatment	Everything is groovy

Figure 23.1 Polyanna's world (ideal world).

Assessed Need

		yes	no
Service Use	yes	Parents or teachers misreport symptoms *Appropriate Service Use* *Unnecessary Service Use*	Reporting error? *Unnecessary Service Use*
	no	Denial, self-reliance, lack of trust, ignorance, expense, inconvenience, fear, transportation, waiting list *Unmet Need* *Appropriate Non-Service Use*	Reporting error? *Appropriate Non-Service Use* *Misclassification of both Need and Service*

Figure 23.2 Reality of need and service use.

shown in Figure 23.2, such as denial of symptoms (even though the informant is willing to report symptoms to an interviewer), self-reliance, a lack of trust in the provider and health care system, ignorance about where to go for treatment, expense, inconvenient location and hours, fear of treatment, not having transportation to the provider and being put on a waiting list for services.

As illustrated in the above discussion, accurate prevalence rates of unmet need are directly related to the reporting of need and service use, and, as described above, because there is disagreement in informant reports there is the potential for misclassification of unmet need. In order to reduce information bias, children should be given the opportunity to report their own feelings and behaviors. Realizing that young children may have cognitive limitations that could affect their ability to respond reliably (Butcher, 1972; Yates, 1990), many of the limitations may be diminished if lengthy assessments, which challenge young children's attention span, are avoided. In addition, assessments that use vocabulary aimed at older children and adults, and boring questionnaire formats need modifying so that a suitable environment is created for younger children in which they feel comfortable and able to give accurate responses. As Zahner (1991) points out, symptoms of depression have been the most unreliable, especially among young children.

Assessing psychopathology in four to eight year olds

Our group has begun to use a battery of assessments that will reduce classification bias by directly assessing children in the youngest age cohort – four to eight year olds – where traditionally, parent caregivers are asked to report on their child's behavior. The battery includes observational measures, cartoon-based measures and a puppet measure. This chapter describes the cartoon-based measures and the puppet measure.

Cartoon-based measures

To facilitate reports of behavior among very young children, pictures, or cartoons, have been used. The pictorial format has been found to focus the attention of children and to stimulate their interest. Thus, pictures minimize having to draw on the child's vocabulary. Cartoons have been used to assess the developmental stages of children (Di Leo, 1977), and have become the 'state of the art' for assessing mental health in very young children. In focus groups, children say they enjoy cartoons because they help them understand the questions better, they can see what is happening to the child in the cartoon, and they are fun.

The Dominic is a standardized, pictorial assessment battery which elicits information necessary to make DSM-III-R- and DSM-IV-based diagnoses in children aged six to eleven (Valla, Bergeron, Berube, Gaudet & St George, 1994). The developer of the cartoon measure, Jean-Pierre Valla, is a child psychiatrist and epidemiologist. The original version contained a representation and name of one child only – Dominic – who was intended to represent both a boy and girl. Valla and colleagues hypothesized that cartoons with pictures of Dominic expressing DSM symptoms, which were presented while the symptom questions were read aloud, would make it easy for the children to understand the behavior and allow young children to report their own feelings.

The original version of Dominic included 26 pictures; later versions became more elaborate with 194 drawings used. In a series of presentations at national and international meetings, Valla and colleagues reported excellent test–retest reliability of diagnoses, and good concurrent validity when Dominic was compared to the K-SADS-E. Although the psychometrics of the instrument were good, the instrument was too lengthy and was later shortened to 20 minutes. The Dominic includes items covering attention deficit hyperactivity disorder, conduct disorder, oppositional defiant disorder, major depressive disorder, separation anxiety disorder, overanxious disorder, and simple phobia.

For use in our study of young children funded by the National Institute of Mental Health (NIMH), the Dominic was modified to show a male and female character, as well as characters of varying ethnic groups. Working with Valla and colleagues, the St. Louis team proposed Dominic, the Caucasian child; Terry, the African American child; Ming of undetermined Asian origin, and Lupe, the Latino/Hispanic child. In order to know which set of cartoons the interviewer needs to use, children are asked to tell the interviewer which cartoon character looks most like them. If they choose Ming, Ming is used throughout the interview. Surprisingly, in our pilot study, children did not necessarily choose the character that portrayed their actual racial or ethnic group. In our study, the cartoon is paper and pencil based; however, there is a computerized version that can be used on a laptop.

The interviewer shows the child each cartoon and reads the question designed to elicit the symptom. For example, for the symptom about sadness, the child is shown the cartoon and the interviewer then asks, 'Are you sad or unhappy most of the time like Ming?' If the child says yes, the interviewer then asks, 'How often do you feel this way?' Children answer using a visual thermometer-type scale that indicates one time, a few times, and lots of times. Since young children have real difficulty with concepts such as duration, clustering, onset and recency, these questions are not asked. Thus, the instrument will not give a formal DSM diagnosis, but rather a count of DSM symptoms.

The Dominic with ethnic cartoons has been evaluated using the test–retest methodology in a study of 37 children in St. Louis and Los Angeles. Preliminary data suggest that several items from the Dominic should be dropped or reworded (only the anxiety and depression scale were used). In some cases, the cartoon itself may have been ambiguous. Kappa values for individual items ranged from 0.19 (do you feel tired nearly every day?) to 0.73 (do you often have bad dreams?).

A second cartoon-based assessment for young children is the VEX-R, Violence Exposure Scale, revised, developed by Fox & Leavitt (1995). This measure is important for assessing the exposure of children as young as four to violence. Dimensions of violence include witnessing and experiencing violence in the context of the home, school and neighborhood. The VEX-R uses 'Chris', a male/female character that looks multicultural. Cartoons show Chris witnessing violence, and Chris being the victim of violence. Items include, among others, slapping, pushing and shoving, use of a weapon, being attacked, dealing drugs, and stealing. Children are given a description of the situation and then asked how many times they have been in the situation that is shown in the cartoon. The answers range from never to lots of times; thermometer-style measuring scales are used to document the responses. Preliminary data show excellent intra-class correlations (ICCs) greater than 75 for the four possible dimensions of the scale (high violence, low violence, witness of violence, and victim of violence).

Puppet measure

Puppets have been used since the 1950s in studies of young children to equalize the expressive abilities of verbal and nonverbal children, as well as inhibited and noninhibited children. Studies have shown that two puppets using a standardized script can enable even the youngest cohort of children to express their feelings and behaviors (Eder, 1990). The Berkeley Puppet Interview (BPI) is a new, innovative method for interviewing young children developed by Ablow & Measelle, with funds from NIMH (Ablow & Measelle, 1993; Measelle, Ablow, Cowan & Cowan, 1998). The aim of the BPI is to cover DSM criteria of depression, anxiety, and conduct and oppositional disorders, and to assess hostility and aggression, inattention, impulsivity, inhibition, body image and enuresis. Use of the BPI in studies that assess identical domains from parents enables investigators to obtain the full complement of data about a child's emotions and behavior. In addition to a symptom scale, there is a self-perception scale, family environment scale, school context scale, teacher scale, and social scale. The use of the BPI requires extensive training, practice interviews, and certification.

The BPI is targeted at children aged four to seven. A trained interviewer, who provides the voices of the puppets, engages the child in a discussion with two identical hand puppets that look like puppy dogs. The puppets, named Iggy and Ziggy, are clearly labeled with name tags. The interviewer introduces the puppets as his or her friends; 'puppets' then introduce themselves to the child and state that they will be talking about themselves, and hope the child will talk about himself/herself.

The puppets express contrasting experiences or emotions and then ask the child about his or her experience or emotions. For example, Iggy says, 'I'm a sad kid' and Ziggy says, 'I'm not a sad kid'. Then Iggy says, 'How about you?' After the child endorses one of the emotions or behaviors, the puppet who expressed that emotion or behavior acknowledges their common experience by saying, 'that's like me' or, 'me too' or, 'I'm a sad kid too.' This acknowledgement is conveyed to the child in a neutral and accepting tone. The interaction between the puppets and the child resembles a discussion between three peers, which is more comfortable and engaging for the child than a standard interview situation.

The test–retest reliability of the BPI has not been established. Efforts are underway, funded by the MacArthur Foundation, to begin a psychometric study of this instrument in three sites: Stanford, Manchester (England) and St. Louis. It is hoped that this instrument can be used in epidemiological studies, in conjunction with the Dominic, to provide investigators with another way to understand the psychopathology of young children.

Future directions

Information about young children's psychopathology benefits from assessments with both children and adults, and use of such instruments in diverse cultures seems feasible because cartoons, pictures and puppets are likely to be universally understood and accepted by young children. Despite this overall perspective, measures of psychopathology in young children are not fully developed, and there are challenges inherent in improving these measures. For instance, to assess these children, we need to facilitate the interest and understanding of children of varying developmental stages, levels of inhibition, and cognitive abilities. Enabling young children to provide self-report information about their feelings and behaviors is critical to the understanding of their psychopathology and need for mental health services. We owe it to ourselves to explore and validate measures that will make this communication possible.

References

Ablow, J.C. & Measelle, J.R. (1993). *The Berkeley Puppet Interview: Administration and Scoring System Manuals.* Berkeley: University of California.

Andrews, V.C., Garrison, C.Z., Jackson, K.L., Addy, C.L. & McKeown, R.E. (1993). Mother-adolescent agreement on symptoms and diagnoses of adolescent depression and conduct disorder. *Journal of American Academy of Child Adolescent Psychiatry,* **32**, 731–8.

Angold, A., Weissman, M. & John, K. (1987). Parent and child reports of depressive symptoms in children at low risk of depression. *Journal of Child Psychology and Psychiatry,* **28**, 901–15.

Bird, H.R., Gould, M. & Staghezza, B. (1992). Aggregating data from multiple informants in child psychiatry epidemiological research. *Journal of American Academy of Child Adolescent Psychiatry,* **31**, 78–85.

Burns, B.J. & Friedman, R. (1990). Examining the research base for child mental health services and policy. *Journal of Mental Health Administration,* **17**, 87–98.

Butcher, H.J. (1972). *Human Intelligence: its Nature, and Assessment.* New York: Harper and Row.

Costello, E.J. (1989). Developments in child psychiatric epidemiology. *Journal of American Academy of Child Adolescent Psychiatry,* **28**, 836–41.

Costello, E.J., Burns, B.J., Angold, A. & Leaf, P. (1993). How can epidemiology improve mental health services for children and adolescents? *Journal of American Academy of Child Adolescent Psychiatry*, **32**, 1106–13.

Di Leo, J.H. (1977). *Child Development: Analysis and Synthesis.* New York: Brunner/ Mazel.

Edelbrock, C., Costello, A., Dulcan, M.K., Conover, N.C. & Kalas, R. (1986). Parent-child agreement on child psychiatric symptoms assessed via structured interviews. *Journal of Child Psychology and Psychiatry*, **27**, 181–90.

Eder, R.A. (1990). Uncovering young children's psychological selves: individual and developmental differences. *Child Development*, **61**, 849–63.

Fox, N.A. & Leavitt, L.A. (1995). Violence Exposure Scale for Children-Revised (VEX-R). www.inform.umd.edu/EDUC/Depts/.Fox/vex.html

Gagnon, C., Vitaro, F. & Tremblay, R.E. (1992). Parent-teacher agreement on kinder-gartner's behaviour problems: a research note. *Journal of Child Psychology and Psychiatry*, **33**, 1255–61.

Horwitz, S., Leaf, P., Leventhal, J., Forsyth, B. & Speechley, K. (1992). Identification and management of psychosocial and developmental problems in community-based primary care pediatric practices. *Pediatrics*, **89**, 1–6.

Lapouse, R. & Monk, M. (1958). An epidemiological study of behaviour characteristics in children. *American Journal of Public Health*, **48**, 1134–44.

Measelle, J.R., Ablow, J.C., Cowan, P.A. & Cowan C.P. (1998). Assessing young children's views of their academic, social and emotional lives: an evaluation of the self-perception scales of the Berkeley Puppet Interview. *Child Development*, **69**, 1556–76.

National Center for Clinical Infant Programs (1994). *Diagnostic Classification: 0 to 3.* Arlington: National Center for Clinical Infant Program.

Offord, D.R., Boyle, M.H., Racine, Y., Szatmari, P., Fleming, J., Sanford, M. & Lipman, E. (1996). Integrating assessment data from multiple informant. *Journal of American Academy of Child and Adolescent Psychiatry*, **35**, 1078–85.

Reich, W. & Earls, F. (1987). Rules for making psychiatric diagnoses in children on the basis of multiple sources of information: preliminary strategies. *Journal of Abnormal Child Psychology*, **15**, 601–16.

Reich, W., Herjanic, B., Welner, Z. & Gandhy, P.R. (1982). Development of a structured psychiatric interview for children: agreement on diagnosis comparing child and parent interviews. *Journal of Abnormal Child Psychology*, **10**, 325–36.

Schwab-Stone, M., Fallon, T., Briggs, M. & Crowther, B. (1994). Reliability of diagnostic reporting for children aged 6 to 11 years: a test-retest study of the diagnostic interview schedule for children-revised. *American Journal of Psychiatry*, **151**, 1048–54.

Valla, J.P., Bergeron, L., Berube, H., Gaudet, N. & St George, M. (1994). A structured pictorial questionnaire to assess DSM-III-R based diagnoses in children 6 to 11 years: development, validity, and reliability. *Journal of Abnormal Child Psychology*, **22**, 403–23.

Verhulst, F.C. & Akkerhuis, G.W. (1989). Agreement between parents' and teachers' ratings of behavioural/emotional problems of children aged 4 to 12. *Journal of Child Psychology and Psychiatry*, **30**, 123–36.

Yates, T. (1990).Theories of cognitive development. In M. Lewis (ed.), *Child and Adolescent Psychiatry*. Baltimore: Williams and Wilkins.

Zahner, G.E. (1991). The feasibility of conducting structured diagnostic interviews with preadolescents: a community field trial of the DISC. *Journal of American Academy of Child Adolescent Psychiatry*, **30**, 659–68.

24

Unmet need in Indigenous mental health: where to start?

Ernest Hunter

Aborigines and Torres Strait Islanders are the most disadvantaged distinct population in Australia. In terms of health status they fare worse, not only by comparison with nonIndigenous Australians, but also when compared to Indigenous populations in similar situations elsewhere. The social justice issues underlying Indigenous ill-health and the consequences for Aboriginal and Torres Strait Islander mental health are emphasized in this chapter. While they are clearly a population with significant unmet mental health needs, health planners are pulled between two fundamental demands. On the one hand is the imperative to address underlying social justice issues. On the other is the pressing need for programs and services to address problems that, in some instances (such as Indigenous suicide), are increasing alarmingly.

> Big brown eyes, little dark Australian boy
> Playing with a broken toy.
> This environment his alone,
> This is where a seed is sown.
> Can this child at the age of three
> Rise above this poverty?
> The walls all cracked and faded, bare.
> The glassless window stare and stare
> Like the half-dead eyes of a dying race
> A sad but strange, compelling place.
> (Davis, 1988)

In his poem, 'Slum Dwelling', Jack Davis poses a question that should be considered by all Australians as an issue not only of social justice but national social responsibility. It is now 30 years since the Commonwealth Referendum of 1967 which provided for de facto 'citizenship' by including Aborigines and Torres Strait Islanders in national census enumerations and allowing for the Commonwealth to legislate in Aboriginal affairs. Unfortunately, much of the Indigenous optimism of those heady days of protest and planning has evaporated in the face of persistent disadvantage. The issue of social justice remains as relevant as ever, emphasized in the late 1980s by the Royal Commission into Aboriginal Deaths in Custody (1991), which focused national attention on the social issues underlying the massive overrepresentation of Aborigines and Torres Strait Islanders in the criminal justice system. A decade later, social justice issues have again been raised with the release of the report of the Human Rights and Equal Opportunity Commission's Inquiry into the Separation of Aboriginal and Torres Strait Islander Children from their Families – 'Bringing them Home' (1997). The Commission examined the history of state-sanctioned intrusion into Indigenous cultural and family life, including the abduction of children to dormitories and foster care, that stopped only recently. It has also begun the long overdue debate on compensation for such systematic injustice.

However, at the same time Australia has been shaken from its postwar social complacency about its relationship with Indigenous and immigrant Australians by the reemergence of right wing political extremism and the prospect of a national election fought on issues of race. Is this coincidence? Whether it is or not, the political climate is clearly consequential for Indigenous affairs and for Indigenous health. When the current Commonwealth government came to power in 1996, one of the first areas targeted for significant funding cuts was Aboriginal affairs. While the health budget was supposedly protected from these cuts, at the end of March 1997 funding for the peak Commonwealth Indigenous agency, the Aboriginal and Torres Strait Islander Commission (ATSIC), was reduced by Aus$440m over three years, amounting to 11% of its operating budget, functionally eliminating, among many others, its community and youth support programs. This further consolidates the problem focus in Indigenous mental health promotion and prevention activities, erasing almost all of what could have been conceived as investments in Indigenous social and emotional wellbeing.

The medical profession's responses to these developments have been, at best, modest. This cannot be attributed to ignorance of the health and circumstances of Aboriginal and Torres Strait Islanders. Most Australian health professionals are now aware of the deplorable health status and entrenched disadvantage experienced by Indigenous populations. In terms of morbidity, mortality, life expectancy, injury, suicide, violence, unemployment, adult and juvenile arrest, incarceration, school retention, substitute care, substance use, adolescent pregnancy, and fetal and infant growth, the health statistics for Australia's Aboriginal and Torres Strait Islander population are uniformly dismal. However, fewer health professionals are aware that not only are these statistics all significantly worse than those for non-Indigenous Australians, but they are also substantially worse than those for indigenous populations living in similar settings elsewhere in the world.

Steven Kunitz (1994) has explored this issue, comparing the rates of morbidity and mortality for indigenous populations in areas of, 'Anglo settler colonialism' (Canada, the USA, New Zealand and Australia). Although there are common features in the patterns of morbidity and mortality across those groups, Australian Aborigines are distinguished by having the worst health status according to almost every measure. A number of correlates emerged in his analysis. Health is worse where no formal treaty has been concluded between the colonizing and indigenous populations, and worse where states and provinces retain responsibility for Indigenous health rather than federal or national governments. In Australia, no credible treaty was ever concluded with indigenous populations, and health has functionally remained the responsibility of States. Ironically, in the nation with the least equitable system of health care for the population as a whole, the USA, indigenous health is comparatively best. By contrast, in Australia, where health care resource allocation is probably least inequitable, Indigenous health is worst. Kunitz (1994) points to the disadvantage of the underprivileged in accessing resources even on a 'level playing field', emphasizing the importance in the USA of a well resourced national program, the Indian Health Service, which specifically addresses the needs of that disadvantaged population – regardless of the slope of the playing field. Meanwhile, as the gap between Indigenous and non-Indigenous longevity elsewhere is narrowing, in Australia it is stagnant, and in some cases it is widening, for instance in the gap between the longevity of Torres Strait Islander women and women nationally.

In terms of Aboriginal and Torres Strait Islander mental health, social disadvantage both undermines wellbeing and compromises the capacity of Indigenous populations to access services or to benefit, as have non-Indigenous Australians, from the health promotion initiatives of recent decades. Adequacy of services is more than providing culturally appropriate services, or assuring physical access. It requires introducing social justice into consideration of resource allocation. In this regard, McDermott, Plant & Mooney (1996, p. 598) have addressed the problems of conceptualizing 'access' and 'need', making the point that, 'these constructs are concerned normally only with horizontal equity (the equal treatment of equals) and not with vertical equity (the unequal treatment of unequals)'. In terms of Indigenous Australia, even this service baseline will require massive additional resources (Tsey & Scrimgeour, 1996) – particularly in such unaddressed areas as Aboriginal and Torres Strait Islander child mental health.

After decades of neglect there is now, fortunately, significant professional interest in the field of Indigenous mental health. Despite the national political tensions in Indigenous affairs, there are the beginnings of a constructive dialogue between Indigenous consumers and mental health professionals, both non-Indigenous and Indigenous. This modest achievement has been realized neither quickly nor easily. Having previously been relegated to the status of silent subjects, Aboriginal and Torres Strait Islander people now contest non-Indigenous theories of Indigenous 'mental health', and have developed holistic hypotheses that combine traditional and appropriated elements (Hunter, 1997). In contrast to the orientation of mainstream mental health systems towards illness, Indigenous workers and critics emphasize the need to support social and emotional wellbeing. Considerations of supporting wellbeing – what might be called mental health public health – must contend with the immediacy of need and the enormity of background social and physical problems in Indigenous communities which blur distinctions between physical and mental health. Indeed, all the major causes of increased Indigenous mortality and morbidity are behavior and thus socio-environmental factors: cardiovascular diseases caused by poor exercise, diet and by smoking, respiratory diseases caused by smoking and alcohol, and accidents and injuries attributed to alcohol. In settings of limited (and contested) resources, the residents have a compromised ability to respond to conventional health promotion interventions. As Spark, Donovan & Howat (1991, p. 11) point out, 'Educational interventions are generally based on the premise that the physical and social environment will support the behavioural changes desired. In the case of remote Aboriginal communities however, the environment frequently inhibits the adoption of the desired changes.'

Indeed, effective interventions for such disadvantaged populations are further compromised by the medicalization of complex social problems, resulting in a focus on risk factors (those factors proximately associated with a particular problem) rather than risk conditions (those conditions of social disadvantage that underlie and predispose) (Hawe, Noort, King & Jordens, in press). The negative consequences of this are most significant for those with the greatest burden of risk – they are at risk both because of their social disadvantage and because they are least likely to benefit from downstream interventions targeted at risk factors. In a financially restricted health system increasingly calling for program 'accountability', disadvantage may be amplified because of the requirement to demonstrate measurable outcomes. Hawe and colleagues (in press) comment that, 'those programs about which we have the strongest evidence for effect, may result in further health inequities. This is because innovative interventions for disadvantaged and minority groups are generally not included among programs considered to have best evidence for effectiveness.'

Clearly, Aboriginal and Torres Strait Islander communities present mental health planners with a complex topography of unmet need. Confronted with the defining social landmarks of this terrain – poverty, overcrowding, unemployment, dismal educational outcomes, etc. – planners must consider the relative priorities they give to addressing underlying social injustice versus improving services. The ethical dimensions of these considerations must be considered, but should not preclude practical action (Hunter & Garvey, in press). As Syme (1997, p. 9) notes, 'insisting only on fundamental and revolutionary social change is dooming us to programs that will take years and generations to take effect. Since it is difficult to implement such major social change, it is easy to ignore inequalities because, they say, nothing can realistically be done about them. Moral outrage about inequalities is appropriate but may be self-indulgent. If we really want to change the world we may have to begin in more modest but practical ways'.

Clearly, it will require both significant social change and immediate pragmatism to effectively address the burden of disadvantage and ill-health experienced by the Indigenous population of Australia. The needs are urgent, not only because of the scale of the problems, which is substantial, but because the situation is, in some very real respects, deteriorating. In the cross-cultural analysis of Kunitz described above, I noted that the measures of Aboriginal and Torres Strait Islander ill-health are worse by almost every conceivable measure – but not all. One notable exception is suicide. The indigenous populations of North America have had elevated suicide rates for many decades, leading the Royal Commission on Aboriginal Peoples (1995) to prepare a special report on suicide in Canadian Aboriginal populations. The Commission found the suicide rate to be two to three times higher among indigenous populations and five to six times higher among Aboriginal youth than among their non-Aboriginal peers. That is somewhat higher than in Australia. However, data from the Australian Institute for Suicide Research and Prevention demonstrates that for the period 1990–1996 in the State of Queensland the suicide rate for Indigenous males was twice that for the non-Indigenous population, and the rate for those aged 15 to 29 was nearly four times higher. This is particularly alarming as up until the 1980s, suicide in Aboriginal populations was extremely uncommon (Hunter, 1993).

We in Australia should take note of the clear parallels with the Canadian experience. The Commissioners there concluded that patterns of self-harm result from, 'a complex mix of social, cultural, economic and psychological dislocations that flow from the past into the present'. In their view, 'suicide is one of a group of symptoms, ranging from truancy and law-breaking to alcohol and drug abuse and family violence, that are in large part interchangeable as expressions of the burden of loss, grief and anger experienced by Aboriginal people in Canadian society' (Royal Commission on Aboriginal Peoples, 1995, p. 2). Furthermore, the Commissioners addressed the same issues of social justice versus practical action that have been raised earlier in this chapter, noting that:

An adequate response cannot be limited either to crisis services in the absence of long-term family and community supports, or to narrowly focused suicide prevention programs without reference to the web of related social problems in which communities may be caught. An adequate response to suicide must entail an overall healing strategy. It must speak to the many forms taken by self-destructive behavior in Aboriginal communities and to its underlying causes. It is not enough to treat desperate individuals and the immediate sources of their despair – although such treatment must be the starting point of a comprehensive suicide prevention strategy.

As well, Aboriginal people must gain the means to address long-standing needs of families and communities and to redress the imbalance of power between themselves and other Canadians from which so much distress flows. (Royal Commission on Aboriginal Peoples, 1995, p. 2)

Ultimately, addressing underlying social injustice and achieving reconciliation between the Indigenous and non-Indigenous populations of this nation will necessarily involve all Australians. Mental health professionals and health planners may both facilitate that process, and help Aboriginal and Torres Strait Islander communities find solutions to the pressing problems of daily existence, by collaborating rather than imposing. They will serve their purposes best by ensuring that social justice for indigenous Australians is prioritized on the national political agenda while, at the same time, providing expertise and energy to the development of innovative solutions to the problems of the moment. To this end, they should strive to resist fatalism and to maintain optimistic about what can be achieved. They might well take a lesson from Indigenous Australians who have sustained hope in the face of over two centuries of oppression in which were sown seeds of anger and despair. At the beginning of this chapter I suggested that Jack Davis's poem presents a challenge rather than simply a statement. Can individual Indigenous children rise above the adversity of their surroundings? Of course they can, Jack Davis and many others demonstrate that. But that is not the point. In Australia this amount of adversity leveled against a population is unique – 'This environment his alone' – only Indigenous Australians can anticipate that most of their children will experience such circumstances. And Davis is very clear about responsibility – the Aboriginal child of three is an 'Australian boy' – it is an Australian story and an Australian responsibility.

References

Davis, J. (1988). Slum Dwelling. In K. Gilbert (ed.), *Inside Black Australia*, Sydney: Penguin Books Australia.

Hawe, P., Noort, M., King, L. & Jordens, C. (in press). Multiplying health gains: the critical role of capacity-building within health promotion programs. *Health Policy*.

Human Rights and Equal Opportunity Commission (1997). *Bringing them Home: Report of the National Inquiry into the Separation of Aboriginal and Torres Strait Islander Children from Their Families*. Canberra: Australian Government Publishing Service.

Hunter, E. (1993). *Aboriginal Health and History: Power and Prejudice in Remote Australia*. Melbourne: Cambridge University Press.

Hunter, E. (1997). Double talk: changing constructions in Indigenous mental health. *Australian and New Zealand Journal of Psychiatry*, **31**, 820–7.

Hunter, E. & Garvey, D. (in press). Mind over matter? Indigenous mental health promotion. *Australian Journal of Health Promotion*.

Kunitz, S.J. (1994). *Disease and Social Diversity: The European Impact on the Health of non-Europeans.* New York: Oxford.

McDermott, R.A., Plant, A.J. & Mooney, G. (1996). Has access to hospital improved for Aborigines in the Northern Territory? *Australian and New Zealand Journal of Public Health,* **20**, 589–93.

Royal Commission into Aboriginal Deaths in Custody (1991). *Final Report.* Canberra: Australian Government Publishing Service.

Royal Commission on Aboriginal Peoples (1995). *Choosing Life: Special Report on Suicide among Aboriginal People.* Ottawa: Canada Communication Group.

Spark, R., Donovan, R.J. & Howat. P. (1991). Promoting health and preventing injury in remote Aboriginal communities: a case study. *Health Promotion Journal of Australia,* **1**, 10–16.

Syme, S.L. (1997). Individual vs. community interventions in public health practice: Some thoughts about a new approach. *Health Promotion Matters,* **2**, 2–9.

Tsey, K. & Scrimgeour, D. (1996). The funder-purchaser-provider model and Aboriginal health care provision. *Australian and New Zealand Journal of Public Health,* **20**, 661–4.

25

Health systems research: a pragmatic model for meeting mental health needs in low-income countries

Vikram Patel

Summary

Mental illness is now recognized as an important cause of morbidity and disability worldwide. In particular, health priorities in low-income countries will need to achieve a balance between communicable and noncommunicable diseases, as alarming rates of depression, problem drinking and other mental disorders are reported in epidemiological surveys. Psychiatric research across different societies has polarized into two schools of thought. The universalist school prescribes that mental disorders are fundamentally the same everywhere and that epidemiological studies can ultimately lead to a body of information for local health workers on how to respond to mental health needs. The cultural relativist school argues that mental disorders are so influenced by culture that research must be conducted within specific cultures in order to make it valid and meaningful to local health workers.

The author argues that neither pole of research has made any significant impact on the understanding of mental disorders by general health workers in low-income countries because of the uneven emphasis placed on either biology or culture. On the other hand, health systems research (HSR) offers a pragmatic model for investigating worldwide mental health problems because of its recognition that mental illness and mental health care are profoundly influenced not only by culture and biology but by the complex interaction of numerous social, political, economic, historical and health service related factors, that is the various components of the health system.

The unique features of HSR, which are rarely incorporated in previous models of research, include: its multidisciplinary nature; the use of a problem-oriented approach as opposed to complex classification systems heavily biased towards European and American nosologies; the focus on locally generated priorities as opposed to multinational agendas; its participatory methodology; the evaluation of its effectiveness on the basis of its impact on health service changes or health worker training changes; and the dissemination of findings in varied, community-friendly formats.

A significant advantage of the HSR approach is that there are likely to be far fewer types of health systems worldwide than there are different cultures. The concept of 'families of health systems' is explored as a way of determining similarities between the health systems of apparently different cultures, and the differences between the health systems of apparently similar cultures. The Primary Mental Health Care Project in Harare, Zimbabwe, is briefly described as an example of HSR in mental health.

Introduction

Mental illness is recognized as one of the commonest and most disabling of all noncommunicable disorders in low-income countries. Meeting the needs of millions in such countries is a complex and difficult task which must take into account the diverse influences which affect the delivery of mental health care, such as the limited extent of health services, poor awareness and associated stigma of mental illness, and economic changes that further restrict resources for the social sector and lead to dramatic changes in income and income inequality. Research offers a useful approach for determining key questions, such as who is most in need of existing health services?; what factors lead to mental illness and how can they be ameliorated?; how can existing health services respond to the needs of the mentally ill?; and what new avenues of development are needed in the health services to meet needs? Arguably, the enormous diversity within and between low-income countries means that research and programs which may be relevant in one region may not necessarily be applicable in another. Despite the growing mountain of research carried out in a variety of settings in low-income countries since the 1970s, the goal of meeting the needs of millions of those with mental health problems remains a distant one. This situation is, at least in part, accounted for by the models adopted in psychiatric research. While these have generated a great deal of academic interest and many scientific publications, they have had a limited impact on the way mental health problems are recognized or managed by communities and primary health services in low-income countries. Indeed, in most countries, mental illness remains a very low priority for health workers, community health programs, policy makers, and funding agencies. This chapter examines the existing models of research and proposes an alternative model, the health systems research (HSR) model, as a way of understanding and meeting the mental health needs of communities in diverse regions in the low-income world. The chapter concludes with a brief account of the Primary Mental Health Care Project in Harare as an example of a research initiative which uses the HSR model.

The etic-emic debate: time to move on?

Research on world mental health problems has followed one of three related methodologies. The 'universalist' or 'etic' approach places singular emphasis on diagnostic groups of mental disorders and the accuracy of diagnostic methods. The process of psychiatric diagnosis begins with the patients' presenting complaints. The health worker then obtains the symptoms and clarifies patterns amongst the complaints and symptoms which lead to the identification of syndromes or clusters of symptoms. In the absence of any reliable physiological, biochemical or anatomical marker for any functional psychiatric disorder, diagnosis ends at the syndromal stage. Diagnostic criteria for syndromes can and do change over time, as is well demonstrated by the regular revisions of international psychiatric classifications; these revisions are considerably influenced by attitudinal, political, and historical factors (Westermeyer, 1985). Historically, universalist studies have suffered several problems. First, case-identification techniques varied from site to site and methods were not standardized. These inconsistencies led to a movement to standardize the process of psychiatric measurement and diagnosis. Standardized interviews that mimic the clinical psychiatric evaluation were developed and have become the criteria for determining 'caseness' in epidemiological investigations. After standardizing the interview schedules in Euro-American cultures, the interviews were subsequently used in other cultures. Most of these subsequent cross-cultural psychiatric investigations relied on implicit, largely untested assumptions: (1) the universality of mental illnesses, implying that regardless of cultural variations, disorders as described in Euro-American classifications occur everywhere; (2) invariance, implying that the core features of psychiatric syndromes are invariant; and (3) validity, implying that although refinement is possible, the diagnostic categories of current classifications are valid clinical constructs (Beiser, Cargo & Woodbury, 1994).

The universalist approach takes the view that mental illness is similar throughout the world, and therefore psychiatric taxonomies, their measuring instruments and models of health care are also globally applicable. There are two dominant systems of psychiatric classification, the ICD and the DSM, which reflect the psychiatric nosologies of Euro-American medicine. These classifications have considerably influenced the practice of psychiatry throughout the world and have virtually become, somewhat inappropriately, textbooks of psychiatry for many low-income countries (Littlewood, 1992). The World Health Organization (WHO) epidemiological studies have used the ICD system of categorizing mental disorders and psychiatric measures developed by Euro-American researchers and are therefore examples of the etic approach.

Problems with the universalist approach arose when cross-cultural researchers pointed out that there was risk of confounding culturally distinctive behavior with psychopathology on the basis of superficial similarities of behavior patterns or phenomena in different cultures. It was argued that the classification of psychiatric disorders largely reflected American and European concepts of psychopathology based on implicit cultural concepts of normality and deviance (Kirmayer, 1989). Some argued that cross-cultural psychiatry should examine the influence of culture itself on mental illness in Euro-American societies, rather than assume that these illnesses are 'natural' and free of any cultural bias (Murphy, 1977). Critics accused the universalist approach of contributing to a worldview which 'privileges biology over culture' (Eisenbruch, 1991) and of ignoring the cultural and social contexts of psychiatric disorders.

The field of medical anthropology has exerted a growing influence on health research, particularly in low-income countries. This influence has seen a shift in paradigms in public health and epidemiology from their unifocal and positivist 'scientific' approach to the recognition that illness is the result of a 'web of causation' which includes the individual's socio-cultural environment (Heggenhougen & Draper, 1990). Medical anthropology was one of the key factors that fuelled the development of the 'emic' approach in cross-cultural psychiatry. At a general level this approach argues that the culture-bound aspects of biomedicine, such as its emphasis on individual medical diseases, limit its universal applicability (Helman, 1991). The emic approach proposed to evaluate phenomena from within a culture and its contexts, aiming to understand its significance and relationship with other elements of that culture. Examples of such studies are more likely to be found in anthropological and social science literature. Studies of community attitudes to mental illness, indigenous classifications of illness and the traditional treatments of mental illness are examples of the emic approach, since they use open-ended unstructured interviews with local informants and aim to describe the local models of illness without imposing Euro-American psychiatric diagnoses on the illness states. Purely emic studies have also drawn their share of criticism, the most fundamental being that they are unable to provide data that can be compared across cultures (Mari, Sen & Cheng, 1989). These studies are usually small in scale and are unable to resolve questions of the long-term course and treatment outcome of an illness (Kirmayer, 1989). The reliability and validity of emic studies are in doubt because of the lack of standardized research methods and the bias introduced by individual researcher's interpretations of their findings. The emic approach has been criticized for not suggesting plausible alternatives, such as a set of principles that would help ensure cultural sensitivity, or models upon which to fashion culturally sensitive nosologies. It is argued that culture is not a static concept; all cultures are constantly evolving and changing and with the increasing influence of Euro-American values and urbanization in many low-income societies, 'traditional' beliefs may not be as rigidly held as is supposed. Furthermore, individuals may have many ideas about their illness, any or all of which may change with time.

Despite the limitations of the etic and emic approaches, they have both contributed immensely to psychiatric theory and epidemiology. For example, the etic approach has proven beyond doubt the existence of most major groups of mental disorders in all cultures, while the emic approach has demonstrated convincingly the powerful influence of cultural beliefs on the way mental health services are used. The etic–emic debate, which has been extensively covered by other authors (Kleinman, 1987; Littlewood, 1990), started the notion that a 'new' cross-cultural psychiatry was needed in which the emphasis lay not on biomedical categories but on the varying contexts of mental illness in different cultures. It was persuasively argued that psychiatric epidemiology needs to blend ethnographic and quantitative techniques, and that symptom-based measures of morbidity derived from local idioms are likely to be more valuable than interviews based on complex biomedical classifications. The new cross-cultural approach has been adopted by numerous authors when describing mental illness in different cultures. It includes the development of assessment measures based on local idioms, such as the Chinese Health Questionnaire (Cheng & Williams, 1986) and the Shona Symptom Questionnaire (Patel, Simunyu, Gwanzura, Lewis & Mann, 1997).

Despite the various merits of existing research, most of the etic, emic and the integrative research studies have had limited impact on the practice of health workers and on the care of those suffering from mental disorders. For example, the author's experience with a depression education program conducted by the City of Harare Health Department revealed that the program led to virtually no change in the recognition of depressive illness in primary care attenders. This example from Zimbabwe showed that nurses were unwilling to use the term depression because its link to mental illness made it stigmatizing, and they were reluctant to diagnose depression because of the lack of staff in primary care clinics, and the lack of convincing data on the management of depression from their health system (Patel, 1996). It is clear that neither culture nor biomedical entities were the only, or indeed even the main, factors that determined the usefulness of mental health research. Indeed, it would be reasonable to argue that by focusing on methodologies that emphasize either biological or cultural variables, or both, mental health problems remain little understood, awareness amongst the community, health policy makers and general health practitioners remains low, and its prioritization by health funders and policy makers a remote objective. Above all, the vast majority of those suffering from mental illness in developing countries remain untreated or treated inappropriately, even though there have been substantial advances recently in psychiatric treatments. One of the key reasons for this failure to link research findings to

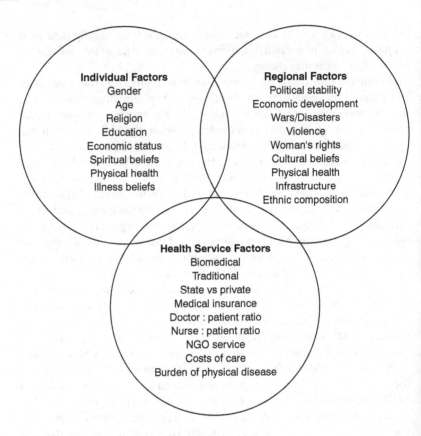

Figure 25.1 Examples of variables that define a health system.

appropriate health service changes is, in the view of this author, the lack of recognition of the profound role played by the health system in the presentation and management of mental disorders.

The health system

A health system has been defined as consisting of three key components: the beliefs about health and illness which influence health-seeking behavior; the health care services in the region; and the socioeconomic, geographical, and political context of those beliefs and institutions. Examples of the main types of variables which together describe the health system are shown in Figure 25.1.

The vast majority of psychiatric research measures only biological or cultural variables. The health system is regarded as being independent.

However, there is abundant evidence from studies of both somatic and psychological illnesses that the system probably plays the most crucial role in explaining the prevalence of diseases and the implementation of successful interventions. Take the case of tuberculosis. Tuberculosis, at the turn of the twentieth century, was very common in Europe, yet it is relatively rare today. This, a classic 'biological' disease, was successfully treated through a combination of new antibiotics, public health interventions to reduce overcrowding and improve hygiene, and sustainable development which brought an increase in living standards of all sections of society, all of which had its basic foundation on an enlightened political leadership and an investment in public health. Despite the availability of antibiotics in low-income countries, tuberculosis is a major killer, not because the cultural beliefs or the biology of the illness are necessarily different, but because the system is entirely different. More recently, the greatest impact of HSR on public health research in low-income countries has been in the area of sexual health and sexually transmitted diseases, particularly acquired immunodeficiency syndrome (AIDS). The literature on this subject is a classic reminder that, even though AIDS is an infectious disease, as is tuberculosis, the key factors influencing its etiology, diagnosis, management and health service implications are those which are defined by the health system. If such biologically well-defined diseases are so profoundly influenced by the health systems in which they occur, then it is clear that the influence of health systems on the ill-defined and multifactorial psychiatric disorders is even greater.

Families of health systems

The health systems model recognizes that different cultures may share a similar health system while similar cultures may have widely different health systems. An example of the former would be the rural health systems of Zimbabwe and those of India, while an example of the latter would be the urban and rural health systems of India. Indeed, in a nation as vast and varied as India, the very notion of a single Indian 'culture' is utterly false. Instead, India may be viewed as a cohesion of several different health systems. The variation in health services, beliefs, political will, women's rights, literacy and other demographic variables is so enormous that to lump India into one category is as fallacious as lumping Africa into a single category – while recognizing that some parts of London are quite different from others! For example, whereas antenatal coverage and infant mortality in some Indian states such as Goa and Kerala are similar to those of countries in Southern Europe, the statistics for the northern states of Bihar and Uttar Pradesh are worse than those of some of the poorest countries in Africa (International Institute for Population Sciences, 1995). The doctor:patient ratio, the awareness of psychiatric disorders, the availability of psychiatric services and the nature of the stigma attached to these vary enormously; most often, it is not the culture per se but the overall economic and educational level of the society which determines these factors.

This does not mean that each health system needs to conduct its own research on every topic. Indeed, it is likely that there are far fewer types of health systems than individual cultures. Thus, it would be possible to devise *families of health systems*. Each health system may be fitted into the closest model and data from that model may then be used to develop appropriate services. Examples of such families of health systems may include:

1. Urban, industrialized settings with extensive and comprehensive biomedical coverage by insurance/social security, e.g., London, Singapore, Sydney, Toronto.
2. Urban, low-income settings with coexisting public and private medical systems and alternative medical systems, e.g., Bombay, Harare, Rio de Janeiro, Jakarta.
3. Rural, low-income settings with minimal public health services but extensive traditional medical systems and community nongovernmental organizations (NGO) health programs, e.g., parts of rural South Asia, South America and Africa.
4. Areas where the health system has disintegrated, with NGOs being the sole or main health care providers, e.g., war zones.
5. Rural, industrialized country settings, with biomedical and alternative medical practitioners, e.g., parts of Europe and North America.
6. Isolated communities, such as tribes in remote regions of Asia and Africa and islanders of small South Pacific and Caribbean islands.

The above list does not aim to be exhaustive but serves as an example of how the apparent endless diversity of cultures may be more pragmatically approached as a smaller number of health systems within which research and service models may be comparable.

Incorporating HSR in psychiatric research

Varkevisser, Pathmanathan & Brownlee (1991) identify the following guidelines for conducting HSR:

1. It should focus on priority problems.
2. It should be action-oriented, i.e., with a clear aim of developing solutions rather than simply identifying problems.
3. It should adopt an integrated multidisciplinary approach.
4. It should have a participatory nature, involving all concerned parties

from inception to dissemination.

5. Its emphasis should be on simple, short-term research designs that yield practical results relatively quickly.

6. It should emphasize cost-effectiveness, favoring low-cost studies that utilize personnel in the course of their daily activities.

7. It should be disseminated in formats that are useful for administrators, decision-makers and the community.

8. The research should *not* be evaluated on the basis of the number of papers published but on its ability to influence policy, improve services and ultimately lead to better health.

Before examining ways in which HSR can be incorporated into psychiatric research, it is worth considering the extent to which existing research methods conform to HSR principles. Universalist strategies have, to date, been conducted largely by tertiary-care-based psychiatrists or multilateral organizations, most of whom have little contact with community or primary health care. Priorities and objectives reflect the needs of psychiatrists and academics rather than those of the health care providers and patients. Medical pluralism is barely recognized at all; for instance, even though a growing proportion of health care in developing countries is provided by private general practitioners, they are rarely included in either the research phases or the dissemination of findings. Culturally relativist studies tend to recognize the role of traditional medicine in many developing countries. However, these studies tend to be academic investigations by ethnographers with small nonrepresentative samples. In neither methodology is there much involvement of health policy makers or primary health workers, nor is there any attempt to disseminate the findings other than through academic journals, most of which are not read in developing countries. There is rarely a follow-up evaluation of the impact of the findings on health service changes, community awareness or changes in the care received by those suffering from mental illness.

HSR can be incorporated into psychiatric research in the following ways:

1. *Incorporating a range of health services variables*: an essential component of any epidemiological or health services research is a comprehensive understanding of the variables that define the health system (see Figure 25.1).

2. *Focusing on priority problems*: priorities need to be determined in consultation with local health care providers and community leaders. For example, rather than devising a new interview for newly developed illness categories, health workers may wish to research how best to manage those people who consult repeatedly for commonly recognized psychological disorders. Examples of priorities in various health systems may include the psychological management of depression, bereavement counseling, the management of domestic or other violence, and problem drinking. Treatment

studies are almost nonexistent in low-income countries and remain the cornerstone of a confident intervention program.

3. *Action-oriented research*: 'problem-oriented' research aims to take the priorities of health workers and the local region and from them devise action-oriented research questions. For example, why are women more likely to be depressed? What form of treatment at primary care can help reduce the duration and severity of depressive illness? What are the health service implications of children who drop out of school? What is the impact of postnatal depression on maternal and child health?

4. *Multidisciplinary approach*: academic psychiatrists, particularly in low-income countries, rarely typify mental health care in their societies. Most societies now have a significant private medical sector, particularly general practitioners, most of whom are not involved in psychiatric research. Public health facilities in many countries, particularly in Africa, are manned mainly by nurses who are alienated from biomedically oriented, doctor-led research. Traditional medical practitioners are similarly ignored, even though they may outnumber biomedical health workers even in urban areas. NGOs play an increasingly important role in community and primary health care initiatives in low-income countries. These agencies tend to focus their activities on communities or groups that are particularly disadvantaged or vulnerable. Examples may include refugees fleeing from conflict zones who are likely to have witnessed violent incidents; homeless children; battered women; impoverished urban slum communities; people with serious illnesses such as AIDS; and the physically disabled. It is immediately apparent that many of these groups are the very ones in whom psychological disorders are likely to be more common than in a general population. Rarely does psychiatry take notice of the rich clinical experiences of health workers in these settings, nor do nonpsychiatric health workers take notice of the exciting advances in psychiatric research. The involvement of these myriad groups of health workers is an essential feature of any successful HSR model.

5. *Participatory methodology*: the vast bulk of psychiatric research in low-income countries is conceptualized and designed in isolation from the front line of mental health care. The participatory approach involves working from within the health system, by becoming part of it and intimately familiar with all its components and participants. Thus, research objectives arise out of direct experience and consultations with the users and beneficiaries of the research itself.

6. *Simple, short-term designs*: an emphasis on simple study designs with clearly set out hypotheses which relate to the priorities established earlier. The results should be of practical significance to health care providers and users.

7. *Cost-effectiveness*: it is likely that the least cost-effective type of psychiatric research is the multinational design. In addition to the high costs for

transporting researchers across the globe to various meeting points, this research is far removed from the principles of HSR. These moneys would be far better used by facilitating and supporting individual research programs in different health systems with objectives that reflect their local priorities and emphasize the use of local resources and skills.

8. *Dissemination*: it is imperative that HSR is published in local journals, newspapers and in cheaply produced reports for free circulation to the concerned target audience. In this context, researchers should recognize the far greater impact of lay and popular magazines for disseminating findings to the wider community and broaden the scope of their activities to include advocacy for mental health issues through the popular media.

9. *Evaluation of research*: here, arguably, is the final test of the usefulness of research. Measuring attitudes and practice at various points of a research and development program is one method of evaluating the broader impact of the research on actual health care. The implementation of health policy changes in the direction of the research findings is the most potent marker of the success of an HSR program.

The Primary Mental Health Care Project (PMHC)

This was a three-year project in primary care in Harare, Zimbabwe (Patel, 1998), which is an example of the use of HSR principles in psychiatric research in low-income countries. Before embarking on research, extensive networking and consultations were held with key health providers, policy makers, academics, and NGOs. A multidisciplinary research team which included representatives of all these bodies was constituted and common mental disorders (CMD) identified as the priority area for the PMHC Project. The research went through sequential phases, beginning with an ethnographic description of concepts of CMD held by primary care providers in Harare (Patel, Musara, Maramba & Butau, 1995). The next study used the concepts to elicit symptoms and explanatory models of primary care attenders with conspicuous CMD (Patel, Gwanzura, Simunyu, Mann & Lloyd, 1995). The idioms were collated into a preliminary questionnaire which was evaluated and a 14-item questionnaire based on these idioms developed as a locally valid measure of CMD (Patel, Siminyu, et al., 1997). This questionnaire, the Shona Symptom Questionnaire, was then used in a case–control investigation of the associations and risk factors of CMD in primary care; many of the risk factors were related to local health system variables (Patel, Todd, et al., 1997). The cohorts of cases and controls were reviewed over a 12-month period leading to the first data on the outcome and incidence of CMD in an African setting (Patel et al., 1998; Todd et al., 1999). The key findings of these studies are described in detail in the individual papers cited above.

In summary, the project led to the eliciting of Shona models of illness (supernatural illness; thinking too much) which resemble CMD, and confirmation of this association quantitatively. We were able to demonstrate that the most discriminatory symptoms of CMD are universal, though some, such as perceptual symptoms, may be unique to the setting of the PMHC. We demonstrated the higher prevalence of CMD in attenders of traditional healers as compared to those of primary health care. Being female, older, poorly educated, impoverished and infertile were identified as key risk factors for CMD. CMD persisted in 40% of cases at the 12-month follow-up. Persistence was associated with higher morbidity scores at recruitment, bereavement and a psychological illness model. The onset rate was 16% for new episodes of CMD. Onset was also associated with higher morbidity scores and bereavement; also belief in witchcraft as a cause of illness and economic problems predicted onset. CMD were strongly associated with disability; indeed, synchrony between disability and CMD was noted during follow-up. Similarly, economic problems were associated with the onset and recovery from CMD.

The key methodologies of the PMHC which demonstrate its adherence to the principles of HSR include an academic collaboration between psychiatrists, community medicine and social scientists, the active participation of primary health care nurses, traditional and faith healers, and general practitioners in the research phases, and dissemination of findings through workshops, and the local media (and journals!). The findings of the PMHC had an immediate bearing on the medical curriculum in Zimbabwe; for example, material relating to spiritual distress and other local idioms were used in teaching medical students about CMD. New programs for debt relief and infertility were recommended, as the study indicated that they have the potential to improve mental health in the population. The exchange of information about the roles of different groups of health care providers was facilitated to increase understanding of the purpose of medical pluralism in primary mental health care in Harare city.

Why HSR for mental health?

There is evidence that the prevalence of CMD such as depressive illness is high in many low-income countries. Studies from diverse settings, ranging from rural Lesotho, the slums of Santiago in South America and the urban general practices of India, reveal prevalence figures of CMD exceeding 30% in community samples and approaching 50% in primary care samples (Araya, Robert, Richard & Lewis, 1994; Hollifield, Katon, Spain & Pule, 1990; Shamasundar, Krishna Murthy, Prakash, Prabhakar & Subbakrishna, 1986). If anything, these figures suggest a rising prevalence over the last 30 years of the twentieth century, although variations in case definition and epi-demiological methods in psychiatry make comparisons difficult. The high and potentially rising prevalence of CMD are of concern for many reasons. First, the social factors known to be linked to these disorders are on the increase throughout low-income countries. The formula for economic devel-opment adopted by most countries is leading to a reduction in public health expenditure, a rising inequality between the rich and poor, increased migra-tion to urban areas with its attendant rise in urban squalor and rapid culture change as the great urban centers take on an international, cosmopolitan flavor. Second, there is the much replicated association between CMD and disability independent of any coexisting physical illness. Thus, those who are already vulnerable because of their gender or social circumstances risk be-coming ill with a disorder that will further disable them and render them less able to cope with the adverse circumstances that they already face. Third, despite epidemiological research from both multinational and local research initiatives, most individuals with a CMD remain undiagnosed and untreated.

In addition to CMD, behavioral health problems, ranging from problem drinking to domestic violence to the impact of war and violence on commu-nities, are of considerable public health significance. Research offers a key opportunity to examine these needs and to offer guidance as to how these may be met within the various constraints that low-income countries face. However, existing methodologies of research, by focusing on disease catego-ries, cultural variables, or both, fail to recognize the crucial role of the health system in influencing the causes of, and potential interventions for, mental illness. HSR provides a practical alternative to the current approaches used when researching mental illness because of its emphasis on a pragmatic, participatory and action-oriented approach to the health issues considered relevant by local health workers.

Leon Eisenberg (1997) wrote that, 'the diseases that afflict men and women are determined by how they live, where they live, with whom they live, what they do and the resources they command,' a definition which is remarkably relevant to health systems. A recent *Lancet* editorial (1997) commented on the need to, 'put public health back into epidemiology' by reorienting the focus of epidemiology towards 'global issues such as war, poverty, and environmental warming and to social aspects of health and disease'. This author agrees entirely with these commentaries; after all, it was changes in the health systems that led to the massive reduction in communicable diseases in industrialized societies, and it is HSR today which is leading the frontline war against the modern epidemics of tuberculosis and AIDS in low-income countries. It is only prudent, therefore, for psychiatric research to reorient its own methods and priorities towards an HSR model in order to meet the mental health needs of low-income countries.

References

Araya, R., Robert, W., Richard, L. & Lewis, G. (1994). Psychiatric morbidity in primary health care in Santiago, Chile. Preliminary findings. *British Journal of Psychiatry*, **165**, 530–2.

Beiser, M., Cargo, M. & Woodbury, M. (1994). A comparison of psychiatric disorder in different cultures: depressive typologies in South-East Asian refugees and resident Canadians. *International Journal of Methods in Psychiatric Research*, **4**, 157–72.

Cheng, T.A. & Williams, P. (1986). The design and development of a screening questionnaire (CHQ) for use in community studies of mental disorders in Taiwan. *Psychological Medicine*, **16**, 415–22.

Eisenberg, L. (1997). A very British kind of social psychiatry. *British Journal of Psychiatry*, **171**, 309–13.

Eisenbruch, M. (1991). From post-traumatic stress disorder to cultural bereavement: diagnosis of Southeast Asian refugees. *Social Science and Medicine*, **33**, 673–80.

Heggenhougen, K. & Draper, A. (1990). *Medical Anthropology and Primary Health Care*. EPC Publication No. 22. London: London School of Hygiene and Tropical Medicine.

Helman, C. (1991). Limits of biomedical explanation. *Lancet*, **337**, 1080–2.

Hollifield, M., Katon, W., Spain, D. & Pule, L. (1990). Anxiety and depression in a village in Lesotho, Africa: a comparison with the United States. *British Journal of Psychiatry*, **156**, 343–50.

International Institute for Population Sciences (1995). *National Family Health Survey (MCH and Family Planning), India 1992-3*. Bombay: IIPS.

Kirmayer, L.J. (1989). Cultural variations in the response to psychiatric disorders and emotional distress. *Social Science and Medicine*, **29**, 327–39.

Kleinman, A. (1987). Anthropology and psychiatry: the role of culture in cross-cultural research on illness. *British Journal of Psychiatry*, **151**, 447–54.

Littlewood, R. (1990). From categories to contexts: a decade of the 'New Cross-Cultural Psychiatry'. *British Journal of Psychiatry*, **156**, 308–27.

Littlewood, R. (1992). DSM-IV and culture: is the classification internationally valid? *Psychiatric Bulletin*, **16**, 257–61.

Mari, J., Sen, B. & Cheng, T.A. (1989). Case definition and case identification in cross-cultural perspective. In P. Williams, G. Wilkinson, & K. Rawnsley (eds.), *The Scope of Epidemiological Psychiatry*, pp. 489–508. London: Routledge.

Murphy, H.B.M. (1977). Transcultural psychiatry should begin at home. *Psychological Medicine*, **7**, 369–71.

Patel, V. (1996). Recognising common mental disorders in primary care in African countries: should 'mental' be dropped? *Lancet*, **347**, 742–4.

Patel, V. (1998). *Culture and Common Mental Disorders in Sub-Saharan Africa: Studies in Primary Care in Zimbabwe* (Maudsley Monograph). Hove: Psychology Press.

Patel, V., Gwanzura, F., Simunyu, E., Mann, A. & Lloyd, K. (1995). The explanatory models and phenomenology of common mental disorder in Harare, Zimbabwe. *Psychological Medicine*, **25**, 1191–9.

Patel, V., Musara, T., Maramba, P. & Butau, T. (1995). Concepts of mental illness and medical pluralism in Harare. *Psychological Medicine*, **25**, 485–93.

Patel, V., Simunyu, E., Gwanzura, F., Lewis, G. & Mann, A. (1997). The Shona Symptom Questionnaire: the development of an indigenous measure of non-psychotic mental disorder in Harare. *Acta Psychiatrica Scandinavica*, **95**, 469–75.

Patel, V., Todd, C.H., Winston, M., Gwanzura, F., Simunyu, E., Acuda, S.W. & Mann, A. (1997). Common mental disorders in primary care in Harare, Zimbabwe: associations and risk factors. *British Journal of Psychiatry*, **171**, 60–4.

Patel, V., Todd, C.H., Winston, M., Gwanzura, F., Simunyu, E., Acuda, S.W. & Mann, A. (1998). The outcome of common mental disorders in Harare, Zimbabwe. *British Journal of Psychiatry*, **172**, 53–7.

Shamasundar, C., Krishna Murthy, S., Prakash, O., Prabhakar, N. & Subbakrishna, D. (1986). Psychiatric morbidity in a general practice in an Indian city. *British Medical Journal*, **292**, 1713–15.

The Lancet (1997). Putting Public Health back into epidemiology. *Lancet*, **350**, 229.

Todd, C., Patel, V., Simunyu, E., Gwanzura, F., Acuda, S.W., Winston, M. & Mann, A. (1999). The onset of common mental disorders in primary care attenders in Harare, Zimbabwe. *Psychological Medicine*, **29**, 97–104.

Varkevisser, C.M., Pathmanathan, I. & Brownlee, A. (1991). *Designing and Conducting Health Systems Research Projects*; Volume 2, Part 1: *Proposal Development & Fieldwork*. Ottawa: IDRC; Geneva: WHO.

Westermeyer, J. (1985). Psychiatric diagnosis across cultural boundaries. *American Journal of Psychiatry*, **142**, 798–805.

26

Disablement associated with chronic psychosis as seen by two groups of key informants: patients and mental health professionals

Charles B. Pull, Arnaud Sztantics, Steve Muller,
Jean Marc Cloos, and Jean Reggers

Summary

Since the early 1980s, a number of surveys have attempted to assess public attitudes to alcohol, drug and mental (ADM) disorders. In most instances, the investigations have focused on finding out the extent of acceptance and rejection of patients with ADM disorders or on the factors that shape these attitudes.

Some of the attitudes relate to patients and their disorders, while others relate to culture. Prominent among the former are the type of disorder and diagnostic labeling (Angermeyer & Matschinger, 1996a), perceived dangerousness, and the severity of disturbance in behavior (Nieradzik & Cochrane, 1985). Prominent among the latter are the age and education of the respondents (Trute, Tefft & Segall, 1989), their personal and social involvement (Ramon, 1979), social relations and social responsibility (Trute et al., 1989), personal experience of mental disorders (Angermeyer & Matschinger, 1996b, 1997), having or not having children (Bowen, Twemlow & Boquet, 1978), being an expert in psychiatry or being a member of the lay public (Angermeyer & Matschinger, 1994).

The present study is not concerned primarily with attitudes towards people who have an ADM disorder, but with the opinions concerning the *disablement* that accompanies such disorders. Two groups of key informants, i.e., a group of patients with an ADM disorder and a group of mental health professionals, were asked their opinion about what people in their society – in this case the country of Luxembourg – think and do when they are confronted with a person who suffers from the consequences of schizophrenia or another chronic psychotic disorder.

The study is part of an ongoing multicenter WHO study examining the consistency of the disablement construct in different cultures.

Method

Key informants were defined as people who, by virtue of their position, know about relevant cultural phenomena. We selected people who were considered to be 'cultural informants', and well informed about the disablement associated with ADM disorders. The patient group included individuals with an ADM disorder that had been present for at least five years and was in either full or partial remission. Patients were selected from the inpatient and outpatient psychiatric units of a general hospital. Patients had to be able to fully understand the language and content of the questionnaire and to be capable of responding to the questions. Mental health professionals were selected to represent the major groups of professionals as well as institutions and organizations working in the field of mental health in Luxembourg. Each of the key informants completed a self-administered questionnaire after being given the following information:

This is a study of how the consequences of having a health condition are thought about and responded to in different places around the world. You are asked to speak for people in your society. We are not asking about what you may know from expert knowledge, nor about your own personal opinions. Rather, we are asking for what you think is true in this society, whether you personally agree with it or not.

In the *first* part of the questionnaire, respondents were given five brief vignettes, each describing a person with a particular health condition. They were asked ten open-ended questions on: specific aspects of that person's behavior that might first attract the attention or notice of others; his/her need for help with daily activities; his/her ability to get a job or get married; as well as his/her entitlement or eligibility regarding assistance from the government. The present study will focus on the answers obtained for the vignette pertaining to people who 'have difficulty with the activities of everyday life because they are bothered by strange thoughts, and sometimes cannot control their actions.'

In the *second* part, respondents were presented with a deck of 17 cards describing different health conditions. They were instructed to rank them from the most disabling to the least disabling condition. The 'most disabling condition' was described as that which would make daily activities very difficult, and the 'least disabling' as that which would not interfere with the activities of everyday life. Thirteen of the 17 conditions were adapted from the 22 indicator conditions used by Murray & Lopez (1996) to measure the burden of disabilities and diseases. One of the conditions included in the list was 'active psychosis', defined as 'being unable to judge what is real such as having delusions, hearing voices, and being unable to speak in clear sentences.'

In the *third* part, the key informants were asked to indicate how surprised people in their culture would be if a person who says that 'there are voices talking to him/her all the time' performed one of ten activities, and how likely it would be that he/she would face barriers or restrictions in attempting to perform such activities.

In the *fourth* part, respondents were asked to give their opinion on the degree of social disapproval or stigma usually encountered by people with various conditions. Participants were asked to use Likert-type scales to assess the level of negative reaction encountered by a person with one of several conditions. The scales ranged from 0 (no social disapproval) to 10 (extreme disapproval). The list of conditions included in particular a condition labeled as chronic mental disorder. Since alcoholism, drug addiction, borderline intelligence, depression and dementia were separately included in the list, the term chronic mental disorder can probably be equated in this instance with chronic psychotic disorder.

The *last* part of the questionnaire pertained to public reaction when people with certain conditions, including various health conditions, appear in public. The six response options were 'people would think there was no issue, and would not pay attention'; 'people would notice, but would not think there was an issue'; 'people would be uneasy about it, but would probably not do anything'; 'people would be uneasy about it and try to avoid the person'; 'people would think it was wrong and might say something about it'; and 'people would think it was wrong and try to stop it.' The six options were subsequently regrouped under the three headings of 'no issue', 'uneasy' and 'wrong'. One of the conditions referred to in this section was chronic mental disorder in a patient who acts out. It is obvious that not all psychotic patients act out and that there are patients with other chronic mental disorders who do. However, given that the concept certainly includes a number of patients with psychosis the results from this section of the questionnaire are also presented in this chapter.

The results were computed for the total group and separately for the patient and the expert group. The significance of differences ($P < 0.01$) between the two groups was determined using chi-squared tests in parts one, three and five; Kruskal–Wallis tests for between-groups effects and Friedman tests for within-group in part two; and multiple one-way analysis of variance (ANOVA) in part four.

Results

A total of 80 key informants, 40 patients with a mental disorder and 40 mental health professionals, completed the questionnaire. Included in the patient group were 13 patients with a psychotic disorder, 15 with a recurrent mood disorder, five with an anxiety disorder, and seven with alcohol or drug dependence. Included in the mental health professionals group were ten medical professionals, ten psychologists and psychiatric nurses, ten social workers and case workers, and ten policy makers or opinion leaders. There were no significant differences between the two groups in terms of age, sex, and years of residence in the country. The two groups did, however, differ in terms of years at school, with the professionals having spent a longer time there than the patients.

The answers from the open-ended questions were grouped according to major similarities in their content. There were no statistically significant differences for any of these questions in the type or frequency of answers provided by professionals and patients.

The first open-ended question was about specific aspects of the person's behavior that might first attract the attention or notice of others. The answers could be related to three major areas of behavior: psychomotor behavior, speech and communication, and physical appearance. Key informants listed aspects of psychomotor behavior (44%), speech or communication (41%), and physical appearance (8%). With the exception of two patients, key informants agreed that a person presenting with psychotic symptoms will attract the attention of others, as soon as the problem is fairly serious. In addition, 87% of the professionals and 77% of the patients mentioned that people with these type of symptoms will attract the attention of others even if their problems are only quite mild.

Abnormalities in psychomotor behavior, physical appearance and speech or communication were listed most frequently as signs that would indicate a person with a psychotic disorder would need help from someone else to do activities of everyday life. Using the same criteria, abnormalities in psychomotor behavior and speech or communication were listed by respectively 65% and 10% of the professionals and 55% and 5% of the patients. Abnormalities in physical appearance were listed significantly more often by professionals (43%) than by patients (15%).

In the opinion of 75% of the professionals and 60% of the patients, the problem would have a major impact on the person's ability to get work. Forty-seven percent of the professionals and 46% of the patients said that the problem would greatly affect the person's ability to get married and have a family. According to the remaining key informants, a fairly serious problem of this sort would have at least some negative effect on the person's ability to get a job or do productive work, as well as to get married and have a family.

When considering the types of problems that a person with psychotic symptoms might experience in his/her daily activities, both professionals and patients list difficulties in interpersonal relationships (55%, 30%), social isolation (43%, 35%), occupational problems (28%, 25%), and problems in basic daily activities (28%, 25%).

About half of the participants (45% of the professionals and 41% of the patients) thought that society would propose government assistance to be implemented for the mentally ill within a year of their problems being noticed. An additional 25% of the professionals and 10% of the patients thought that people in their society would favor social assistance in such cases if the problem lasted more than one year. According to the answers of the remaining key informants (25% of the professionals and 52% of the patients) – subsumed under 'other' – people in their society would favor assistance under certain conditions, e.g., if the problem was chronic or recurrent or if rehabilitation had been tried without success.

According to 51% of the professionals and 65% of the patients, the fact that the person's problem might be related to something he/she had had from birth would have an impact on how others thought of the problem and how the person was regarded. About half of the key informants (43% of the professionals and 50% of the patients) thought that people in their society would more easily accept a problem of this kind if it could be linked to a cause that had been present from birth. Finally, 38% of the professionals and 43% of the patients thought that people in their society would more easily accept a problem of this kind if it could be linked to a road accident. An additional 25% of the key informants said that the problem might be more easily accepted if the person had had no personal responsibility in such an accident.

According to 58% and 55% of the professionals and patients, people in their society would think that a person with this kind of problem should get social assistance from the government if the problem was serious. According to an additional 33% and 20% of professionals and patients, entitlement to social assistance would depend on various factors, such as severity of symptoms or handicaps. Three professionals (8%) and eight patients (20%) considered that people in their society would not favor any kind of assistance in such cases.

There was no significant difference in the way the patients and professionals ordered 17 health conditions, ranked from most disabling to least disabling. Overall, and in either group separately, active psychosis was considered the third most disabling condition, preceded only by quadriplegia and dementia. In particular, active psychosis was considered more disabling, by both professionals and patients, than any other physical disorder included in the list, such as blindness, paraplegia, deafness, or infection with human immunodeficiency virus (HIV), as well as any other ADM disorder such as depression, drug addiction, alcoholism, and mental retardation (Figure 26.1).

Table 26.1 presents the percentage of key informants who think that people would be surprised (or very surprised) if a person hearing voices performed the various activities listed, and that it would be likely (or very likely) that they would face barriers or restrictions in attempting to perform such activities. The majority of patients and professionals responded that people

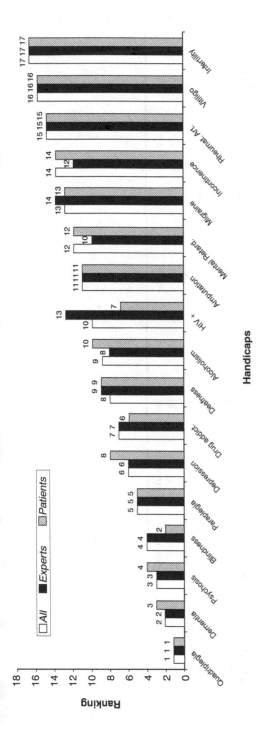

Figure 26.1 Disablement ranks: ordering from the most disabling (lowest rank) to the least disabling (highest rank).

Table 26.1. Percentage responding that those in their culture would be surprised or very surprised if a person hearing voices performed the activity, and percentage responding that barriers and or restrictions would probably or very likely be placed on such a person

Activity	All (n = 80)		Professionals (n = 40)		Patients (n = 40)	
	Surprised	Barriers	Surprised	Barriers	Surprised	Barriers
Keeping things tidy	28	28	30	28	25	28
Using public transportation	18	40	18	43	18	38
Being in love	33	56	40	58	25	55
Having sex (as part of a relationship with someone)	30	59	38	63	23	55
Actively taking on parenting roles	73	92	80	93	65	90
Actively taking part in community fairs and festivals	36	64	33	70	40	58
Managing own money	39	69	38	65	40	73
Getting an apartment or somewhere to live	31	63	38	65	25	60
Keeping a full-time job	58	70	60	68	55	73
Being elected/named to a position in local government	92	95	98	100	85	90

in their culture would be surprised or very surprised if such a person was nominated or elected to a position in local government, kept a full-time job, or took on parenting roles. In both groups, a minority of participants said people would express surprise about such people using public transportation, keeping things tidy, being in love, having sex, actively taking part in community fairs, managing their own money, or getting an apartment. More professionals than patients volunteered that people in their culture would be surprised if such a person was in love, had a sexual relationship with someone, actively took on parenting roles, or got an apartment or somewhere to live, but none of these differences was statistically significant.

With the exception of keeping things tidy and using public transportation, the majority of both professionals and patients volunteered that it was likely that people would place restrictions or barriers on such a person if he or she wanted to perform any of the other activities. In particular, almost all the participants in either group mentioned that it was likely that there would be such restrictions or barriers for being elected to a position in local government, actively taking on parenting roles, managing one's own money, keeping a full-time job, getting an apartment in which to live or even taking part in community affairs. There were no statistically significant differences between the two groups of key informants for any of the items under investigation.

Mean ratings of social disapproval are presented in Table 26.2, for the total sample and separately for the two groups of key informants. Mean ratings for social disapproval show that people who are blind, those in wheelchairs, and those with borderline intelligence are met with the least amount of social disapproval, while those with an alcohol problem, a criminal record for burglary, those who do not take care of their children and those with a drug problem are disapproved of most. Someone labeled as having a chronic mental disorder (and as mentioned earlier, most probably chronic psychotic disorder in this case) received an overall social disapproval rating of 5.62, with a rating of 6.02 from the professionals and 5.24 from the patients. Overall, this rating of social disapproval ranks a person with chronic psychotic disorder with people who cannot hold down a job or who suffer from leprosy or dementia.

Table 26.3 presents the rank order of the mean ratings for public reaction to people with various health conditions appearing in public. In the opinion of both groups of key informants people pay attention when a person with a chronic psychotic disorder appears in public. According to the vast majority of the participants (73%) in either group (80% of the professionals and 67% of the patients), people will feel uneasy when such a person appears in public, for instance on a bus, in a store or a market. In addition, a significant proportion (15%) of the professionals and patients volunteer that people in

Table 26.2. Degree of social disapproval/stigma: ordering from least stigmatized condition (lowest rank) to most stigmatized (highest rank)

Health condition	All (n = 80)			Professionals (n = 40)			Patients (n = 40)		
	Rank	Mean	SD	Rank	Mean	SD	Rank	Mean	SD
Blind	1	1.23	1.68	1	1.03	1.21	2	1.42	2.04
Wheelchair bound	2	1.38	1.84	2	1.47	1.83	1	1.29	1.87
Borderline intelligence	3	3.12	2.28	3	3.03	2.34	3	3.21	2.24
Obese	4	3.16	2.24	4	3.00	1.71	4	3.32	2.66
Depression	5	3.61	2.22	5	3.56	1.98	5	3.66	2.45
Inability to read	6	3.89	2.68	6	3.64	2.59	7	4.13	2.78
Facial disfigurement	7	4.09	2.89	7	4.53	2.91	6	3.68	2.84
Cannot hold down a job	8	5.50	2.11	8	5.61	1.90	10	5.39	2.32
Chronic mental disorder	9	5.62	2.70	10	6.02	2.81	9	5.24	2.56
Leprosy	10	5.76	3.42	9	6.00	3.61	11	5.53	3.25
Dementia	11	5.91	2.98	11	6.14	3.04	8	5.68	2.95
Dirty and unkempt	12	6.69	2.52	12	6.64	2.37	14	6.74	2.69
Homeless	13	6.78	2.81	15	6.92	2.93	13	6.66	2.72
HIV positive	14	6.97	2.59	13	6.64	3.05	12	7.29	2.05
Alcoholism	15	7.70	2.21	14	7.58	2.13	16	7.82	2.30
Criminal record for burglary	16	7.78	2.07	16	8.00	1.93	15	7.58	2.20
Does not take care of their children	17	8.01	2.10	17	8.03	2.08	17	8.00	2.16
Drug addiction	18	8.93	1.66	18	9.22	1.49	18	8.66	1.77

Table 26.3. Percentage responding 'people would think there was *no issue*', 'people would be *uneasy* about it', and 'people would think it was *wrong*' to person with the given health condition appearing in public

Health condition	All (n=80)			Professionals (n=40)			Patients (n=40)		
	No issue	Uneasy	Wrong	No issue	Uneasy	Wrong	No issue	Uneasy	Wrong
A person in a wheelchair	59	41	0	65	35	0	52	48	0
Woman 8 months pregnant	99	0	1	100	0	0	98	0	2
Someone who is blind	68	31	1	63	35	2	73	27	0
A person who is intellectually 'slow'	46	53	1	43	57	0	50	48	2
Someone with a face disfigured by burns	35	59	6	30	63	7	40	55	5
An obese person	76	10	14	78	5	17	75	15	10
Chronic mental disorder	11	73	15	5	80	15	18	67	15
Someone who is dirty and unkempt	10	51	39	12	48	40	8	55	37
Someone who is visibly drunk	4	40	56	0	30	70	8	50	42
Someone who is visibly under the influence of drugs	3	41	56	0	40	60	5	42	53

their society would consider the presence of such patients in public places as 'wrong'.

Discussion

In the present investigation, two groups of key informants were asked to give their opinion on what people in their culture think about a person with chronic psychosis and about how such a disorder affects that person's life. The results show that there are very few significant differences between the answers given by the two groups of key informants. This finding suggests that professionals and patients with an ADM disorder share the same information concerning the way in which such disorders, in particular psychotic disorders, are perceived in their society.

On the whole, the results show that psychotic disorders are viewed as highly disabling by people in Luxembourg. According to professionals and patients, people in Luxembourg would frequently think that a person with this type of disorder is unable to do some of the things a 'normal' person can do, and they might even try to put some restrictions or barriers in place to prevent him or her from doing some activities.

In addition, the results suggest that psychotic disorders continue to be accompanied by a high degree of stigma, since both professionals and patients indicate that people with a psychotic disorder would be an 'issue' in their society, and that he or she would meet with a high degree of social disapproval and negative reaction.

Finally, the results suggest that there still is no parity between people suffering from a physical illness and those presenting with an ADM disorder. In general, people with physical or cognitive disorders and disablements are reported to encounter less stigma and discrimination against social participation than those with ADM disorders, and particularly those with psychotic disorders.

It should be noted that the results may have been influenced by the fact that the participants were not asked to give their personal opinion but to speak for people in their society.

It should also be pointed out that although the composition of the two groups of respondents in this investigation is similar to that of the population of professionals in the field of ADM disorders and of people presenting with an ADM disorder, neither group meets the criteria of a truly representative sample.

Conclusion

The results from this investigation with key informants provide some indication about current opinion on the disablements associated with psychotic disorders. According to mental health professionals and patients with a mental disorder, patients with a psychotic disorder are easily recognized by other people. Their disorder is viewed as a highly disabling condition. Most people consider that such people can barely live independently from other people. They are viewed as being unable to perform most activities of daily life and as requiring considerable social assistance. Other people are likely to place restrictions or barriers on them because of their condition. In addition, most people will feel ill-at-ease in their company and would prefer to avoid them. On the whole, both professionals and patients in this investigation volunteered that the needs of psychotic patients were many and that few of them were currently met by our society.

References

Angermeyer, M.C. & Matschinger, H. (1994). Lay beliefs about schizophrenic disorders: the results of a population survey in Germany. *Acta Psychiatrica Scandinavica, Supplementum*, **382**, 39–45.

Angermeyer, M.C. & Matschinger, H. (1996a). The effect of labelling on the lay theory regarding schizophrenic disorders. *Social Psychiatry and Psychological Epidemiology*, **31**, 316–20.

Angermeyer, M.C. & Matschinger, H. (1996b). Social distance of the population toward psychiatric patients. *Gesundheitswesen, Supplementum*, **1**, 18–24.

Angermeyer, M.C. & Matschinger, H. (1997). Social distance towards the mentally ill: results of representative surveys in the Federal Republic of Germany. *Psychological Medicine*, **27**, 131–4.

Bowen, W.T., Twemlow, S.W. & Boquet, R.E. (1978). Assessing community attitudes toward mental illness. *Hospital and Community Psychiatry*, **29**, 251–3.

Murray, C.J.L. & Lopez, A.D. (eds.) (1996). *The Global Burden of Disease: a Comprehensive Assessment of Mortality and Disability from Diseases, Injuries and Risk Factors in 1990 and Projected to 2020*. Cambridge, MA: Harvard University Press.

Nieradzik, K. & Cochrane, R. (1985). Public attitudes towards mental illness-the effects of behaviour, roles and psychiatric labels. *International Journal of Social Psychiatry*, **31**, 23–3.

Ramon, S. (1979). The meaning attached: attitudes towards the mentally ill. *Mental Health and Society*, **5**, 164–82.

Trute, B., Tefft, B. & Segall, A. (1989). Social rejection of the mentally ill: a replication study of public attitude. *Social Psychiatry and Psychiatric Epidemiology*, **24**, 69–76.

27

The assessment of perceived need

Graham Meadows, Ellie Fossey, Carol Harvey, and
Philip Burgess

Individuals make active decisions in pursuing patient careers, usually with choice as to whether they become consumers. Therefore, perceived need is relevant to an assessment of the dynamics of a service delivery system. The Australian National Survey of Mental Health and Well-Being collected data about these perceptions and decisions, which required a new questionnaire to be devised. This chapter presents something of the history of incorporation of this perspective into needs assessment, then describes the development of the instrument for the Australian Survey.

The major focus of this book is to encourage us to look closely at what constitutes need. We are all preoccupied with the prevalence of mental health disorders in populations. However, estimating prevalence is not the same as quantifying need. There are people who can be diagnosed but do not have mental health needs, and there are people who have needs, but who do not meet criteria for diagnosis. The concept of need has been difficult to define (Johnson, Thornicroft, Phelan & Slade, 1996; Marshall, 1994; Stevens & Gabbay, 1991). The notion of perceived need highlights the subjective and socially negotiated aspects of the nature of need (Slade, 1994a). Perceived need, then, can be seen as being closely linked with perceptions of mental health care, barriers to care, and the prevalence of untreated disorders.

An individual's perceptions of what is appropriate treatment may influence the acknowledgement of a problem. Whilst many of us may feel comfortable with the model of psychiatric care in which a patient comes with a problem, asks for a solution, and trusts advice enough to act upon it, help-seeking may not be predicated on such a model. However, individuals may not seek help from such a professional unless they have some clearly formulated ideas about either the nature of a particular problem, or what help they need. To illustrate, consider the differential use of alternative practitioners and doctors. If a person feels the need for discussion, and some sort of support and intervention to address what they conceive to be an imbalance in their life forces, then this person may be more likely to seek help from an alternative practitioner than from a doctor. Individuals who feel they need medications for their ill-health may be more likely to go to a doctor.

Hence, individuals are not necessarily passive recipients of expert-derived care, rather they make active choices in their own lives. Current models of mental health care delivery increasingly emphasize the role of the individual as an active consumer, influenced by the development of consumer empowerment movements. The shift from institutional to community care allows individuals greater autonomy in help-seeking (Slade, 1994b). Szasz & Hollander (1956) proposed different models of the doctor–patient relationship, including activity–passivity, guidance–cooperation and mutual participation. Increasingly, with deinstitutionalization and the active consumer movement, the experience of delivering mental health care is moving towards the participative end of this spectrum. Thus, need may be defined differently in relation to these other concepts, models of mental health care delivery, and according to whose perspective is reflected (Slade, 1994a, b).

This variation in the conceptualization of need has been mirrored in the development of needs assessment tools. Recently it has been increasingly recognized that rates of disorder are an insufficient basis for assessing need for services (Bebbington, 1990; Johnson et al., 1996). This has led to various developments, including the incorporation of the consumer's or patient's point of view into the assessment of needs in recognition that need is, at least in part, subjectively defined. Marshall articulated this concept within the Cardinal Needs Schedule (Marshall, 1994; Marshall, Gath & Lockwood, 1995). Marshall argues that, at least in some circumstances, for a need to be judged as cardinal the individual must acknowledge, realize, or at least accept that the need for help exists. This he terms the criterion of 'cooperation'. This can be challenged in some circumstances in which need is judged as present, even if the individual does not accept it. An extreme example is an individual with psychotic illness who 'needs' compulsory treatment and may well not wish to accept it. For such circumstances, Marshall and colleagues propose two further criteria concerned with carer stress and severity for defining cardinal needs. However, when approaching needs assessment in community-based samples, such conditions and circumstances will be rare. Other recently developed instruments such as the Camberwell Assessment of Need (Phelan et al., 1995; Slade, Phelan, Thornicroft & Parkman, 1996) have also been designed to incorporate the consumer perspective into the assessment of needs.

The methodology of the Australian National Survey of Mental Health and Well-Being includes a community survey of mental disorders, with estimation of accompanying disability and need, among a probability sample of 10,000 of the Australian population. As we embarked upon this survey, we did so in the context of this rapidly developing field of needs assessment. It seemed appropriate from an early point in the design of the survey to try and include the perception of the consumer, or potential consumer, into the assessment of need. However, there was no immediately accessible tool that could be readily incorporated into such a survey instrument. At the core of the survey questionnaire is the Composite International Diagnostic Interview (CIDI). A number of the other instruments included in the survey instrument are tools that were elaborated and devised elsewhere. To assess the dimension of perceived need in the context of the survey, a new tool had to be designed.

In developing this tool, we have gone through an interesting investigation of the conceptual issues and difficulties of constructing questionnaires in this area. Early in its development, we role-played various designs and came across some problems. One was that, in many designs, individuals would find it very difficult to define themselves as having a need if that need was already met. As a result, it becomes difficult to differentiate between individuals who have a met need and individuals who have no need. In the course of the questionnaire design for the National Survey, we have to some degree overcome this problem by first finding out service use, followed by the experience of particular interventions, and then assessing need. We then had to address the issue of creating an equivalent questionnaire for assessing the need of individuals who had not used services.

The outcome is the Perceived Need for Care Questionnaire, a tool with a four-stage design. We begin with questions about service use. Following this, if there is service utilization, we question the individual about the types of interventions they have received. Then, if they have received interventions, they are asked whether those interventions were adequate to meet their needs for this type of help. If the interventions have not met their needs for this type of help, the individual is asked about possible barriers to care in order to identify the reasons why this need was not fully met.

To find out about the unmet need of individuals who reported not using mental health services, they were asked about any mental health problems that they had described earlier in the interview. The following statement is made, 'Earlier on in the interview you mentioned that you had mental problems, such as the following (mental health problems from the CIDI) but you didn't mention getting any help from any health professional. Were there any types of help which you needed in the last year but did not get?' At this point the individual is presented with a list of possible types of help. If they endorse any of these types of help as being needs that had not been met, then they are presented with a series of statements about barriers to care, from which reasons why those needs were not met may be ascertained.

To illustrate the operation of the questionnaire, we present below the sequence of responses from one imaginary survey participant. The following clinical vignette characterizes our notional respondent.

A man in his thirties, self-employed, has recently been through an episode of depression. He was treated by an empathic and skilled general practitioner who prescribed him a good dose of medication. During his illness his productivity was reduced, and he lost substantial income from his self-employed business. Therefore he has not felt able to spend the money to complete the prescribed course of medications.

The following sequence of questions reflects the course of the questionnaire in this context. The questions follow the section of the survey that inquires about service utilization, and that has elicited this participant's history of health consultations and any hospitalizations.

Which of these forms of help did you receive from those (consultations and/or hospital admissions), for any problems with your mental health?
- Information about mental illness, its treatments, and available services ✓
- Medicine or tablets ✓
- Psychotherapy - discussion about causes that stem from your past
- Cognitive-behavioral therapy - learning how to change your thoughts, behaviors and emotions
- Counseling - help to talk through your problems ✓
- Help to sort out housing or money problems
- Help to improve your ability to work, to use your time in other ways

You mentioned that you received
- Information about mental illness, its treatments, and available services

Do you think you got as much of this kind of help as you needed?
NO   YES ✓

You mentioned that you received
- Medicine or tablets

Do you think you got as much of this kind of help as you needed?
NO ✓YES

Why didn't you get more of this help? Please choose the main or the single reason which most closely applies.
- I preferred to manage myself
- I didn't think anything more could help
- I didn't know how or where to get help

- I was afraid to ask for help, or of what others would think of me if I did
- I couldn't afford the money ✓
- I asked but didn't get the help
- I got help from another source _____

You mentioned that you received
- Counseling – help to talk through your problems

Do you think you got as much of this kind of help as you needed?
NO   YES ✓

You mentioned that you did not receive
- Help to sort out housing or money problems

Do you think you needed this type of help?
NO   YES ✓

Why didn't you get this help? Please choose the main reason, or the single reason which most closely applies.
- I preferred to manage myself
- I didn't think anything more could help
- I didn't know how or where to get more help
- I was afraid to ask for more help, or of what others would think of me if I did ✓
- I couldn't afford the money
- I asked but didn't get the help
- I got help from another source _____

You mentioned that you did not receive
- Help to improve your ability to work, to care for yourself or to use your time

Do you think you needed this type of help?
NO ✓   YES

The data gained for this individual generated by the instrument would be:

Information: met need.
Drugs: partially met need.
Psychotherapies: met need.
Social interventions: unmet need.
Skills training: no need.

For Drugs and Social interventions (where there is a need and it is not fully met) barrier items apply; the barriers are finance and stigma, respectively.

The Perceived Need for Care Questionnaire is an instrument that can be delivered in some two minutes in a population-based survey. It is a way of incorporating a participant-orientated assessment of needs into such a survey. The categories have good to very good reliability. A homo/hetero trait homo/hetero method approach to construct validity (Streiner & Norman, 1989) lent support to the categories. Analysis of extreme groups also supports the view that the constructs within the instrument are valid.

When one has collected the data on perceived need, the question of how to use it arises. As stated at the beginning of this chapter, the concept of perceived need overlaps with a number of other ideas such as literacy, demand and want. Hence, the dataset could be analyzed from a number of different perspectives. This dataset could be used to adjust prevalence figures to other estimates of unmet need.

We will propose a series of categories of need within the survey. There will be a core group of individuals who suffer from degrees of disorder that, by their very nature, would clearly be indicative of having a need for mental health care. Disorders such as severe depression, the psychotic disorders, and severe anxiety disorders and their associated disabilities are clearly within the target groups for public mental health services and should be priorities in terms of delivering care. In this context, the attitude of the individual is relatively less significant for identifying cases of need.

At the other end of the spectrum, an individual with a mild social phobia who does not have significant associated disabilities, and does not express a need for any kind of care, is another matter. Although such individuals may be able to benefit from help, they are not within the primary target group for mental health services, at least in Australia. Their loss of productivity and their degree of distress or impairment is relatively small. In this context of estimating service needs, and with limited health care resources, it may be legitimate to argue that such individuals are not in a group that should be aggressively targeted for intervention. In particular, if they do not want an intervention, then perhaps their autonomy should be respected and the intervention should not be pressed upon them. A characteristic of previous large-scale epidemiological surveys has been the very high rates of generation of this type of disorder. This dataset of perceived need will allow such results from the Australian Survey to be qualified.

The described instrument for assessing perceived need relies on a particular conception of need, which is based on an internal cognitive process that occurs in an individual seeking help. The individual must acknowledge having some kind of mental health problem, which forms the basis for some kind of action on their part. At this point the individual may form an idea that they have some kind of need for mental health care. Having recognized this need, the individual may then act upon it, making some behavioral

Table 27.1. Perceived need for specific interventions

| Intervention | Level of perceived need | | | | |
	No need	Unmet need	Partially met need	Met need	Barriers*
Information	95	24	8	15	32
Drugs	104	8	1	22	9
Psychotherapies	71	35	9	28	44
Social interventions	116	6	1	11	7
Skills training	100	19	2	14	21

*Potential numbers for 7 barriers to accessing specified intervention.

Table 27.2. Perceived barriers to care: summarized data for partially met and unmet need

| Intervention | Barriers to accessing the specified intervention | | | | | | | |
	SR	U	LA	S	F	NR	AP	Total
Information	6	0	10	4	3	6	2	31
Drugs	2	2	0	1	1	2	1	9
Psychotherapies	12	3	9	5	10	1	3	43
Social interventions	1	0	0	0	1	2	0	4
Skills training	3	5	6	3	0	3	1	21
Column total	24	10	25	13	15	14	7	

Note: SR, self reliance; U, unawareness; LA, lack of access; S, stigma; F, finance; NR:, non-response; AP, alternative provision.

change in terms of help seeking, based on how the need is viewed. For such individuals to come to the attention of services, they, or someone else, need to declare their problem to such services. Hence we move through a model of perceived need in which the individuals first realize that they have a mental health problem, and then that they must take some action. They may then seek care. Whether the need for care is met through a satisfactory interaction with some provider of care or not will then depend on other variables, both external and internal. Within this context, we come to the notion of barriers to care, illustrated in the earlier vignette.

The data obtained from the Australian National Survey of Mental Health and Well-Being allow us to qualify downwards estimates of unmet need as judged by the prevalence of untreated disorders. Disorders associated with low levels of disability, in which there is no significant danger to life or limb, of self or others, should be qualified by some perception of need on the part of the individuals before being regarded in administrative terms and by targeting surveys as cases of prevalent disorders.

The Survey also gives useful information on the barriers to care. The barriers and types of service delivery were chosen in view of studies of consumers' views of mental health services, such as that conducted by Mind in the UK (Rogers, Pilgrim & Lacey, 1993). Thus, the items reflect the kinds of things that consumers commonly report they need from mental health services, or the kinds of issues that tend to stop them from getting what they need.

The illustrative dataset from the tool that we have created is presented in Tables 27.1 and 27.2. This is a dataset from the first wave of the reliability study, which was carried out at the Clinical Research Unit for Anxiety Disorders, Sydney. It is reassuring that each cell of the perceived needs grid is filled, as is each column of the barrier items. Lower numbers in the barriers items were expected because individuals only respond to them if they also declare partially met or unmet needs. This suggests that the categories had appropriate coverage.

Readers may be interested in pondering these figures. The kind of information that this tool produces might be useful to people running services, in establishing the degree to which people attending their service understand themselves as having a mental health need. In addition, the tool has a measure of satisfaction: the degree to which met need is fulfilled might be used to predict satisfaction with services, and quality of life. Information such as this, constructed around the notion of met need, may well present a way of gaining useful quality assurance information about services, as well as useful information for national services' planning and resource allocation.

In summary, the definition and construct of need is complex. Nonetheless, in modeling the realities of clinical practice, it is being increasingly recognized that it is important to incorporate the patient's or the potential consumer's views when defining what such needs should be. By using an instrument which, by virtue of a moderately complex questionnaire design, can deliver this information, we have demonstrated that it is possible to estimate perceived need within the context of a survey. We and future designers incorporating this type of instrument into their surveys shall have to explore the meanings of these datasets. The reporting of the National Survey of Mental Health and Well-Being will be the first substantial opportunity to do this.

References

Bebbington, P.E. (1990). Population surveys of psychiatric disorder and the need for treatment. *Social Psychiatry and Psychiatric Epidemiology*, **15**, 33–40.
Johnson, S., Thornicroft, G., Phelan, M. & Slade, M. (1996). Assessing needs for mental health services. In G. Thornicroft & M. Tansella (eds.), *Mental Health*

Outcome Measures, pp. 217–26). Berlin: Springer-Verlag.

Marshall, M. (1994). How should we measure need? Concept and practice in the development of a standardized assessment schedule. *Philosophy, Psychiatry, Psychology*, 1, 27–36.

Marshall, M.H.L., Gath, D.H. & Lockwood, A. (1995).The Cardinal Needs for Care Schedule – a modified version of the MRC Needs for Care Schedule. *Psychological Medicine*, 25, 605–17.

Phelan, M., Slade, M., Thornicroft, G., Dunn, G., Holloway, F., Wykes, T., Strathdee, G., Loftus, L., McCrone, P. & Hayward, P. (1995). The Camberwell Assessment of Need (CAN): the validity and reliability of an instrument to assess the needs of people with severe mental illness. *British Journal of Psychiatry*, 167, 589–95.

Rogers, A., Pilgrim, D. & Lacey, R. (1993). Experiencing psychiatry: users' views of services. In J. Campling (ed.), *Issues in Mental Health* (1st edition). London: Macmillan.

Slade, M. (1994a). Needs assessment; involvement of staff and users will help to meet needs. *British Journal of Psychiatry*, 165, 293–6.

Slade, M. (1994b). Needs assessment: who needs to assess? *British Journal of Psychiatry*, 165, 287–92.

Slade, M., Phelan, M., Thornicroft, G. & Parkman, S. (1996). The Camberwell Assessment of Need (CAN): comparison of assessments by staff and patients of the needs of the severely mentally ill. *Social Psychiatry and Psychiatric Epidemiology*, 31, 109–13.

Stevens, A. & Gabbay, J. (1991). Needs assessment needs assessment. *Health Trends*, 23, 20–3.

Streiner, D.L. & Norman, G.R. (1989). *Validity Health Measurement Scales. A Practical Guide to their Development and Use*, pp. 106–25. Oxford: Oxford University Press.

Szasz, T. & Hollander, M.H.A. (1956). A contribution to the philosophy of medicine. A.M.A. *Archives of Internal Medicine*, 97.

28

Public knowledge of and attitudes to mental disorders: a limiting factor in the optimal use of treatment services

Anthony F. Jorm, Mattias Angermeyer, and Heinz Katschnig

The distribution of treatment services in the population is determined not only by the planning of health administrators and service providers, but also by the wishes of the public for particular kinds of services. Unfortunately, the public's beliefs about mental disorders and their treatment do not always correspond with those of service providers. This chapter reviews national surveys of public knowledge and attitudes towards mental disorders carried out in Australia, Germany, and Austria. Putting the results of these surveys together, it can be concluded that while the public believe that mental disorders can be treated, their views on the effectiveness of various treatments differ greatly from those of mental health professionals. The public are very negative about pharmacological treatments, but more positive about psychotherapy and alternative treatments. Many believe that psychotherapy is effective for psychotic and organic mental disorders. There is also a widespread stigma against those who suffer from a mental disorder. These beliefs may affect the sorts of help the public seek for mental disorders and may adversely affect adherence to some types of interventions. Any attempt at top-down planning of the distribution of mental health services will run into difficulties if it conflicts with the public's beliefs about treatment. A more feasible approach may be to encourage a diversity of effective interventions which consumers can choose from, according to their beliefs about treatment.

A major assumption of this book is that treatment services could be more rationally distributed in the population if we took account of data on prevalence, disablement, treatment effectiveness, and the direct and indirect costs of mental disorders. The implicit view is that planning from the top by health administrators and service providers could provide a rational solution to the problem of distributing scarce treatment services. However, we will present data in this chapter to show that any attempt to distribute services rationally must also consider public knowledge and attitudes towards mental disorders and their treatment.

The view that the distribution of services is a top-down process is not unusual. Psychiatric epidemiologists have traditionally viewed people who experience mental disorders as rather passive recipients of help. An example is the popular Pathways to Care model of Goldberg & Huxley (1980, 1992). According to this model, there are four filters operating between a person in the community with a mental disorder and their admission to a psychiatric ward. The first filter is 'illness behavior' which determines whether the individual will seek help in primary care. The second is the general practitioner's ability to detect the mental disorder. The third filter is whether the general practitioner will make a referral to specialist mental health services, and the final filter is whether the specialist services will admit the individual to a psychiatric ward. In this model, the individual with a mental disorder is seen as a largely passive recipient of the decisions of medical practitioners, with little active role other than to take the initial step of seeking help. The Pathways to Care model does not allow for the possibility that the knowledge and attitudes of the person with the mental disorder may also be a major factor in determining whether they pass through each of the filters and what treatment they receive at each stage.

An alternative view is that people with mental disorders have a role as important as that of the service providers in determining what services they receive. For people with severe mental disorders, the knowledge and attitudes of family and friends may also play a significant role and, of course, people with mental disorders are influenced by the attitudes of the broader society in which they live. There are a range of knowledge and attitudinal factors that might influence help seeking, including ability to recognize the problem as a mental disorder, knowledge of services available, beliefs about the effectiveness and risks of various sorts of treatments, beliefs about causes of the problem, and stigmatizing attitudes.

In this chapter we present data on public knowledge and attitudes from three national surveys, in Australia, Austria, and Germany. We will then compare the results to those from other surveys and discuss the implications for the optimal distribution of mental health services.

The three national surveys

Surveys of nationally representative samples have been carried out in Australia, Germany, and Austria. Each survey involved household interviews in which the participants were presented with case vignettes of hypothetical people with mental disorders. Attitudes and knowledge were assessed in relation to the cases described. Table 28.1 summarizes the methods of each survey.

Table 28.1. Comparison of the methods of the three surveys

Methodological characteristic	Australian survey	Austrian survey	German survey
Year of survey	1995	1991	1990
Sample size	2031	1443	3098
Response rate	85%	Quota sample: rate unknown	72% in west, 67% in east
Age groups surveyed	18–74 years	15+ years	18+ years
Case vignettes presented	1. Depression	1. Depression	1. Major depressive disorder
	2. Schizophrenia	2. Anxiety/Panic	2. Panic disorder with
		3. Psychosis	agoraphobia
		4. Dementia	3. Schizophrenia
Topics covered in interview	1. Recognition of disorders	1. Knowledge of services	1. Recognition of disorders
	2. Treatment	2. Treatment	2. Treatment
	3. Prognosis	3. Prognosis	3. Causes
	4. Causes and risk factors	4. Social distance	4. Prognosis
	5. Stigmatizing attitudes		5. Attitudes to drugs and
			psychotherapy
			6. Social distance

The following are examples of case vignettes used in each of the three surveys.

Australian survey - schizophrenia (male version)

John is 24 and lives at home with his parents. He has had a few temporary jobs since finishing school but is now unemployed. Over the last six months he has stopped seeing his friends and has begun locking himself in his bedroom and refusing to eat with the family or to have a bath. His parents also hear him walking about his bedroom at night while they are in bed. Even though they know he is alone, they have heard him shouting and arguing as if someone else is there. When they try to encourage him to do more things, he whispers that he won't leave home because he is being spied upon by the neighbor. They realize he is not taking drugs because he never sees anyone or goes anywhere.

Austrian survey - delusion of persecution/psychosis

Imagine that a person, who has led a normal life until recently, begins hearing voices, believes he is persecuted and talks in a confused way.

German survey - schizophrenia (male version)

Imagine that you hear the following about an acquaintance with whom you occasionally spend your leisure time. Within the past months, your acquaintance appears to have changed. More and more, he retreated from his friends and colleagues, up to the point of avoiding them. If someone managed to involve him in a conversation, he would address only one single topic: the question as to whether some people had the natural gift of reading other people's thoughts. This question became his sole concern. In contrast with his previous habits, he stopped taking care of his appearance and looked increasingly untidy. At work, he seemed absent-minded and frequently made mistakes. As a consequence, he has already been summoned to his boss. Finally, your acquaintance stayed away from work for an entire week without an excuse. Upon his return, he seemed anxious and harassed. He reports that he is now absolutely certain that people cannot only read other people's thoughts, but that they also directly influence them. He was however unsure who would steer his thoughts. He also said that, when thinking, he was continually interrupted. Frequently, he would even hear those people talk to him, and they would give him instructions. Sometimes, they would also talk to each other and make fun of whatever he was doing at the time. The situation was particularly bad at his apartment, he claimed. At home, he would really feel threatened, and would be terribly scared. Hence he had not spent the night at his place for the past week, but rather he had hidden in hotel rooms and hardly dared to go out.

Details of the Australian survey can be found in Jorm et al. (1997*a*, *b*, *c*, *d*, *e*). Details of the German survey can be found in Angermeyer, Däumer & Matschinger (1993) and Angermeyer & Matschinger (1994, 1996*a*, *b*, *c*).

There have also been several subsequent German surveys that have dealt with similar issues and these have been used to track changes in attitudes over time (e.g., Angermeyer & Matschinger, 1995, 1996d, 1997; Matschinger & Angermeyer, 1996). The results of the Austrian survey are available as a research report (Katschnig, Etzersdorfer & Muzik, 1993).

Overview of the results

Recognition of disorder

Only the Australian survey examined the public's ability to recognize mental disorders. Respondents were asked what they thought was wrong with the person described in the vignettes. For the depression vignette, 39% mentioned the term depression and 22% mentioned stress. For the schizophrenia vignette, only 27% mentioned schizophrenia and a further 26% mentioned depression. Although only a minority of respondents used the conventional psychiatric labels, most recognized a mental health problem of some sort. Physical disorders were mentioned by only 11% for the depression vignette and only 2% for the schizophrenia vignette.

Knowledge of services available

Only the Austrian survey examined whether respondents knew about various services. While 85% knew the nearest psychiatric hospital and 51% the nearest practising psychiatrist, only 12% knew about a new mental health facility in the neighborhood (which partly reflects the lack of such facilities at the time when the survey was carried out) and 4% knew the number of the Austrian crisis hotline.

Beliefs about professions that provide help

In the Australian survey, respondents were asked to rate the likely helpfulness of a range of people, both professional and nonprofessional. For the depression vignette, the groups most likely to be rated as helpful were general practitioners (83%), counselors (74%), close friends (73%), close family (70%), telephone counseling services (53%), psychiatrists (51%) and psychologists (49%). For the schizophrenia vignette, the highest ratings were for counselors (81%), general practitioners (74%) and psychiatrists (71%). Admission to a psychiatric ward was rated as harmful by 72% for depression and by 51% for schizophrenia.

In the Austrian survey, when respondents were asked what they would do if a family member suffered from various mental disorders, the most popular response was to talk to them. Professional help from general practitioners, psychiatrists, psychologists, and psychiatric hospitals was mentioned much less frequently. Even for the psychotic individual, the specialist mental health services were only mentioned by a minority (psychiatrist 38%, psychologist 18% and psychiatric hospital 9%). Even general practitioners did not enjoy the same popularity as in Australia (mentioned by only 11% for depression and 15% for psychosis). The German survey did not ask about helping professions.

Beliefs about pharmacological treatments

All three surveys examined beliefs about pharmacological treatments and found negative opinions. In Australia, more people saw pharmacological treatments as harmful than as helpful. For the depression vignette, 29% believed antidepressants would be helpful, while 42% thought they would be harmful. For the schizophrenia vignette, 23% believed that antipsychotics would be helpful, while 34% thought they would be harmful.

In the German survey, respondents were asked to rate a range of treatments as recommended or not recommended. Drug treatments were recommended by only 32% in the western part of Germany and 29% in the east. The reason most often given for not recommending drugs was their side-effects, particularly the risk of addiction. Other common arguments were that drugs provide only symptomatic treatment and that they are ineffective.

In the Austrian survey, only a minority of respondents believed that mental disorders respond 'exclusively' or 'mainly' to pharmacotherapy. The percentages with this belief were 20% for the depression vignette, 27% for anxiety, 27% for dementia and 35% for psychosis. Respondents were also given an attitude scale on psychotropic medication, which revealed strongly negative attitudes. It was widely believed that drugs lack efficacy because they do not deal with the roots of the problem, that they have more risks than benefits (e.g., dependence), and that they are prescribed for the wrong reasons (e.g., to avoid talking about problems, to make people believe things are better than they are, as a straight jacket).

Beliefs about psychotherapy

In all three surveys, the public's beliefs about psychotherapy were, by contrast, predominantly favorable. In Australia, psychotherapy was regarded as helpful for depression by 34% and harmful by 13%. For schizophrenia, it was regarded as helpful by 55% and harmful by only 7%.

The results were similar in Germany. Over half of the respondents in both the west and east of Germany recommended psychotherapy as the treatment of choice. The argument most often given to support this choice was that psychotherapy can determine and treat the causes of the disorder. As in Australia, psychotherapy was rated more highly for schizophrenia than for depression. Psychoanalysis was the favored form of psychotherapy in the western part of Germany, while group therapy was favored in the east. Behavior therapy and family therapy were ranked third and fourth respectively in both parts of Germany.

In Austria, most respondents believed that mental disorders respond 'exclusively' or 'mainly' to psychotherapy. This was true for all disorders: depression (80%), anxiety (73%), psychosis (65%), and dementia (73%). The strong belief in the effects of psychotherapy on dementia are particularly surprising. Various psychological treatments were also amongst those which respondents believed should be used more frequently: talking with the therapist (56%), behavior therapy (34%) and psychoanalysis (28%).

Beliefs about alternative treatments

The term 'alternative treatment' is used here to mean any treatments which are frequently used outside the mainstream health professions or are self-administered. All three surveys found that such treatments had a more positive image than standard pharmacological treatments.

In Australia, 57% of the public believed that 'vitamins, minerals, tonics or herbal medicines' are helpful for depression, and 34% for schizophrenia. Other treatments which were frequently believed to be helpful were: getting out and about more; becoming more physically active; courses on relaxation, stress management, meditation or yoga; reading self-help books; cutting out alcohol altogether; and a special diet or avoiding certain foods. These alternative treatments were more often favored than both psychotherapy and pharmacological treatments.

In Germany, 32% of respondents in the west and 29% in the east recommended natural remedies. Similarly, 28% and 23% respectively recommended meditation or yoga. However, there was an almost equal percentage who were against these alternative treatments. Although the alternative treatments were more often recommended than pharmacological treatments, they were less often recommended than psychotherapy.

In the Austrian survey, beliefs about the effectiveness of alternative treatments were not assessed. However, respondents were asked about whether they thought certain treatments should be used more frequently. More frequent use of yoga/meditation was advocated by 38%, relaxation by 55% and self-help groups by 38%.

Beliefs about prognosis

All three surveys asked about prognosis with and without treatment. In the Australian survey, 80% thought the person with depression would recovery fully after receiving help. Without help, however, 56% believed the person would get worse and only 5% believed in a full recovery. Beliefs were similar for schizophrenia: 69% believed that help would result in full recovery, but without help 75% believed the person would get worse and only 3% thought there would be full recovery.

In Germany, the public similarly thought that the prognosis of schizophrenia would be poor if the disorder was allowed to take its 'natural course'. Most expected a chronic progressive course or a chronic stable state. However, with optimal treatment the general belief was that there would be remission, although possibly with relapse.

In Austria too, respondents overwhelmingly believed that professional treatment would result in remission (either with or without later relapse), while without treatment they believed the result would much more often be no change or deterioration. According to the opinion of 55% of the respondents, leaving depression untreated would result in a chronic or deteriorating course, while 96% thought that professional treatment would lead to remission. For anxiety, the figures were similar (62% chronic or deteriorating without treatment, 97% remission with treatment). It is astonishing that the responses to the psychosis and dementia vignettes showed a similar pattern: 72% chronic for untreated psychosis, and 88% remission for professionally treated psychosis; 85% chronic for untreated dementia, and 59% remission for treated dementia. Even allowing for the fact that the effects of psychiatric treatment were greatly over-rated, the relative differences between treatment and nontreatment are still remarkable.

Beliefs about causes and risk factors

Only the Australian and German surveys asked about this issue. The Australian public considered that social environmental factors were likely causes of both depression and schizophrenia. The factors most commonly endorsed were 'day-to-day problems such as stress, family arguments, difficulties at work or financial difficulties', 'some recent traumatic event such as bushfires threatening your home, a severe traffic accident or being mugged' and 'problems from childhood such as being badly treated or abused, losing one or both parents when young or coming from a broken home'. Similarly, the risk factors most often endorsed were being unemployed, divorced/separated, poor or young. Genetic factors were less commonly believed to be causes, although more so for schizophrenia than for depression.

The German public had similar beliefs. For schizophrenia, psychosocial stress was the most frequently believed cause. This was measured by questions on 'difficulties in partner or family relationship', 'work difficulties', and 'stressful life event'. Next in popularity were biological factors (brain diseases, heredity, constitutional weakness), intrapsychic factors (lack of will power, expecting too much of oneself, unconscious conflict), and socialization (grown up in a broken home, lack of parental affection, overprotective parents). Work from a subsequent German survey carried out in 1993 confirmed these findings. For schizophrenia and depression, psychosocial stress factors were most often believed to be causes. By contrast, for border-line personality disorder, causes within the individual were chosen more often.

Stigmatizing attitudes

All three surveys investigated attitudes towards people with mental disorders. In the Australian survey, the public were asked to say how the person in the vignette would be in the long-term after receiving help. Responses were more often positive than negative for characteristics such as being violent, drinking too much, having a good marriage and understanding others feelings. These positive responses are congruent with the findings summarized above, i.e., that the public believe that treatment will produce a good outcome. However, when asked if the person in the vignette would be discriminated against by others in the community (again, after treatment), 54% thought the person with depression would be, and 75% thought so for schizophrenia.

In Germany, there have been repeated surveys charting changes in social distance over recent years. In these surveys, the public were asked whether they would be willing to enter into various relationships with people who suffer from a mental disorder. The most rejected group were the alcohol dependent, followed by those with schizophrenia, then narcissistic personality disorder, panic disorder with agoraphobia, and those with major depression were the least rejected. While 35% rejected having an alcohol-dependent person as a neighbor, only 13% rejected a person with major depression. However, 79% rejected an alcohol-dependent person for child care, and 52% rejected a person with major depression. Because of the repeated attitude surveys in Germany, it has been possible to assess the effect of two events when a person with schizophrenia attacked a politician. Both events were accompanied by widespread media coverage. Following these attacks, social distance from the mentally ill increased and they were more likely to be seen as 'dangerous' and 'unpredictable'.

The Austrian survey included some questions on social distance and on propensity to violence. Most members of the Austrian public agreed that people with a mental disorder should participate in community life (88% for anxiety and depression, 83% for dementia), with the lowest agreement being for people with psychosis (66%). The main reason for being against partici-pation was that it would be too difficult for the person affected, but for psychosis another common reason was that it would be too dangerous for the community. Half the public believed that mentally ill people tend to violence. When asked what they would do if a flat for ex-psychiatric patients was established in their neighborhood, most said they would do nothing (68%), rather than help or welcome (19%), or try to prevent it or move away (12%).

Comparison of public and professional beliefs

Only the Australian survey compared public and professional beliefs. Postal surveys were carried out with national samples of general practitioners, psychiatrists and clinical psychologists. There was substantial agreement among the three professions about what interventions are effective for depression and schizophrenia, but big differences from the public. The professionals were much more likely to believe that antidepressants are helpful for depression, and antipsychotics and admission to a psychiatric ward are helpful for schizophrenia. Conversely, the public were more likely to believe that vitamins and minerals and special diets are helpful for both depression and schizophrenia, and that reading self-help books is helpful for schizophrenia.

Although the public beliefs in Germany and Austria were not directly compared to those of mental health professionals, it appears likely that there are major discrepancies, particularly in beliefs about the effectiveness of various treatments and about the causes of mental disorders.

Effects of age, education and contact with mental disorders

The effects of these variables are interesting because they suggest possibilities for change in knowledge and beliefs. Age group differences may be due to cohort effects and, if so, suggest the direction in which beliefs may move in the future, while education and contact with mental disorders suggest ways of producing change. In the Australian survey, there were few age differences, but younger people were more positive about psychological interventions for depression. In Germany, social distance for people with mental disorders was found to increase across age groups. In Austria, older people were more likely to believe that mentally ill people are violent.

With education, the Australian survey found that the better educated were more favorable to psychological interventions for both depression and schizophrenia, and to medical interventions for schizophrenia. In Germany, the better educated were more in favor of psychotherapy and alternative treatments, and more opposed to pharmacological ones for all disorders. The better educated also responded with less social distance to those with a mental disorder. Similarly, in Austria, the better educated were less likely to believe that mentally ill people are violent.

In Australia, contact with mental disorders, either in oneself or others, had little effect. However, those who said that they had suffered from a problem like that in the schizophrenia vignette were more negative to medical interventions. In Germany, those who had themselves received pharmacological treatment were more negative about this form of treatment, while those who had received psychotherapy had a clear preference for this treatment. It was also found that contact with mental disorders decreases social distance.

Conclusions from the three surveys

Putting the results of these surveys together, we can conclude the following:

1. The public have very negative views about the benefits and risks of pharmacological treatments.
2. The public have much more positive views on psychotherapy, many even believing it is effective for psychotic and organic mental disorders.
3. Alternative treatments are seen as effective more often than pharmacological ones.
4. The public believe that prognosis of mental disorders is poor without treatment, but very good with treatment.
5. Public beliefs about treatment differ greatly from those of mental health professionals.
6. There is a widespread stigma against those who suffer from a mental disorder.
7. Although age, education and contact with mental disorders influence attitudes, the effect is small.

Comparison with other studies

Several national surveys of the public in other countries can be compared with the three described here. There has been an Irish national survey of public attitudes to depression (McKeon & Carrick, 1991). Depression was seen as treatable by 73%, with the treatments most frequently nominated being counseling, medication and talking to someone close. Stress and bereavement were most frequently identified as the cause of depression. Only 43% agreed that people who have suffered from depression can be trusted to mind children.

A survey was carried out in the USA as part of the Depression Awareness Recognition and Treatment (DART) program (Regier et al., 1988). The American public was found to have good knowledge of the mood symptoms of depression, but not of psychomotor changes. It was generally believed that treatment would help, but only 12% said they would take medication for depression, while 78% said they would live with it until it passed. Deterrents to seeking treatment were the cost and a fear of a negative impact on the person's employment situation.

A similar survey was carried out in the UK in connection with the Defeat Depression Campaign (Priest, Vize, Roberts, Roberts & Tylee, 1996). When asked whom they would consult for depression, 60% nominated their general practitioner, but the same proportion thought that it would be embarrassing to consult a general practitioner for depression, mainly because he/she would see them as unbalanced or neurotic (50%) or would be annoyed by it (23%). The most favored treatment was counseling (91%), compared with 16% for antidepressants. Only 46% considered antidepressants to be effective, and 78% thought they were addictive. Psychosocial stressors were most commonly seen as the cause of depression.

Implications for the optimal distribution of services

The good news from the surveys is that the public believe in the treatability of mental disorders. The bad news is that their beliefs about how these disorders should be treated are often very different from the beliefs of service providers. *This finding has profound implications for service providers and planners.* A rational approach to service planning based purely on prevalence, disablement, treatment effectiveness, and the costs of illness might have limited success if it does not concur with the beliefs of consumers. Take major depression as an example. There is evidence that this disorder is common and highly disabling, there are meta-analyses showing that antidepressants are an effective treatment, and this treatment can be implemented at relatively low cost. The solution would appear to be simple. However, the public are skeptical about the benefits of antidepressants and suspicious of their side-effects. Whatever the efficacy of antidepressants in controlled trials, their effectiveness in practice and their impact on public health may be more limited. The public would prefer psychotherapy or counseling, which is unfortunately much more expensive, and not all forms of which have been demonstrated to be effective in meta-analyses of controlled trials.

What can be done to bring a closer alignment of public and professional beliefs? There is reason to believe that public beliefs and attitudes can be changed, although this is not easy to achieve. The discrepancy between public and professional beliefs in itself testifies that beliefs can be changed, because health professionals start out as members of the public and it is their professional training that changes their opinions. The effects of age, education and contact with mental disorders have also been investigated and show small effects. Age group differences may represent cohort effects and suggest the direction in which attitudes will move in the future. The effects of education and contact suggest that greater knowledge can have some influence on beliefs and attitudes. There is also evidence that attitudes can change in a negative direction in response to intense media reporting of violence from mentally ill individuals (Angermeyer & Matschinger, 1995), implying that positive change might also be possible if appropriate events were reported. There have been only a few large-scale attempts to change beliefs and attitudes. An early experiment on reducing stigma in a single community had no effect (Cumming & Cumming, 1957), but this has not deterred the development of national public education campaigns in some countries. There have been national campaigns to change public beliefs about depression in the USA and UK, and to change stigmatizing attitudes in Australia. The United Kingdom Defeat Depression campaign has been the best evaluated, with national surveys both before and after. This evaluation showed some small changes in beliefs and attitudes after three years (Corrado & Aronstam, 1995). For example, the belief that antidepressants are a very or fairly effective treatment increased from 46% to 51%, while the belief that they are very addictive decreased from 58% to 51% (although there was a corresponding increase in the percentage who thought they were fairly addictive). It seems likely from the limited evidence available that major changes in public beliefs and attitudes may take generations rather than years to achieve.

The other possibility for reducing the discrepancy between public and professional beliefs is to bring the professionals more in line with the public. This may seem a strange suggestion given the limitations of public beliefs. However, it may be possible to promote mental health interventions that are both consistent with public belief systems and effective. For example, with depression there are effective interventions consistent with various belief systems: medical (antidepressants, electroconvulsive therapy), psychological (cognitive-behavioral therapy, interpersonal psychotherapy), and alternative (physical exercise, and the herb St. John's Wort). A widening of professional beliefs to encompass a broader range of interventions may help to reduce the gap with the public. Indeed, there is evidence that this is occurring in Australia, with younger mental health professionals endorsing a wider range of interventions as helpful than older ones (Jorm et al., 1997c). If this age difference represents a cohort effect, it will help reduce the public–professional gap in the future.

Conclusion

A top-down rational approach to the planning of mental health services will run into difficulties if it conflicts with public beliefs about treatment. Conversely, a bottom-up approach in which the supply of services is completely driven by consumer demand would also be unwise, because is would encourage the use of services with limited effectiveness. It may be preferable to have an 'interactive' approach in which there are both top-down and bottom-up influences. Such an approach would supply a diversity of treatments so that consumers can choose those which fit in with their beliefs about treatment. However, the diversity of treatments needs to be constrained to ensure that scarce public resources go towards the more effective approaches within each belief system. It may also be possible to change public beliefs about treatments to bring them in closer correspondence with professional beliefs, but this should be seen as a very long-term process.

References

Angermeyer, M.C. & Matschinger, H. (1994). Lay beliefs about schizophrenic disorder: the results of a population survey in Germany. *Acta Psychiatrica Scandinavica*, 89, 39–45.

Angermeyer, M.C. & Matschinger, H. (1995). Violent attacks on public figures by persons suffering from psychiatric disorders: their effect on the social distance towards the mentally ill. *European Archives of Psychiatry and Clinical Neuroscience*, 245, 159–64.

Angermeyer, M.C. & Matschinger, H. (1996a). The effect of diagnostic labelling on the lay theory regarding schizophrenic disorders. *Social Psychiatry and Psychiatric Epidemiology*, 31, 316–20.

Angermeyer, M.C. & Matschinger, H. (1996b). The effect of personal experience with mental illness on the attitude towards individuals suffering from mental disorders. *Social Psychiatry and Psychiatric Epidemiology*, 31, 321–6.

Angermeyer, M.C. & Matschinger, H. (1996c). Public attitude towards psychiatric treatment. *Acta Psychiatrica Scandinavica*, 94, 326–36.

Angermeyer, M.C. & Matschinger, H. (1996d). Relatives' beliefs about the causes of schizophrenia. *Acta Psychiatrica Scandinavica*, 93, 199–204.

Angermeyer, M.C. & Matschinger, H. (1997). Social distance towards the mentally ill: results of representative surveys in the Federal Republic of Germany. *Psychological Medicine*, 27, 131–41.

Angermeyer, M.C., Däumer, R. & Matschinger, H. (1993). Benefits and risks of psychotropic medication in the eyes of the general public: results of a survey in the Federal Republic of Germany. *Pharmacopsychiatry*, 26, 114–20.

Corrado, M. & Aronstam, S. (1995). *New MORI Survey Finds General Public Informed but Stigma still Exists: Results of Second MORI Poll on Attitudes Towards Depression.* London: MORI.

Cumming, E. & Cumming, H. (1957). *Closed Ranks: An Experiment in Mental Health Education.* Cambridge, MA: Harvard University Press.

Goldberg, D. & Huxley, P. (1980). *Mental Illness in the Community: the Pathway to Psychiatric Care.* London: Tavistock.

Goldberg, D. & Huxley, P. (1992). *Common Mental Disorders: a Bio-social Model.* London: Routledge.

Jorm, A.F., Korten, A.E., Jacomb, P.A., Christensen, H., Rodgers, B. & Pollitt, P. (1997a). 'Mental health literacy': a survey of the public's ability to recognise mental disorders and their beliefs about the effectiveness of treatment. *Medical Journal of Australia*, 166, 182–6.

Jorm, A.F., Korten, A.E., Jacomb, P.A., Christensen, H., Rodgers, B. & Pollitt, P. (1997b). Public beliefs about causes and risk factors for depression and schizophrenia. *Social Psychiatry and Psychiatric Epidemiology*, 32, 143–8.

Jorm, A.F., Korten, A.E., Jacomb, P.A., Rodgers, B. & Pollitt, P. (1997*c*). Beliefs about the helpfulness of interventions for mental disorders: a comparison of general practitioners, psychiatrists and clinical psychologists. *Australian and New Zealand Journal of Psychiatry*, 31, 844–51.

Jorm, A.F., Korten, A.E., Jacomb, P.A., Rodgers, B., Pollitt, P., Christensen, H. & Henderson, S. (1997*d*). Helpfulness of interventions for mental disorders: beliefs of health professionals compared with the general public. *British Journal of Psychiatry*, 171, 233–7.

Jorm, A.F., Korten, A.E., Rodgers, B., Pollitt, P., Jacomb, P.A., Christensen, H. & Jiao, Z. (1997*e*). Belief systems of the general public concerning the appropriate treatments for mental disorders. *Social Psychiatry and Psychiatric Epidemiology*, 32, 468–73.

Katschnig, H., Etzersdorfer, E. & Muzik, M. (1993). Nicht nur eine minderwertige Gesundheit – eine Untersuchung über die Einstellung der österreichischen Bevölkerung zu psychisch Kranken und zur Psychiatrie. *Abschlussbericht an den FWF*. Vienna

Matschinger, H. & Angermeyer, M. C. (1996). Lay beliefs about the causes of mental disorders: a new methodological approach. *Social Psychiatry and Psychiatric Epidemiology*, 31, 309–15.

McKeon, P. & Carrick, S. (1991). Public attitudes to depression: a national survey. *Irish Journal of Psychological Medicine*, 8, 116–21.

Priest, R.G., Vize, C., Roberts, A., Roberts, M. & Tylee, A. (1996). Lay people's attitudes to treatment of depression: results of opinion poll for defeat depression campaign just before its launch. *British Medical Journal*, 313, 858–9.

Regier, D.A., Hirschfeld, R.M.A., Goodwin, F.K., Burke, J.D., Lazar, J.B. & Judd, L.L. (1988). The NIMH depression awareness, recognition, and treatment program: structure, aims, and scientific basis. *American Journal of Psychiatry*, 145, 1351–7.

Part V

Unmet need: conclusion

29

A personal overview

John R.M. Copeland

You will have read in the preceding chapters about the problems facing those who attempt to provide health and social services to older and younger people, the special problems of primary care, and the particular problems in developed and in deprived countries. From these chapters, strong messages emerge that are relevant to the questions posed in other parts of this book.

First, there is likely to be a rapid increase in the prevalence of certain diseases soon, for example dementia. Second, there is still a massive unmet need for treatment amongst sufferers of treatable diseases everywhere, but especially in developing countries. Third, the principal problem is a shortage of money and human resources: too little money to treat everyone whom the services consider should be treated, or would benefit from treatment; and too few trained staff to undertake the treatment, should it be available. We should recognize that part of that shortage of human resources is because professionals have approved long and expensive training programs for their students who, in consequence, are expensive to employ. Some, it has to be said, use their time in a manner inappropriate to their training. For example, does a doctor, in cash-limited times, have to be trained in anatomy, physiology, biochemistry, and the physical signs of inguinal hernia to practise psychotherapy? I doubt it.

Psychiatrists have long believed that part of the problem of their overburden exists because primary care physicians persist in doing a poor job. Primary care physicians appear either not to recognize mental illness or, if they do, not to treat it well. In spite of campaigns in the UK by the Royal Colleges of Psychiatrists and General Practitioners, such as the Defeat Depression initiative, there has been little substantial change in practice behavior. Are general practitioners as bad as they seem? I think not. It is more likely that in their practice they have too little time to recognize psychiatric illness, especially as much of it is concealed as physical illness. To do so requires a higher degree of psychiatric sophistication and experience than most general practitioners can be expected to possess. Psychiatrists tend to underestimate the difficulties of a busy primary care practice.

Conscientious primary care clinicians are over-burdened and as a consequence too many patients go untreated or are sent on to secondary care. It is now fashionable in many countries for psychiatrists to treat outpatients in local health centers. As a consequence, however laudable this practice, and there is much to be said in its favor, psychiatrists have become stressed and isolated from one another, wasting endless hours in traffic jams. Can this be a cost-effective method of maximizing our resources?

Psychiatrists are expensive to produce: they have a long training. Can there ever be enough psychiatrists to cope with the potential need? In the UK alone, it is said that there are currently over four hundred vacant consultant psychiatric posts. Again we must ask, if that is happening in a developed country, how can developing countries afford to train enough psychiatrists and how can they be trained adequately with the increasing service pressures? Pressures on teachers will ensure that many posts are not good training experiences.

Having read this far in the book you cannot fail to have received the message that everywhere in the world there is inequality and lack of resources. We are told that there is only rudimentary health care in some rural areas of a developed country like Australia. What then must be done? Or can be done?

Medicine must come into the real world and it must stop playing professional games. Most of us came into the business of medicine to relieve suffering. This is not just a problem for psychiatry, but for medicine as a whole. However, psychiatry has the opportunity to lead the way, as it has done in the past.

This is a book on epidemiology. Can epidemiology help solve our problems? Many purchasers of services may have to stop wasting time, and give up thinking that they can accurately estimate the needs of the community. They must understand that it is very difficult, if not impossible, to translate community needs into personal needs for planning. Personal needs are complex and too dependent on interacting and ever-changing contextual circumstances. Epidemiology can provide only a coarse indication of this state of affairs, but there are things it can do. It can provide a broad assessment of community unmet need, as several contributors have pointed out. It can draw comparisons between communities both to reveal different quantities and qualities of need, and to identify unusual or inappropriate service provision. It may also discover risk factors for disease, suggesting packages for intervention and prevention. It can point out those whom the services have failed and suggest reasons and remedies.

Nevertheless, even when the provision for potential need has been broadly assessed, it is important to ask the question, 'How far is planning sensible or possible?' There are too many social variables, new illnesses, new and expensive treatments, new political fashions, too many managers who must be seen to be changing policies whether the policies are good or bad, and of course earthquake, famine, flood, tornadoes and all forms of political and armed unrest. Such examples would seem to make planning services little better than forecasting the economy or predicting the long-range weather outlook. Everything is constantly shifting.

We know that over-planning delays implementation and is outdated before it is completed. We remember Karl Popper's (1957) concept of piecemeal social engineering. What possible solution do we have to these problems?

In primary care it seems, developing countries can no longer afford to rely on the doctors who are said to treat the majority of mental illness. This has been implied in other chapters in this book. We now have good screening methods for the most common psychiatric illnesses. These methods can be adapted to make them highly sensitive at the expense of some specificity, so that they can be used by trained health workers. We need to provide mental health workers with new tools by efficiently applying new technology. In the age of Mr Bill Gates and the World Wide Web, it is surprising that, so far in this book, computers have been mentioned only fleetingly. We have many computer diagnostic methods for psychiatric illness which could be adapted to clinical use. Doctors may dislike computers, but other health professionals are not averse to them. Such methods do not need expensive training. If nurses are in short supply, other intelligent workers can be trained to use computerized diagnostic and treatment protocols and thus effectively monitor and direct the management of uncomplicated cases, and assess their outcome probably at least as well as most doctors, at least at the primary care level. This should dramatically reduce the many referrals to psychiatric community clinics.

I include in the diagnostic process, of course, measures of disability and severity, social supports and other essential information for case management. Such computerized treatment protocols could be made sensitive to local conditions. Updated algorithms could be regularly provided, with accessible information on drug complications and interactions and, finally, give clear directions of when to refer to the supervising clinician.

As for secondary care, similar but more sophisticated computer methods for admission and monitoring procedures would be required for clinic and ward use. Fewer junior medical staff would be required in outlying hospitals and they could be trained in specialty centers of high quality. We would probably not need more psychiatrists and yet we could solve many of our staffing problems. Psychiatrists would be able to concentrate on a smaller number of patients whom the computer was unable to help. Such methods would provide better statistics for monitoring health care both within and between health districts and generally provide better value for money.

Yet who is to be treated, and can we provide treatment for all who would benefit or feel that they require it? How do we decide which cases we can and cannot afford to treat? No society can afford to treat everyone who wishes to be treated, and many societies can only afford to treat the very ill. Purchasers will eventually set cash limits, but will they have the courage, or will they be allowed by their political masters to try to agree on a hierarchy of disease priority with community health teams? We would all have our own hierarchical system. Below, I present my off-the-cuff, back-of-the-envelope suggestion. I present it as an 'Aunt Sally', which in Britain is a fairground character which onlookers are encouraged to knock down by throwing hard objects. No doubt you will disagree with the details, but some hierarchy must be negotiated and set.

Top priority

1. Severe social disruption due to psychiatric disorder.
2. All acute psychotic episodes – socially disruptive (self, family, community).
3. All acute psychotic episodes – not socially disruptive.
   Chronic psychosis – socially disruptive.
4. All remaining cases of recent-onset major illness.
   Chronic psychosis – not socially disruptive.
5. Acute neurotic illness.

Low priority

6. Chronic neurotic illness.
   Other nonsocially disruptive psychiatric disorders.

In short, most of us agree that no health service can provide unlimited care. It has to prioritize, however uncomfortable that may be to politicians, and however much they may wish to shift the burden of that responsibility onto others. At the moment, doctors and other health workers are left to make these decisions, and although I believe they do it reasonably successfully they should not have to carry this burden on their own. Many such decisions are political rather than medical, and society must take collective responsibility.

To sum up, we should, in my view, aim to cut the costs of mental health care and improve its quality by computerizing clinical psychiatry as much as possible for the majority of straightforward psychiatric problems, thus avoiding the inevitable variation and lapses in human behavior. Computers are increasingly more sophisticated and portable. They are cheaper than doctors and, dare one say it, more reliable, in the sense of being consistent, although it is true, more easily stolen. This would give the clinical team more time to care for their more challenging patients. Care is a rapidly disappearing concept from our health services and is vanishing from our hospitals. If you do not believe me, have yourself admitted for a night to any ordinary ward in a local hospital.

The politicians should set society's priorities but the clinical team must nevertheless argue forcibly if it believes the priorities are wrong. Their arguments for an adequate provision of health services will be backed by the ammunition provided by the epidemiologists.

Let us have a little less planning and fewer top-down decisions. The experienced clinical team is best suited to know, assess and respond quickly to need. Its judgement should be informed by periodical population assessment, placing it in the best position to explore new provisions for unmet needs. The clinical teams should lead in advising the managers and purchasers, and vigorously present their case. The old system where clinicians and nurses led the health services was not a bad system in itself. After all, it functioned on dedication and massive good will. Managers have eroded that good will at enormous financial cost. It failed because it was unmonitored and unresponsive to the need for cash limits. The clinical teams must therefore function within these limits and be judged by stringent outcome measures.

Unless we automate our methods, make our services better and cheaper, and are prepared to share our expertise among a wider circle of health workers, we shall fail our communities and we will lose out to that uncomfortable and alien invention, 'commercial managed care'. Care that is managed, not primarily for the benefit of patients, nor to improve existing methods of treatment and provision of services, nor to innovate new methods of care by ploughing back profits, but so that shareholders can increase their financial gain from other people's suffering. I do not believe that any civilized society wants that. I don't.

Reference

Popper, K.R. (1957). *The Poverty of Historicism.* London: Routledge.

30

Conclusion: the central issues

Scott Henderson

It is only towards the end of the present millennium that mental disorders have come to take their place in health care. The burden they place on communities is now irrefutable. Psychiatric epidemiology has played a vital part in two ways in the process of achieving greater recognition for the needs of people with mental disorders. The use of epidemiological information for advocacy stands separately from scientific studies of what determines the onset and course of mental disorders. The problem of unmet need straddles both advocacy and science.

Until the first half of the twentieth century, people with more severe disorders were sent to specially built hospitals; and it was not recognized that a range of disabling mental disorders was also to be found in the general population. Epidemiology helped to change this. The community-based surveys pioneered by research psychiatrists such as Brugger (1933) in Germany, Srole, Langner, Michael, Opler & Rennie (1962) and the Leightons (Leighton, Harding, Macklin, Hughes & Leighton, 1963) in North America, Taylor & Chave (1964) in Britain, Hagnell & Öjesjö (1975) in Sweden, Dube (1968) in India, and Krupinski & Stoller (1971) in Australia helped to persuade policy makers that a sizeable fraction of the general population had clinically significant psychiatric symptoms and that these were accompanied by disablement of some economic significance. In retrospect, it is now possible to see that attitudes and beliefs about the needs of people with mental disorders have changed considerably during the later decades of the twentieth century. Indeed it was only in the second half of the twentieth century that psychiatry began to take a more appropriate place in medical education, and that the first professors of psychiatry were appointed in most medical schools.

Mental disorders are different from most other medical conditions, such as cardiovascular disease, cancer or infectious diseases. In industrialized countries, only a relatively small fraction of these common medical disorders remains unrecognized: that is, most cases reach health services. Unlike mental disorders, about half of them are *not* misdiagnosed in general practice, and the majority are appropriately treated. Unlike mental disorders, those most severely afflicted by cardiovascular disease, cancer or infectious diseases do want treatment and are likely to accept it when this is offered. Clearly, epidemiology has done much to advance the care of the mentally ill by demonstrating both the extent of such morbidity and that it has received short shrift in most communities; but epidemiology has at the same time opened a Pandora's box of problems for providing adequate mental health services. We have assembled information here to allow the situation to be assessed from a global perspective.

The cone of morbidity

Unmet need can occur at each of the three levels traditionally used in psychiatric epidemiology: the general population; primary care or general practice; and mental health services (Figure 30.1). Goldberg & Huxley's (1980) concept of filters helps us understand how people may move up the cone towards different levels of care. This model can now be further developed. Our contributors show that there are many variables that determine whether symptomatic people reach services, and that even then their needs may remain unmet. This is shown as the upward arrows in Figure 30.1. Then some people move down the cone, and again there are filters influencing this movement.

Of the three levels, the most energetic efforts should be deployed in primary care and general practice. Michael Shepherd (1987) gave powerful reasons why this is so. A great deal has yet to be done in continuing education and the introduction of innovative administrative arrangements. It is through these that general practitioners can contribute much more effectively to the recognition, the management and the prevention of mental disorders.

Estimation of unmet need for services is one of the most important tasks of psychiatric epidemiology. This is for only one reason: to provide information that can be presented to politicians and health administrators, nationally and globally, to bring about better care for mental disorders. However, in trying to estimate unmet need, epidemiologists have come against a problem of outstanding attractiveness for scientific endeavor. Quite simply, this is how one can identify *people who are really sick* whether or not they have reached the health services. Of the people with an unmet need for mental health care, most of them must currently be symptomatic, or will probably become so soon. However, it has recently become clear that not all people who are symptomatic in a general population need some form of health or social care. That is, SYMPTOMS $\neq$ NEED.

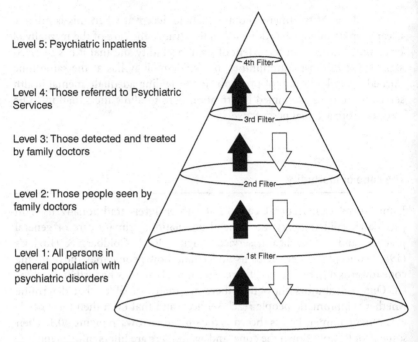

Level 5: Psychiatric inpatients

Level 4: Those referred to Psychiatric Services

Level 3: Those detected and treated by family doctors

Level 2: Those people seen by family doctors

Level 1: All persons in general population with psychiatric disorders

Figure 30.1 Where needs may be unmet.

The exaggerated estimate (EE) problem

Our contributors agree that estimates of the one-year or one-month prevalence of the main mental disorders, as found in several large population samples in industrialized countries, are far greater than a realistic estimate of the numbers needing health care (Frances, 1998; Regier et al., 1998; Spitzer, 1998). This is what we call the exaggerated estimate (EE) problem in psychiatric surveys of general populations. The prevalence rates are much too high. Whatever the reasons for this, the estimates we have are likely to be *underestimates* using the current methods. This is because of selective nonresponse in psychiatric surveys, a topic that is discreetly neglected in polite interchanges (Cox, Rutter, Yule & Quinton, 1977; Gove, McCorkel, Fain & Hughes, 1976; Kessler, Little & Groves, 1995; Williams & Macdonald, 1986). Most of the large surveys have response rates of around 80% or less; they are never better than that. So nothing is known about the 20% of the sample who were not examined. Yet they are likely to have a higher level of psychiatric morbidity than those who agreed to be examined and interviewed. Kessler et al. (1995) say that the National Comorbidity Survey (NCS) estimates had to be corrected by an increase of about 10% for anxiety and depressive disorders, to allow for the morbidity of those not interviewed. So the published prevalence values are likely to be *underestimates*, at least of people who, when examined with one of the current survey instruments, meet the international diagnostic criteria.

Here lies the scientific challenge. What distinguishes those who are *really sick* amongst that larger number of people who have enough symptoms to meet recognized diagnostic criteria, *but are less important for planning and funding services*. Because of the EE problem, being a case according to ICD-10 or DSM-IV in a general population survey no longer means that person is *really sick*. We think that there are at least three reasons causing the EE problem, and any one of them may be true:

1. The case-finding instruments may have too low a threshold, especially when in the hands of interviewers who are not clinicians.
2. Some people may have many symptoms, but these are largely *manageable, either to self or to others* in daily life, as Foulds once proposed but was not taken seriously by epidemiologists. Much too little is known about these noncomplaining cases (Foulds, 1972; Foulds & Bedford, 1977).
3. Symptoms and disablement may be nonlinearly related.

Answers to these three propositions are urgently needed. In Ministries of Health across the world, and in influential international bodies such as the World Bank and the World Health Organization, it is now fairly well accepted that resolving mental disorders is important for human health and well-being, and that, economically, they are far from being trivial. So epidemiologists are now being asked to produce *believable estimates* of unmet need. This can be done only by removing the clinically nonsignificant from the now-familiar prevalence values. In our opinion, one approach is to subtract that fraction of the estimates that are *not also associated with substantial disablement in daily life*. That is, for administrative purposes, we only need consider those people whose symptoms – regardless of whether they meet the international criteria – are demonstrably linked to *handicap in role performance* within the home, the workplace and that individual's wider social environment. When we have that estimate, stripped of exaggeration, epidemiology will have data that may reasonably be used to drive service administration.

The EE problem is causing difficulties in another area of epidemiological research. Although this is outside the topic of the book, it illustrates the widespread consequences of developing international research instruments that are not perfectly valid. If the standardized interviews currently used in general population studies incorrectly identify people as 'cases', then etiological research is likely to be seriously disadvantaged. This applies in any case–control study where an unknown proportion of 'cases' are not real cases. It applies whether the candidate causal factors are exposures from the person's social environment, clinical history, or genetic polymorphisms – each are candidates in the complex web of aetiology. *If the phenotype is incorrectly established, the search for causes will be jeopardized.*

The world cannot wait for the development of yet another standardized psychiatric interview, even if it were more valid than its predecessors. Instead, it is not beyond our wit to use the data already to hand, which for some countries include data on disablement as well as symptoms and officially sanctioned diagnoses. Such data can yield believable estimates of unmet need. This seems to us the best way to go.

Rationalism and its anti-Hippocratic heresy

Until now, resources have been allocated only to a small extent by rationally derived methods. The most disabled have rarely been accorded priority, but much emphasis has been placed on replacing hospital-based by community services. Kessler (Chapter 5) now proposes a solution. He challenges the notion that some derived expression of need should be the means of arranging the mentally ill in a hierarchy. He advocates that a ratio be examined instead, saying that, 'Need is implicitly defined in terms of impairment. This is an important focus, but it is inadequate for making decisions about the appropriateness of intervention. Instead, an intervention should be considered appropriate *if, and only if, its expected benefits clearly exceed the sum of its direct costs and expected risks.* There is no necessary relationship between level of need and appropriateness of intervention,' (authors italics). This position is very much in line with contemporary thinking of economic rationalism. The decision to treat or not to treat is to be determined by a ratio. But is it morally defensible? Is it likely to be what clinicians will actually practise when deciding on an individual patient's ration of treatment? One answer is that clinicians may no longer be those who decide: it will be the Government or a commercial organization who will, or will not, pay for it. This goes beyond evidence-based medicine, because it introduces cold financial arithmetic as the arbiter. The prospect is awesome. If no treatment of demonstrable efficacy is available, then no treatment may be paid for. If there is an effective treatment, it may be authorized only if, 'its expected benefits clearly exceed the sum of its direct costs and expected risks' (Kessler, Chapter 5). Such rationalism is heresy against the principles of medicine.

For patients who are both very disordered in mind and very disabled in daily life but who are not to be treated, what is an acceptable professional response? At best, we can hope that some clinicians will be able to continue behaving as they have for many centuries. Nevertheless, there must be some professional obligation to interpret the verdict of economic rationalism so as not to induce hopelessness and further demoralization.

Then suppose that an effective treatment is available but will cost more than leaving the condition untreated? Are we to understand that Governments or commercial organizations may not fund such treatment? That would mean that the patient pays or goes untreated. We should hope that not too many clinicians will be found who will agree to practise medicine under such rationalist restraints. Countries with such a system face difficult times: unmet need may reach new levels, at least until treatments emerge that are both scientifically and financially effective. As Whiteford (Chapter 2) concisely puts it, '. . . the challenge for governments is to influence the allocation of scarce resources on a rational basis to optimize the health status of the population for both humane and economic reasons'. We must hope that an acceptable balance between the humane and the economic will prevail.

References

Brugger, C. (1933). Psychiatrische ergebnisse einer medizinischen, anthropolischen, und soziologischen behölkerungunstersuch. *Zeischrift für Neurologie*, **146**, 489.

Cox, A., Rutter, M., Yule, B. & Quinton, D. (1977). Bias resulting from missing information: some epidemiological findings. *British Journal of Preventive and Social Medicine*, **31**, 131–6.

Dube, K.C. (1968). Mental disorder in Agra. *Social Psychiatry*, **3**, 139–43.

Foulds, G.A. (1972). *Personality and Personal Illness*. London: Social Science Paperback.

Foulds, G.A. & Bedford, A. (1977). Personality and coping with psychiatric symptoms. *British Journal of Psychiatry*, **130**, 29–31.

Frances, A. (1998). Problems in defining clinical significance in epidemiological studies. *Archives of General Psychiatry*, **55**, 119.

Goldberg, D.P. & Huxley, P. (1980). *Mental Illness in the Community: the Pathway to Psychiatric Care*. London: Tavistock Publications.

Gove, W.R., McCorkel, J., Fain, T. & Hughes, M.D. (1976). Response bias in community surveys of mental health: systematic bias or random noise? *Social Science and Medicine*, **10**, 497–502.

Hagnell, O. & Öjesjö, L. (1975). A prospective study concerning mental disorders of a total population investigated in 1947, 1957 and 1972. The Lundby Study. *Acta Psychiatrica Scandinavica*, **263**, 1–11.

Kessler, R.C., Little, R.J.A. & Groves, R.M. (1995). Advances in strategies for minimizing and adjusting for survey nonresponse. *Epidemiologic Reviews*, **17**, 192–204.

Krupinski, J. & Stoller, A. (1971). *The Health of a Metropolis*. Melbourne: Heinemann Educational Australia.

Leighton, D.C., Harding, J.S., Macklin, D.B., Hughes, C.C. & Leighton, A.H., (1963). Psychiatric findings of the Stirling County Study. *American Journal of Psychiatry*, **119**, 1021–26.

Regier, D.A., Kaelber, C.T., Rae, D.S., Farmer, M.E., Knauper, B., Kessler, R.C. & Norquist, G.S. (1998). Limitations of diagnostic criteria and assessment instruments for mental disorders. *Archives of General Psychiatry*, 55, 109–15.

Shepherd, M. (1987). Mental illness and primary care. *American Journal of Public Health*, 77, 12–13.

Spitzer, R.L. (1998). Diagnosis and need for treatment are not the same. *Archives of General Psychiatry*, 55, 120.

Srole, L., Langner, T.S., Michael, S.T., Opler, M.K. & Rennie, T.A.C. (1962). *Mental Health in the Metropolis*, Volume 1. The Mid-town Manhattan Study. New York: McGraw Hill.

Taylor, L. & Chave, S. (1964). *Mental Health and Environment.* London: Longmans.

Williams, P. & Macdonald, A. (1986). The effect of non-response bias on the results of two-stage screening surveys of psychiatric disorder. *Social Psychiatry*, 21, 182–6.

Index

Note: page numbers in *italics* refer to figures and tables.